Palliative Care in Oncology

Bernd Alt-Epping • Friedemann Nauck

Editors

Palliative Care in Oncology

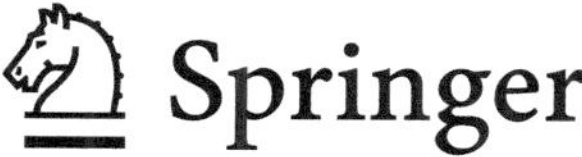 Springer

Editors
Bernd Alt-Epping
Department of Palliative Medicine
University Medical Center
Göttingen
Germany

Friedemann Nauck
Department of Palliative Medicine
University Medical Center
Göttingen
Germany

ISBN 978-3-662-51298-2   ISBN 978-3-662-46202-7   (eBook)
DOI 10.1007/978-3-662-46202-7

Springer Heidelberg New York Dordrecht London

Printed on acid-free paper

Springer is part of Springer Science+Business Media (www.springer.com)

A Palliative Care Revolution

Irene, a 59-year-old patient with cancer of the breast and bone metastases at a London cancer hospital, ruminated on care, treatment, death and bereavement.
She began with

> This is a wonderful place….they have a cure for everything

and ended with

> They are just going to get me through to Christmas….and then decide what to do with me. I'm worried about Bill looking after himself.

I just listened. She took just *6 min* to tell me her story.
Two months later, after her death, her husband, Bill, told me,

> She was so thin, her wedding ring fell off – that hurt. She told me it hurt to hug her … I couldn't even hug her.

The generic palliative care skills of trust building, full attention, listening, reflecting back, open questions and well-paced interspersing of information giving and inquiry were just some of the skills used to coax out what was most worrying for Irene and later her bereaved husband. The skills are almost invisible.

This is one patient's narrative. Narrative medicine encourages us to listen and tease out patients' stories to reach the pain in whatever dimension the patient and those close to them are experiencing it. O'Brien, quoting Elwyn and Gwyn (1999), reminds us, 'for all the science that underpins clinical practice, practitioners and patients make sense of the world by stories' (O'Brien 2013).

Cicely Saunders turned patient narratives and stories into a philosophy and practice of 'total care' for dying people, which revolutionised the care of people with advanced cancer and other conditions with the opening of St Christopher's Hospice, London. The story that founded modern palliative care happened over 60 years ago. The founding patient (Clark 2002, p 273), who inspired the young Cicely Saunders, then a social worker having had to abandon a career in nursing, was David Tasma, a 40-year-old Polish Jewish refugee who was dying of cancer of the rectum, which was inoperable and obstructive, for which he had a colostomy. His symptoms were pain and vomiting. He was a patient at St Thomas' Hospital, London, when Cicely, driven to improve the experience of people who were dying, spoke with him about her vision to build a place away from a noisy acute ward where people could die in peace and dignity. Cicely Saunders had 28 conversations with David Tasma (Gunaratnam 2013).

At the relatively advanced age of 33, Cicely Saunders started to train in medicine, having been advised by a senior doctor that it was 'the doctors who abandon the dying'. She then carried out her groundbreaking research: the recording of 1,100 patients talking about their experiences of pain; the only methodology, she told me, was *listening* to patients (Oliviere 2000). From that evolved the concept of 'total' pain and the concept of holistic care, i.e. 'total care' for body, mind and spirit delivered by a multi-professional team.

David Tasma died on 25 February 1948, having said to Cicely, 'I want what is in your mind and in your heart'. She took that to be an invitation to mean everything of the mind 'research, learning and full scientific rigour always matched with the friendship of the heart' (Saunders 2000) that humanity needed for good care of the dying. He died and left her £500 in his will, declaring that he would not be in her dream of a home where people would die, but he would be *'a window in your home'*.

Cicely Saunders founded 'the home around the window', St Christopher's in South London, in 1967, and the window at the original entrance to the hospice is dedicated to David Tasma. People come from around the world to see it. For Cicely Saunders, the window was an important symbol of openness – a call to openness to others and to the world. This openness extends to our professional practice, to our patients, to the families with whom we work, to those whom we train and to ourselves and our colleagues but also to future challenges (Saunders 2000). David Tasma was well qualified to be the founding patient of palliative care. He was experiencing multiple social and spiritual problems of learning a new language, housing and financial needs and employment and searching to make sense in his illness shortening his young life. He also represents disadvantaged patients: minority ethnic and refugee-status and minority communities needing to access good palliative care. So the opening of St Christopher's hailed a revolution in the care of oncology patients with advanced conditions. The vast majority of palliative care until recent years was for cancer patients. From its inception, palliative care involved the trinity of care, research and education.

So what was the nature of the revolution that one woman inspired by David Tasma and many other patients led?

Barbara Monroe, the current Chief Executive, states that this revolution included

- Meticulous attention to symptom control
- Life, not just death
- Health, not just illness
- Possibilities as well as problems
- The whole individual, not just the physical body
- Families and communities
- Care beyond death into bereavement
- Multi-professional teams and volunteers

- Does not deny suffering – offers support
- Supports coping
- The belief that a little goes a long way (Monroe B, 2010, personal communication)

Forty-six years on, St Christopher's continues to innovate and to evolve modern palliative care and end-of-life care services as contexts have changed.

This book aims to integrate and push forward the knowledge base for palliative care in oncology. The book's comprehensive approach will prove useful for clinical practice including vital elements of good symptom control, good communication at all levels and good family support. Congratulations to the editors, whose expertise in palliative care is renowned and who have collected a number of prestigious contributors in this volume. They open a window for those who wish to learn and gain new vistas in palliative care.

Prof. Ventafrida (2000), one of the founders of the European Association of Palliative Care (EAPC), stated at the very first EAPC Research Congress in Berlin in 2000 that

> Palliative medicine is only part of palliative care: 50 %.

> The other 50 % is the holistic approach. Both make up palliative care.

Integrating good palliative care with oncology raises many challenging questions. This book holds some of the answers.

London, UK   David Oliviere

References

Clark D (2002) Cicely Saunders. Founder of the hospice movement. Selected Letters 1959–1999. Oxford University Press, Oxford

Gunaratnam Y (2013) Death and the Migrant: bodies, borders, care. Bloomsbury Academic, London

O'Brien T (2013) The potential of social work in the multi-professional team. A personal perspective. EAPC Congress, Prague

Oliviere D (2000) A voice for the voiceless. Interview with Dame Cicely Saunders. EJPC 7(3):102–105

Saunders C (2000) The evolution of palliative care. Patient Educ Couns. 41(7):7–13

Ventafrida V (2000) Plenary address. EAPC first EAPC Research Congress, Berlin

Contents

Part IV Pharmacological Aspects

Part V Policy and Structures

Part VI Ethical Aspects

Part VII Perspectives

Contributors

Bernd Alt-Epping, MD Department of Palliative Medicine, University Medical Center, Göttingen, Germany

Joseph Anthony Arthur, MD Department of Palliative Care and Rehabilitation Medicine, The University of Texas M.D. Anderson Cancer Center, Houston, TX, USA

Claudia Bausewein, MD, PhD, MSc Department of Palliative Medicine, University of Munich, Munich, Germany

Stephen A. Bernard, MD University of North Carolina, Chapel Hill, NC, USA

Charmaine L. Blanchard, MPhil Pall Med Wits Centre for Palliative Care, University of the Witwatersrand, Gauteng Centre of Excellence for Palliative Care, Chris Hani Baragwanath Academic Hospital, Johannesburg, South Africa

Eduardo Bruera, MD Department of Palliative Care and Rehabilitation Medicine, The University of Texas M.D. Anderson Cancer Center, Houston, TX, USA

Stephen R. Connor, PhD Worldwide Palliative Care Alliance, Fairfax Station, VA, USA

Liliana de Lima International Association for Hospice and Palliative Care, Houston, TX, USA

John E. Ellershaw, MA, FRCP Marie Curie Palliative Care Institute Liverpool, Liverpool, UK

Steffen Eychmüller, MD Center for Palliative Care, University Hospital Inselspital, Bern, Switzerland

Norbert Frickhofen, MD Department of Hematology, Medical Oncology and Palliative Care, HSK, Dr. Horst Schmidt Klinik, Wiesbaden, Germany

Jan Gaertner, MD Palliative Care Center of Excellence for Baden-Württemberg (KOMPACT), Baden-Württemberg, Germany

Department of Palliative Medicine, Comprehensive Cancer Center
Freiburg – CCCF, University Medical Center Freiburg, Freiburg, Germany

Matthias Gründel, PhD Department of Haematology/Oncology, University
Medical Center, Göttingen, Germany

Clemens Friedrich Hess, MD, PhD Department of Radiotherapy and Radiation
Oncology, University Medical Center, Göttingen, Germany

Andrea Hille, MD Department of Radiotherapy and Radiation Oncology,
University Medical Center, Göttingen, Germany

Karin Hohloch, MD Department of Haematology and Oncology, University
Medical Center, Göttingen, Germany

Birgit Jaspers, DMSc Department of Palliative Medicine, University Medical
Center, Göttingen, Germany

Department of Palliative Medicine, University Hospital, Bonn, Germany

Stein Kaasa, MD, PhD Department of Cancer Research and Molecular
Medicine, Faculty of Medicine, European Palliative Care Research Centre (PRC),
Norwegian University of Science and Technology (NTNU), Trondheim, Norway

St. Olavs Hospital, Trondheim University Hospital, Trondheim, Norway

Cancer Clinic, St. Olavs Hospital, Trondheim University Hospital,
Trondheim, Norway

Andrew F. Khodabukus, BSc, MBChB Royal Liverpool and Broadgreen
University Hospitals NHS Trust, Liverpool, UK

Philip J. Larkin, PhD, MSc School of Nursing, Midwifery and Health Systems,
UCD Health Sciences Centre, University College Dublin, Dublin, Ireland

Our Lady's Hospice and Care Services, Dublin, Ireland

Jon Håvard Loge, MD, PhD Department of Cancer Research and Molecular
Medicine, Faculty of Medicine, European Palliative Care Research Centre (PRC),
Norwegian University of Science and Technology (NTNU), Trondheim, Norway

Regional Centre for Excellency in Palliative Care, South-East Norway, Oslo,
Norway

University Hospital, Oslo, Norway

Bernd-Oliver Maier, MD, MSc St. Joseph's Hospital, Wiesbaden, Germany

Anja Mehnert, PhD Department of Medical Psychology and Medical Sociology,
University Medical Center, Leipzig, Germany

Friedemann Nauck, MD Department of Palliative Medicine, University Medical
Center, Göttingen, Germany

Christoph Ostgathe, MD Department of Palliative Medicine, University Hospital, Erlangen, Germany

Richard A. Powell, MD Global Health Researcher, Nairobi, Kenya

M.R. Rajagopal, MD Pallium India, Trivandrum, Kerala, India

Trivandrum Institute of Palliative Sciences Trivandrum, Trivandrum, Kerala, India

Constanze Rémi, MSc Department of Palliative Medicine, University of Munich, Munich, Germany

Jan Schildmann, MD Institute for Medical Ethics and History of Medicine, Ruhr University Bochum, Bochum, Germany

Thomas J. Smith, MD Department of Oncology, Johns Hopkins Sidney Kimmel Comprehensive Cancer Center, Baltimore, MD, USA

Theresa Stehmer, PharmD Department of Pharmacy, Duke University Hospital, Durham, NC, USA

Daniela Weber, MSc Department of Palliative Medicine, University Medical Center, Göttingen, Germany

Eva C. Winkler, MD, PhD Medical Oncology, Program for Ethics and Patient-Oriented Care in Oncology, National Center for Tumor Diseases (NCT), University of Heidelberg, Heidelberg, Germany

Jürgen Wolf, MD, PhD Department I of Internal Medicine, Centre for Integrated Oncology (CIO), University of Cologne, Cologne, Germany

Hendrik A. Wolff, MD Department of Radiotherapy and Radiation Oncology, University Medical Center, Göttingen, Germany

Part I

Oncology and Palliative Care:
Disease Specific Perspectives

Disease-Specific Oncology – Disease-Specific Palliative Care

Joseph Anthony Arthur and Eduardo Bruera

Content

Cancer is a unique disease which requires special attention to the affected patients and families right from the time of diagnosis. It is a major cause of death in the world and therefore it elicits grave apprehension and concern among many people. In the United States, it is the second most common cause of death, exceeded only by heart disease, and accounts for nearly one of every four deaths. It is estimated that in 2013, about 35 % of all cancer patients will die and 65 % will survive cancer.

Cancer patients undergoing treatment develop peculiar physical, psychological, social, and spiritual needs that require a multidimensional approach to address them (American Cancer Society 2013). Even among those who attain cure, many develop a variety of debilitating treatment-related and disease-related symptoms which can be quite distressing and detrimental to their quality of life. Although the goal of curing and eradicating cancer is laudable, it is quite evident that this has not been achievable in a significant number of patients. Many patients have to learn to deal with the enormous symptom burden until their demise. The overemphasis on the cure for cancer sometimes further obscures our perception of the needs and demands of the unfortunate ones. It is therefore important for clinicians to approach them having the background knowledge of such special needs and to appropriately acknowledge them in clinical practice.

The presentation of palliative care cases can be disease specific, just like in many other medical cases. The disease trajectory, symptom profile, and the needs of cancer patients may be different from those of non-cancer cases. Even among cancer

J.A. Arthur, MD (✉) • E. Bruera, MD
Department of Palliative Care and Rehabilitation Medicine, The University of Texas M.D. Anderson Cancer Center, Houston, TX 77030, USA
e-mail: jaarthur@mdanderson.org; ebruera@mdanderson.org

© Springer-Verlag Berlin Heidelberg 2015
B. Alt-Epping, F. Nauck (eds.), *Palliative Care in Oncology*,
DOI 10.1007/978-3-662-46202-7_1

cases, there may be differences based on specific disease types and patient demographics such as age, gender, and ethnicity. The delivery of palliative care interventions may therefore vary based on these differences.

In a study done assessing the symptom profile of patients with advanced cancer and those with advanced non-cancer diseases like chronic obstructive pulmonary disease (COPD) and chronic heart failure (CHF) and cirrhosis, it was found that the prevalence of common symptoms was equally high in both cancer and non-cancer with an average of 10.33 ± 3.86 symptoms (Tranmer et al. 2003). However, the type of symptoms varied in cancer patients compared with non-cancer patients. Pain, nausea, unpleasant taste, vomiting, and constipation were found to be more common among cancer patients than non-cancer patients. Shortness of breath and cough were generally more common in non-cancer patients. There were no significant differences in the prevalence of psychological symptoms between the two groups (Tranmer et al. 2003). In another study, the ten most prevalent cancer-related symptoms were pain, easy fatigue, weakness, anorexia, lack of energy, dry mouth, constipation, early satiety, dyspnea, and greater than 10 % weight loss (Walsh et al. 2000). Symptom prevalence was independently affected by age, gender, and performance status.

Different cancer types may have different symptom profiles (Table 1.1). For example, patients with head and neck cancer, lung cancer, and other cancers with predominant lung involvement have more dyspnea. Those with gynecological and gastrointestinal malignancies frequently develop bowel obstruction, nausea, vomiting, and abdominal pain (Tranmer et al. 2003). Patients with gynecological malignancies are most likely to have access to palliative care, probably because of the relatively high symptom burden among them, coupled with the relatively limited systemic therapy options in resistant cases. Contrary to this, those with hematological malignancies are least likely to be referred to palliative care. Similar studies have shown that hematological malignancy patients were more likely to receive aggressive therapy at the end of life (Hui et al. 2010), die in an intensive care unit (Delgado-Guay et al. 2009), and have late palliative care referral (Fadul et al. 2007). This is despite the fact that there is no significant difference in the symptom burden between solid tumor patients and hematological malignancy patients (Fadul et al. 2008). The actual reasons for this occurrence are unclear. However, possible reasons include the following: the disease appears relatively more curable with available therapies even in advanced stages (Cheson 2002; McGrath and Holewa 2007; Hampton 2007), patients with the disease can decline very rapidly (Hampton 2007; Mander 1997) thereby possibly narrowing the window of opportunity for palliative care interventions, and there are difficulties in predicting the course of events with hematological malignancies (Glare et al. 2003; Auret et al. 2003; McGrath 2001). Younger patients were more likely to have access to palliative care (Hui et al. 2012), more likely to have higher symptom expression and reporting (Bernabei et al. 1998; Ahmed et al. 2004), and more likely to pursue aggressive measures than older patients. Married couple were also more likely to have access to palliative care (Hui et al. 2012), probably because the spouse provides extra and immediately available support for the patient regarding issues at the end of life.

Table 1.1 Examples of common oncologic disease types and their associated symptoms/issues

Disease	Physical	Psycological	Social	Spiritual / existential	Advance care planning
Gastrointestinal	Anorexia, Nausea, Vomiting, constipation, Bowel obstruction Abdominal pain, Fatigue	Anxiety Depress on Grief and bereavement Adjustment disorder Addictive behavior Psychotic manifestations	Family conflicts Caregiver distress Financial situation Cultural variations Racial disparities Social support system	Religious affiliation Existential distress Loss of meaning Lack of self-worth Loss dignity Hopelessness	Code Status Living will OOH DNR[a] MPOA[b]
Head & neck	Dyspnea Oral pain Dysphagia Fatigue				
Lung	Dyspnea Cough Pain Fatigue				
Gynecological	Bowel obstruction Anorexia, Nausea, Vomiting Constipation Pain Fatigue				
Breast	Pain Fatigue Delirium				
Hematological	Pain Fatigue Bleeding Frequent infections Delirium				

[a]Out of hospital do not resuscitate order
[b]Medical power of attorney discussion

There are also distinct differences between the disease trajectory of cancer and common non-cancer diseases (Fig. 1.1). Dementia disease course is that of a slow, steady, and progressive decline which may be interrupted by periods of cognitive and functional decline usually from acute infections like pneumonia and urinary tract infections (Wolfson et al. 2001; Xie et al. 2008; Walsh et al. 1990). When patients recover from each acute event, they then establish a new baseline cognitive and functional status which is usually lower than the one prior to the illness. They eventually die from those complications. This disease course is also common with old age and stroke. It is estimated that the median life expectancy of most forms of dementia patients is about 4–7 years in many studies (Wolfson et al. 2001; Xie et al. 2008; Walsh et al. 1990). The exceptions are dementias due to Huntington's disease and Creutzfeldt–Jakob disease which have a relatively shorter life expectancy.

The disease trajectory of end-stage chronic obstructive pulmonary disease is marked by frequent periods of episodic exacerbations followed by incomplete recovery with the administration of rescue treatments like supplemental oxygen, bronchodilators, steroids, and antibiotics. This type of disease course poses a significant challenge to the timing of transition into a more palliative mode of care because these acute interventions transiently give the patients a false sense of

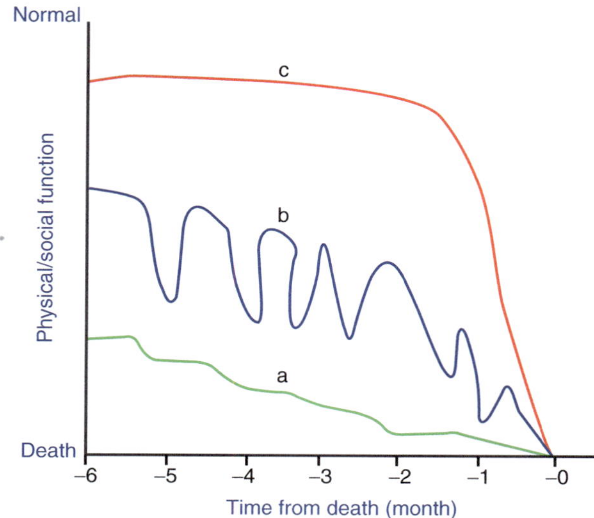

Fig. 1.1 Disease trajectories over the last 6 months of life for patients with (*a*) dementia, (*b*) chronic obstructive pulmonary disease (COPD) and cardiac heart failure (CHF), and (*c*) cancer (Adapted with permission from RAND Health; Lynn and Adamson 2003)

recovery and improvement, thereby attenuating the true grave and poor prognostic picture of their disease. The disease trajectory of heart failure is similar to COPD with periods of decompensation and recovery close to the prior functional status. They usually die from complications of the disease but this is very unpredictable, compared to cancer (Goldstein and Lynn 2006; Lunney et al. 2002, 2003). Also, significant advancements in the management of heart failure tend to obscure the actual disease trajectory. Interventions like cardiac transplantation, ICD (implantable cardioverter–defibrillator) implantation, and left ventricular assist device are known to improve quality of life and increase survival.

In contrast, the disease trajectory of cancer is one in which the patient functions well with the disease for a prolonged period of time (months to years) until the late stages (usually the last 6 weeks) when he declines rapidly. It is more predictable than the other disease courses (Morris et al. 1986; Lunney et al. 2002, 2003). The main indicators of the rapid decline include poor performance status; symptoms such as weight loss, anorexia, breathlessness, or confusion; and laboratory abnormalities such as high white cell count, lymphocytopenia, hypoalbuminemia, and elevated lactate dehydrogenase or C-reactive protein.

There is always the persistent desire among clinicians, patients, and their families to better understand the cancer disease trajectory and predict the course of events. For the patients and their families, this has key implications in planning the medical care, making very important time-dependent decisions, and generating the best goals of care. It guides the physician to provide the most appropriate form of care, thereby avoiding overtreatment and undertreatment, and informs him during the decision-making process of assisting a patient to transition from cure-oriented care to a palliative mode of care with more emphasis on quality of life. A survey conducted among American physicians revealed that they regularly encounter situations that require prognostication (Christakis and Iwashyna 1998). They do not feel well prepared for such situations and perceive them as stressful and difficult. There is the belief among physicians that patients might judge them adversely if they make errors in their prediction.

Various differences were observed among physicians regarding their views about the concept of being "terminally ill" (Christakis and Iwashyna 1998). This demonstrates a relative lack of understanding in this area of medicine. We need to understand certain concepts about prognostication. First, prognostication should not erroneously be seen as a static phenomenon but rather a dynamic one which is subject to revision as the disease evolves and new issues arise. Second, prognostication transcends beyond just predicting death or survival to also involve the ability to predict and provide answers regarding inevitable events related to disease progression or recurrence, functional status, drug toxicity, or health-care cost demands (Fries and Ehrlich 1981). Third, the factors used to predict survival in the late stages of the disease are different from those used in the early stages. Diagnostic, pathological, and treatment-related prognostic factors are more useful in early-stage cancer, whereas performance status, the anorexia–cachexia syndrome, systemic inflammation, lymphocytopenia, poor quality of life, and psychosocial factors are more useful during the late stages of the disease (Glare et al. 2008). Of all the prognostic factors studied, performance status is the one most extensively studied. The Karnofsky Performance Scale (KPS) (Evans and McCarthy 1985; Viganò et al. 2000; Loprinzi et al. 1994; Mor et al. 1984), the Australian modification of the KPS (AKPS) (Abernethy et al. 2005; Nikoletti et al. 2000), the Palliative Performance Scale (PPS) (Anderson et al. 1996), and the Eastern Cooperative Oncology Group Performance Status (ECOG-PS) Scale (Loprinzi et al. 1994; Dewys et al. 1980; Rosenthal et al. 1993) are examples of performance status tools which have all been shown to be predictive of survival in advanced cancer patients. Symptoms such as anorexia and/or weight loss (Loprinzi et al. 1994; Wachtel et al. 1988; Vigano et al. 1999; Bruera et al. 1992), dyspnea (Pirovano et al. 1999; Morita et al. 1999; Escalante et al. 2000; Llobera et al. 2000), and cognitive failure (Bruera et al. 1992; Llobera et al. 2000; Morita et al. 1999; Maltoni et al. 1995) have been consistently shown to be predictors of poor survival in advanced cancer patients. Interestingly, neither pain (Bruera et al. 1992) nor opioid use (Portenoy et al. 2006; Maltoni et al. 1999) was considered to be a predictor of poor survival. Quality of life measures (Ganz et al. 1991; Addington-Hall et al. 1990; Langendijk et al. 2000) and laboratory parameters such as leukocytosis, neutrophilia, lymphocytopenia, low serum pseudocholinesterase, low serum albumin, and elevated proteinuria have also been found to predict poor survival (Maltoni et al. 1997).

Prognostication involves two components: foreseeing (coming up with the prediction) and foretelling (communicating the prediction). There are two ways to come up with a prognosis. It is either by using clinical judgment as commonly done in clinical practice or by using statistical methods. It has been shown that using statistical tools is superior to using clinical judgment (Steyerberg and Harrell 2002). There is therefore a consensus on the use of both parameters in predicting survival (Hampton 2007). Examples of available statistical tools include the Palliative Prognostic Score (Mander 1997) (consists of the KPS score, symptoms, white cell count, lymphocyte percentage, and clinical prediction of survival), the Palliative Performance Index (Glare et al. 2003) (consists of the PPS score, oral intake, edema, dyspnea, and delirium), and the Cancer Prognostic Score (Auret et al. 2003) (a 7-item scale consisting of liver and lung metastases, functional performance status, weight loss, edema, delirium, fatigue, and ascites). There are also links to some web-based prognostic tools available online which may be used (Sinclair 2007).

In summary, just as the presentation of oncologic cases can be disease specific, so do palliative care cases. However, certain symptoms are generally prevalent in most cancer patients irrespective of the cancer type. This is likely because cancer patients are polysymptomatic. A cancer patient may experience symptoms mainly related to the particular organ system but may also exhibit symptoms involving other organ systems. It is also known that although there may be some differences in the physical symptoms, the psychological, social, and spiritual needs of these patients are invariably similar. These multiple physical, psychosocial, and spiritual dimensions of palliative care symptomatology may occur at any phase during the disease trajectory, and palliative care services need to be available throughout this period. The ultimate goal of palliative care is to deliver care that is patient specific rather than disease specific. Therefore personalized evaluation and management is the key to the delivery of a successful palliative intervention.

The ability to understand the disease trajectory and to predict the outcomes of disease conditions is of paramount importance to clinicians, patients, and their families. Regrettably, the concept of prognostication is not well understood even among clinicians. One reason is because the factors used to predict survival in the late stages of the disease are different from those used in the early stages. More effort and research is needed in order to better understand this vital aspect of palliative care.

References

Abernethy A, Shelby-James T, Fazekas B, Woods D, Currow D (2005) The Australia-modified Karnofsky Performance Status (AKPS) scale: a revised scale for contemporary palliative care clinical practice [ISRCTN81117481]. BMC Palliat Care 4(1):7

Addington-Hall JM, MacDonald LD, Anderson HR (1990) Can the Spitzer Quality of Life Index help to reduce prognostic uncertainty in terminal care? Br J Cancer 62(4):695–699

Ahmed N, Bestall JC, Ahmedzai SH, Payne SA, Clark D, Noble B (2004) Systematic review of the problems and issues of accessing specialist palliative care by patients, carers and health and social care professionals. Palliat Med 18(6):525–542

American Cancer Society (2013) Cancer Facts & Figures 2013. American Cancer Society, Atlanta

Anderson F, Downing GM, Hill J, Casorso L, Lerch N (1996) Palliative performance scale (PPS): a new tool. J Palliat Care 12(1):5–11

Auret K, Bulsara C, Joske D (2003) Australasian haematologist referral patterns to palliative care: lack of consensus on when and why. Intern Med J 33(12):566–571, doi:490 [pii]

Bernabei R, Gambassi G, Lapane K, Landi F, Gatsonis C, Dunlop R, Lipsitz L, Steel K, Mor V (1998) Management of pain in elderly patients with cancer. SAGE Study Group. Systematic Assessment of Geriatric Drug Use via Epidemiology. JAMA 279(23):1877–1882, doi:joc71977 [pii]

Bruera E, Miller MJ, Kuehn N, MacEachern T, Hanson J (1992) Estimate of survival of patients admitted to a palliative care unit: a prospective study. J Pain Symptom Manage 7(2):82–86

Cheson BD (2002) Hematologic malignancies: new developments and future treatments. Semin Oncol 29(4 Suppl 13):33–45

Christakis NA, Iwashyna TJ (1998) Attitude and self-reported practice regarding prognostication in a national sample of internists. Arch Intern Med 158(21):2389–2395. doi:10.1001/archinte.158.21.2389

Delgado-Guay MO, Parsons HA, Li Z, Palmer LJ, Bruera E (2009) Symptom distress, interventions, and outcomes of intensive care unit cancer patients referred to a palliative care consult team. Cancer 115(2):437–445. doi:10.1002/cncr.24017

Dewys WD, Begg C, Lavin PT, Band PR, Bennett JM, Bertino JR, Cohen MH, Douglass HO Jr, Engstrom PF, Ezdinli EZ, Horton J, Johnson GJ, Moertel CG, Oken MM, Perlia C, Rosenbaum C, Silverstein MN, Skeel RT, Sponzo RW, Tormey DC (1980) Prognostic effect of weight loss prior to chemotherapy in cancer patients. Eastern Cooperative Oncology Group. Am J Med 69(4):491–497

Escalante CP, Martin CG, Elting LS, Price KJ, Manzullo EF, Weiser MA, Harle TS, Cantor SB, Rubenstein EB (2000) Identifying risk factors for imminent death in cancer patients with acute dyspnea. J Pain Symptom Manage 20(5):318–325

Evans C, McCarthy M (1985) Prognostic uncertainty in terminal care: can the Karnofsky index help? Lancet 325(8439):1204–1206. doi:http://dx.doi.org/10.1016/S0140-6736(85)92876-4

Fadul N, Elsayem A, Palmer JL, Zhang T, Braiteh F, Bruera E (2007) Predictors of access to palliative care services among patients who died at a Comprehensive Cancer Center. J Palliat Med 10(5):1146–1152. doi:10.1089/jpm.2006.0259

Fadul NA, El Osta B, Dalal S, Poulter VA, Bruera E (2008) Comparison of symptom burden among patients referred to palliative care with hematologic malignancies versus those with solid tumors. J Palliat Med 11(3):422–427. doi:10.1089/jpm.2007.0184

Fries JF, Ehrlich GE (1981) Prognosis: contemporary outcomes of disease. The Charles Press Publishers, Bowie

Ganz PA, Lee JJ, Siau J (1991) Quality of life assessment. An independent prognostic variable for survival in lung cancer. Cancer 67(12):3131–3135

Glare P, Virik K, Jones M, Hudson M, Eychmuller S, Simes J, Christakis N (2003) A systematic review of physicians' survival predictions in terminally ill cancer patients. BMJ 327 (7408):195–198. doi:10.1136/bmj.327.7408.195, 327/7408/195 [pii]

Glare P, Sinclair C, Downing M, Stone P, Maltoni M, Vigano A (2008) Predicting survival in patients with advanced disease. Eur J Cancer 44(8):1146–1156. doi:http://dx.doi.org/10.1016/j.ejca.2008.02.030

Goldstein NE, Lynn J (2006) Trajectory of end-stage heart failure: the influence of technology and implications for policy change. Perspect Biol Med 49(1):10–18

Hampton T (2007) New blood cancer therapies under study. JAMA 297(5):457–458. doi:10.1001/jama.297.5.457, 297/5/457 [pii]

Hui D, Elsayem A, Li Z, De La Cruz M, Palmer JL, Bruera E (2010) Antineoplastic therapy use in patients with advanced cancer admitted to an acute palliative care unit at a comprehensive cancer center: a simultaneous care model. Cancer 116(8):2036–2043. doi:10.1002/cncr.24942

Hui D, Kim SH, Kwon JH, Tanco KC, Zhang T, Kang JH, Rhondali W, Chisholm G, Bruera E (2012) Access to palliative care among patients treated at a comprehensive cancer center. Oncologist 17(12):1574–1580. doi:10.1634/theoncologist.2012-0192, theoncologist.2012-0192 [pii]

Langendijk H, Aaronson NK, de Jong JM, ten Velde GP, Muller MJ, Wouters M (2000) The prognostic impact of quality of life assessed with the EORTC QLQ-C30 in inoperable non-small cell lung carcinoma treated with radiotherapy. Radiother Oncol 55(1):19–25

Llobera J, Esteva M, Rifa J, Benito E, Terrasa J, Rojas C, Pons O, Catalan G, Avella A (2000) Terminal cancer. Duration and prediction of survival time. Eur J Cancer 36(16):2036–2043

Loprinzi CL, Laurie JA, Wieand HS, Krook JE, Novotny PJ, Kugler JW, Bartel J, Law M, Bateman M, Klatt NE (1994) Prospective evaluation of prognostic variables from patient-completed questionnaires. North Central Cancer Treatment Group. J Clin Oncol 12(3):601–607

Lunney JR, Lynn J, Hogan C (2002) Profiles of older medicare decedents. J Am Geriatr Soc 50(6):1108–1112. doi:10.1046/j.1532-5415.2002.50268.x

Lunney JR, Lynn J, Foley DJ, Lipson S, Guralnik JM (2003) Patterns of functional decline at the end of life. JAMA 289(18):2387–2392. doi:10.1001/jama.289.18.2387289/18/2387 [pii]

Lynn J, Adamson D (2003) Rand Corporation., Living well at the end of life: adapting health care to serious chronic illness in old age; white paper; Santa Monica CA; RAND; WP-137:iii, 19p. http://www.semeg.es/docs/docum/Rand_Health_White_Paper.pdf

Maltoni M, Pirovano M, Scarpi E, Marinari M, Indelli M, Arnoldi E, Gallucci M, Frontini L, Piva L, Amadori D (1995) Prediction of survival of patients terminally ill with cancer. Results of an Italian prospective multicentric study. Cancer 75(10):2613–2622

Maltoni M, Pirovano M, Nanni O, Marinari M, Indelli M, Gramazio A, Terzoli E, Luzzani M, De Marinis F, Caraceni A, Labianca R (1997) Biological indices predictive of survival in 519 Italian terminally ill cancer patients. Italian Multicenter Study Group on Palliative Care. J Pain Symptom Manage 13(1):1–9

Maltoni M, Nanni O, Pirovano M, Scarpi E, Indelli M, Martini C, Monti M, Arnoldi E, Piva L, Ravaioli A, Cruciani G, Labianca R, Amadori D (1999) Successful validation of the palliative prognostic score in terminally ill cancer patients. Italian Multicenter Study Group on Palliative Care. J Pain Symptom Manage 17(4):240–247

Mander T (1997) Haematology and palliative care: an account of shared care for a patient undergoing bone marrow transplantation for chronic myeloid leukaemia. Int J Nurs Pract 3(1): 62–66

McGrath P (2001) Dying in the curative system: the haematology/oncology dilemma. Part 1. Aust J Holist Nurs 8(2):22–30

McGrath P, Holewa H (2007) Special considerations for haematology patients in relation to end-of-life care: Australian findings. Eur J Cancer Care (Engl) 16(2):164–171. doi:10.1111/j.1365-2354.2006.00745.x

Mor V, Laliberte L, Morris JN, Wiemann M (1984) The Karnofsky performance status scale: an examination of its reliability and validity in a research setting. Cancer 53(9):2002–2007. doi:10.1002/1097-0142(19840501)53:9<2002:AID-CNCR2820530933>3.0.CO;2-W

Morita T, Tsunoda J, Inoue S, Chihara S (1999) Survival prediction of terminally ill cancer patients by clinical symptoms: development of a simple indicator. Jpn J Clin Oncol 29(3):156–159

Morris JN, Suissa S, Sherwood S, Wright SM, Greer D (1986) Last days: a study of the quality of life of terminally ill cancer patients. J Chronic Dis 39(1):47–62. doi:http://dx.doi.org/10.1016/0021-9681(86)90106-2

Nikoletti S, Porock D, Kristjanson LJ, Medigovich K, Pedler P, Smith M (2000) Performance status assessment in home hospice patients using a modified form of the Karnofsky Performance Status Scale. J Palliat Med 3(3):301–311. doi:10.1089/jpm.2000.3.301

Pirovano M, Maltoni M, Nanni O, Marinari M, Indelli M, Zaninetta G, Petrella V, Barni S, Zecca E, Scarpi E, Labianca R, Amadori D, Luporini G (1999) A new palliative prognostic score: a first step for the staging of terminally ill cancer patients. Italian Multicenter and Study Group on Palliative Care. J Pain Symptom Manage 17(4):231–239

Portenoy RK, Sibirceva U, Smout R, Horn S, Connor S, Blum RH, Spence C, Fine PG (2006) Opioid use and survival at the end of life: a survey of a hospice population. J Pain Symptom Manage 32(6):532–540. doi:10.1016/j.jpainsymman.2006.08.003

Rosenthal MA, Gebski VJ, Kefford RF, Stuart-Harris RC (1993) Prediction of life-expectancy in hospice patients: identification of novel prognostic factors. Palliat Med 7(3):199–204

Sinclair C (2007) Prognosis Links. Pallimed: a Hospice & Palliative Medicine blog. http://prognosis.pallimed.org/. Accessed 31 Mar 2014

Steyerberg EW, Harrell FE Jr (2002) Statistical models for prognostication. Symptom research: methods and opportunities. National Institute of Health, Bethesda

Tranmer JE, Heyland D, Dudgeon D, Groll D, Squires-Graham M, Coulson K (2003) Measuring the symptom experience of seriously ill cancer and noncancer hospitalized patients near the end of life with the memorial symptom assessment scale. J Pain Symptom Manage 25(5):420–429

Vigano A, Bruera E, Suarez-Almazor ME (1999) Terminal cancer syndrome: myth or reality? J Palliat Care 15(4):32–39

Viganò A, Dorgan M, Buckingham J, Bruera E, Suarez-Almazor ME (2000) Survival prediction in terminal cancer patients: a systematic review of the medical literature. Palliat Med 14(5):363–374

Wachtel T, Allen-Masterson S, Reuben D, Goldberg R, Mor V (1988) The end stage cancer patient: terminal common pathway. Hosp J 4(4):43–80

Walsh JS, Welch HG, Larson EB (1990) Survival of outpatients with Alzheimer-type dementia. Ann Intern Med 113(6):429–434. doi:10.7326/0003-4819-113-6-429

Walsh D, Donnelly S, Rybicki L (2000) The symptoms of advanced cancer: relationship to age, gender, and performance status in 1,000 patients. Support Care Cancer 8(3):175–179

Wolfson C, Wolfson DB, Asgharian M, M'Lan CE, Østbye T, Rockwood K, Hogan DB (2001) A reevaluation of the duration of survival after the onset of dementia. N Engl J Med 344(15):1111–1116. doi:10.1056/NEJM200104123441501

Xie J, Brayne C, Matthews FE (2008) Survival times in people with dementia: analysis from population based cohort study with 14 year follow-up. BMJ 336(7638):258–262. doi:10.1136/bmj.39433.616678.25

Oncological and Palliative Care for Patients with Lung Cancer and Patients with Breast Cancer: Two Opposite Ends of a Spectrum

2

Norbert Frickhofen

Contents

2.1   Different Patients

2.1.1   The Patient with Lung Cancer

Robert H. was a 68-year-old patient who presented with a recent onset of cough. He used to work in an office. He was married and had two children and two grandchildren. He used to smoke heavily (80 pack-years) until age 60, when his best friend died from pneumonia after suffering from chronic obstructive pulmonary disease (COPD) for many years. Robert was concerned about having lung cancer,

N. Frickhofen, MD
Department of Hematology, Medical Oncology and Palliative Care,
HSK, Dr. Horst Schmidt Klinik, Ludwig-Erhard-Str. 100, D-65199 Wiesbaden, Germany
e-mail: norbert.frickhofen@helios-kliniken.de

© Springer-Verlag Berlin Heidelberg 2015
B. Alt-Epping, F. Nauck (eds.), *Palliative Care in Oncology*,
DOI 10.1007/978-3-662-46202-7_2

but he dismissed this possibility because he had not smoked a single cigarette for 8 years. He only talked to his doctor after persisting coughs and 3 months of dispute with his wife. A diagnosis of stage IIIA adenocarcinoma of the lung with compression of the right lower bronchus by mediastinal lymph nodes was made. Molecular workup of the biopsy did not reveal EGFR mutation, ALK translocation, or other findings that would qualify for molecular targeted treatment. He rejected being included in a phase III trial of chemoradiotherapy. Since he was otherwise in good health, he received preoperative treatment with platin-based chemotherapy followed by right bilobectomy and postoperative radiotherapy to the mediastinum.

Fifteen months later, Robert complained about right upper quadrant pain. Multiple liver metastases, an adrenal mass, and two asymptomatic brain lesions were discovered; there was no evidence of disease in the thorax. In a family conference, the patient was informed about the incurability of the disease. Treatment options including palliative care were discussed. He strongly opposed palliative care and agreed to participate in a randomized phase II trial with chemotherapy with or without an experimental, orally administered tyrosine kinase inhibitor. During treatment he suffered from loss of appetite and fatigue and had to be hospitalized twice for fever of unknown origin. Treatment was discontinued after three cycles for progression of the adrenal mass, new brain lesions, and poor tolerability of the treatment. He received whole brain irradiation. His functional status declined during radiotherapy. After repeated discussions and recommendation of organizing palliative care, he rejected further contact with medical professionals and returned home. Two months later the patient came to the emergency room for uncontrolled vomiting. He was dehydrated, had lost 5 kg of body weight, and was unable to walk without help. He was transferred to the palliative care unit, consented to limiting care for symptom control and died 11 days later, 2.5 years after the initial diagnosis and 8 months after the diagnosis of metastatic disease.

2.1.2 The Woman with Breast Cancer

Iris N. was a 36-year-old woman[1] when a mass in her right breast was discovered in 1994. At that time, she was married, had an 8-year-old daughter, and worked part-time in a bakery. She was in excellent health, worked out regularly, and neither drank nor smoked. A node-positive invasive ductal adenocarcinoma (NST) stage IIB, grade 2, estrogen receptor positive/progesterone receptor negative was being diagnosed. She decided for mastectomy followed by adjuvant anthracycline-based chemotherapy. Adjuvant radiotherapy was not considered to be indicated after mastectomy. Amenorrhea developed during chemotherapy. She stopped anti-hormonal treatment after 7 months for severe, uncontrollable flushing.

---

[1] This manuscript is limited to women with breast cancer. Men comprise only about 1 % of patients with breast cancer, and data and recommendations are derived from small series and expert opinion.

Five years later, a relapse confined to the thoracic wall was detected, again estrogen receptor positive, but also HER2 positive. The mass was resected, followed by radiotherapy and tamoxifen. One year later, asymptomatic bone and liver metastases were discovered. The bone lesions were irradiated, and after 6 months of chemotherapy, which was well tolerated, liver metastases were no longer visible. During subsequent treatment with an aromatase inhibitor and bisphosphonates, liver metastases recurred 6 months after chemotherapy. She received chemoimmunotherapy with a taxane and the newly approved anti-HER2 drug trastuzumab. Complete remission was achieved in the liver (bone metastases stable), which lasted for more than 2 years. During this time, Iris was treated with trastuzumab infusions as an outpatient without any adverse effects. While liver metastases were well controlled, metastatic disease of a supraclavicular lymph node developed in 2003. During the following 10 years, the patient experienced multiple relapses in the liver (with several complete remissions after treatment), locoregional lymph nodes, and bone. She eventually developed pulmonary and peritoneal metastases. All this could be controlled with surgery, radiotherapy, cytotoxic chemotherapy, anti-HER2 treatment, and anti-hormonal agents. Three regimens were delivered in the context of a clinical trial. During these 10 years, she experienced 5.8 years without any anticancer therapy or with only anti-hormonal and bisphosphonate treatment that did not interfere with her daily activities. The longest time without interruption by surgery, radiotherapy, or chemotherapy was 34 months (10/2005–08/2008). She only stopped working in the bakery in 2012. Iris is now, 10/2013, still in a good physical condition, and she awaits the decision of the tumor board on how to best treat her progressive metastases in the lungs and in the abdomen (peritoneum and omentum). She was repeatedly asked whether she were still willing to be treated. She was always surprised by this question since she was doing well and since "the doctors always found a solution in the past."

2.2 Different Diseases, Different Treatment Options

2.2.1 Patient and Disease Characteristics Are Different

The two cases described above are real cases. They have been selected because they illustrate typical patient and disease characteristics and commonly observed courses (Table 2.1).

Robert presented at a typical age of patients with lung cancer. Frequent relapse of locoregional disease and poor results of the treatment of advanced disease are a sad reality both in non-small cell lung cancer (NSCLC) (85 % of cases) and in small cell lung cancer (SCLC) (15 %). In metastatic NSCLC the median survival of patients with good performance status is 8–11 months (Ramalingam et al. 2011). Clinical trials report a median survival of 1,420 months, but this reflects patient selection and is not mirrored in cancer registries (see Sect. 2.2.2). The mean survival times of patients with SCLS are even shorter; this is the less common and typically more aggressive form of lung cancer. Most patients with metastatic SCLC survive only 8–10 months despite treatment (Planchard and Le 2011).

Table 2.1 Characteristics of patients with lung cancer and breast cancer

	Lung cancer	Breast cancer
Incidence (cases/100,000) USA, whites, incl. Hispanics, 2009[a]	75 (men)/55 (women)	127
Estimated deaths (cases/100,000) USA, 2013[a]	63 (men)/40 (women)	22
Median age at diagnosis[a]	70	61
Etiology	90 % due to smoking	Mostly unknown
	10 % unrelated to smoking	10 % hereditary
Stage at diagnosis[a]	40 % early stage, curable	95 % early stage, curable
	60 % metastatic, incurable	5 % metastatic, incurable
Proportion of patients with localized disease (stage I–III) who relapse with incurable, systemic disease	60 % (NSCLC)	20–30 %
	90 % (SCLC)	
Response of metastatic disease to first-line treatment[a]	30 (10–70) % (NSCLC)[c]	30 (20–80) %[c]
	80 % (SCLC)	
5-year overall survival: Central and northern Europe[b] USA[1]	12–15 % 17 %	84–85 % 89 %
5-year survival with locoregional disease, lymph node negative/positive[a]	54 %/26 %	99 %/84 %
5-year survival with metastatic disease[a]	4 %	24 %

Unless stated otherwise, data are given for NSCLC and SCLC combined. Basic epidemiologic data and overall survival data are derived from the SEER database 2003–2009 (SEER 2013)[a] and EUROCARE-5, northern and central Europe population (De Angelis et al. 2014).[b] Stage-adjusted survival is depicted in Fig. 2.1; 5-year survival data in Table 2.1 and Fig. 2.1 differ because they are derived from different databases. High-response data represent results of treatment with targeted drugs[c]

Iris was younger than most patients with breast cancer. However, patients of this age are commonly observed in cancer clinics. About 6 % of breast cancer occurs in women younger than 40 years (Cardoso et al. 2012b). A long history of metastatic disease – not always as long as in this case – that can be controlled with multiple treatment modalities is the rule rather than the exception in breast cancer (Mauri et al. 2008). Advanced breast cancer is often a chronic relapsing disease, in obvious contrast to metastatic lung cancer, which can only be controlled for a short period of time.

About 90 % of the patients with lung cancer have a history of smoking cigarettes. The risk of lung cancer increases with the duration and the intensity of smoking ("pack-years"). In a British study with data up to 1990, men who continuously smoked since young adulthood, who did not die for other causes and reached the age of 75, had an absolute risk of dying from lung cancer of about 16 %; the risk was 10 % in women (Peto et al. 2000). A more detailed study of middle-aged British women with data up to 2011 demonstrated a 21 fold increased risk of dying from lung cancer within a 12-year observation period. Two-thirds of all deaths of smokers in their 50s, 60s, and 70s were caused by smoking, including nonmalignant pulmonary disease, vascular disease, and other cancers. Smoking women lose at least 10 years of their lifespan compared with nonsmokers (Pirie et al. 2013). Low-dose CT screening decreases the risk of elderly smokers of dying from lung cancer by about 20 %, but this strategy is debated (Aberle et al. 2013). The strong association with smoking is a heavy psychological burden for smokers with lung cancer.

The cause of breast cancer is usually unknown. Induction by external agents such as radiotherapy to the chest is well described. It is a real problem for women treated as children or young adults (Kenney et al. 2004), but these patients are rare in clinical practice. About 10 % of women with breast cancer have hereditary breast cancer, mostly due to defective gene repair systems. Mutations in the breast cancer-1 or breast cancer-2 genes (BRCA-1/BRCA-2) are the main causes of hereditary cancers. Women carrying these mutations have a risk of breast and ovarian cancer of about 60 % up to the age of 70 (Mavaddat et al. 2013). In these women, not to have cared for genetic analysis or – if they are known to carry the mutation – not to have participated in early detection programs may cause distress. Similar thoughts may plague women with sporadic breast cancer who did not regularly undergo screening mammography.

With a median age of 70 years and a history of smoking, most patients with lung cancer start with a disadvantage already based on their personal characteristics. The chance of age-related deterioration of organ function is significantly higher in a 70-year-old patient with lung cancer than in a 60-year-old woman with breast cancer. Renal function and hearing both decrease with age and may prevent use of important drugs like cisplatin. Cardiac function decreases with age. It may not allow treatment with cardiotoxic drugs and cause unacceptable fluid retention during chemotherapy. Other diseases such as diabetes and liver disease are more common in older patients and raise concern with drug metabolism and drug interaction. Chronic lung disease may limit radiotherapy planning. Smoking significantly aggravates organ damage and adds specific risks due to chronic obstructive lung disease and generalized vascular disease. Cognitive and sensory impairments may affect adherence to treatment plans. All these factors are making lung cancer patients more vulnerable to treatment and may thereby limit treatment options irrespective of the cancer itself (Hoffe and Balducci 2012; Ou et al. 2009; Puts et al. 2014).

Social networks, financial aspects, and patient preferences influence treatment options and treatment choices more than most physicians are aware of. Older patients are more often living alone and have a less developed network of relatives and friends than younger patients. Having a partner is a major determinant of treatment success with respect to early diagnosis, adherence to treatment, coping with cancer, and many other aspects of a life-threatening disease such as cancer (Aizer et al. 2013). Patient preferences vary according to age and type of disease. A widowed male patient with lung cancer has a different way of reasoning than a mother of small children with breast cancer.

Most women with breast cancer do not present with as many adverse cofactors as patients with lung cancer. They are on average younger, have a lower smoking-associated comorbidity, and usually have a much better developed social network than patients with lung cancer.

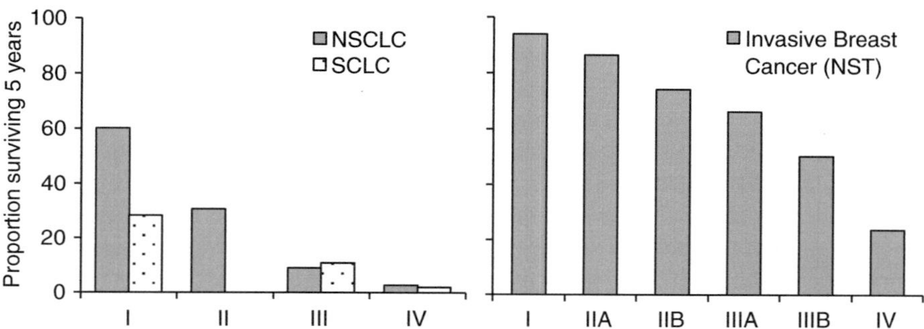

Fig. 2.1 Stage-specific 5-year overall survival of patients with lung cancer (*left*) and breast cancer (*right*) derived from the Tumorregister München, Germany (Tumorregister München 2013). Lung cancer survival is shown separately for non-small cell lung cancer (NSCLC, $n=9,300$) and small cell lung cancer (SCLC, $n=1,874$); stage II SCLC survival is not depicted since fewer than 10 patients were at risk at 5 years. Breast cancer survival data are based on 37,000 women. All stages according to UICC 6th edition

2.2.2 Treatment Options and Treatment Results Are Different

More than 80 % of patients with lung cancer die within 5 years, whereas more than 80 % of patients with breast cancer survive 5 years (Table 2.1). Cancer is the main reason for dying in patients with lung cancer, whereas many women with breast cancer die from causes unrelated to their cancer.

The tragedy of *lung cancer* is that early diagnosis is rare and that even patients with early-stage disease frequently relapse and die from lung cancer.

About 40 % of patients with NSCLC have a tumor confined to the chest at diagnosis (stage I–III). Most of these patients are treated with curative intent. This has to include surgery and in many patients also adjuvant chemotherapy and radiotherapy. However, survival at 5 years is only about 60 % for stage I, 31 % for stage II, and 9 % for stage III (Fig. 2.1) (Tumorregister München 2013). Only about 25 % of the patients with SCLC are diagnosed with cancer confined to the chest (Ignatius Ou and Zell 2009). Surgery of SCLC is only recommended in very early stages. Most patients are treated with definitive chemoradiotherapy. Survival is even poorer than in NSCLC: only 21–38 % of the patients with stage I SCLC, 18–38 % with stage II, and 9–13 % with stage III survive 5 years ((Shepherd et al. 2007) and Fig. 2.1). Adjuvant radiotherapy to the chest reduces local relapse in both NSCLC and SCLC but has only marginal effects on survival. Adjuvant radiotherapy of the brain is usually recommended for patients with SCLC, since it prevents or delays relapse in the brain and may prolong survival even in advanced disease (Slotman et al. 2008). Adjuvant chemotherapy is standard for treatment of patients with resected NSCLC and SCLC. It increases overall survival after surgery with or without radiotherapy by 4–5 % in both types of lung cancer (Arriagada et al. 2010; Planchard and Le 2011). The small benefit of adjuvant treatment must always be kept in mind when counseling patients. This is particularly important for patients with comorbidities.

About 60 % of the patients with NSCLC have metastatic, stage IV disease at diagnosis. Overall, only 3 % (Tumorregister München 2013) of these patients survive 5 years; in surgical series the percentage is 10–15 (Goldstraw et al. 2007). About 75 % of the patients with SCLC have metastatic disease at presentation, and their 5-year survival is only 1–4 % (Ignatius Ou and Zell 2009; Shepherd et al. 2007). Results have significantly improved in molecular defined subgroups of NSCLC (see below), but otherwise progress in the treatment of patients with lung cancer has been frustratingly slow (De Angelis et al. 2014; Owonikoko et al. 2013).

Radiotherapy is used in both types of lung cancer to control local disease and ameliorate symptoms in advanced disease. Palliative chemotherapy has different roles in NSCLC and SCLC. In NSCLC, it primarily controls lung cancer symptoms. Survival is only prolonged by 2–4 months compared to best supportive care. This corresponds to an increase in the 12-month survival by about 10 % (Zhong et al. 2013). In SCLC, palliative chemotherapy is very effective in inducing remission. About 80 % of patients with metastatic disease respond to treatment. However, response lasts for only 5–6 months (Planchard and Le 2011). In both types of lung cancer, the effect of palliative chemotherapy dramatically decreases with further lines of treatment (de Jong et al. 2006; Massarelli et al. 2003).

In patients with *breast cancer*, the situation differs completely. Most women are diagnosed at an early stage and can be cured (Table 2.1). Breast cancer-specific survival is improving in developed countries since about 1990, a combined effect of early diagnosis and better treatment results (Desantis et al. 2014).

About 95 % of women with breast cancer have disease confined to the breast with or without spread to locoregional lymph nodes. Depending on the biological characteristics of the cancer and the extent of nodal involvement, 70–100 % of the women can be cured by surgery and adjuvant hormonal or chemotherapy with or without radiotherapy (Table 2.1 and Fig. 2.1) (Goldhirsch et al. 2013; Tumorregister München 2013).

Twenty to thirty percent of patients with early-stage disease experience a relapse. If it is confined to the initial site of surgery, it can often be cured by combined modality treatment. Cure of oligo-metastatic relapse is more controversial (Pagani et al. 2010). Most patients with disseminated distant metastases eventually die from progressive breast cancer.

Metastatic breast cancer at initial diagnosis or at relapse is usually fatal. Treatment with hormonal agents controls the disease in about 70 % of the patients, including 20–50 % remissions. With conventional cytotoxic regimens, disease control can also be achieved in about 70 % of the patients with 10–35 % remissions after mono-therapy and 30–60 % after multi-agent chemotherapy. Chemotherapy is thus more effective in breast cancer than in lung cancer (Pentheroudakis et al. 2008). In a large series of patients with metastatic breast cancer treated with hormonal agents and conventional cytotoxic drugs, 3 % of all patients remained in complete remission for more than 5 years (Greenberg et al. 1996).

Molecular targeted therapy is a new option both for patients with lung cancer and breast cancer. Results of clinical trials with these drugs receive much attention in the media and raise hopes in patients and among experts (Patel et al. 2014). There are Internet sites such as www.mycancergenome.org where everybody can check the availability of specific treatment options for almost every type of cancer and get into contact with sites all over the world that offer clinical trials with these drugs. Providers of palliative care have to be aware of these new treatment options, since results with targeted drugs can be very impressive even in patients with advanced disease and poor performance status.

Targeted therapy – also referred to as "personalized therapy" – makes news especially in lung cancer. The reason for the publicity is the surprising efficacy in a few patients against the background of very poor results of conventional treatment modalities in the great majority of the patients with lung cancer. About 10 % of the patients with adenocarcinoma of the lung have activating mutations in the gene for the epidermal growth factor receptor 1 (EGFR). Response to EGFR inhibitors like gefitinib and the duration of response are about doubled compared with chemotherapy, and alleviation of symptoms occurs much faster. Higher efficacy is not compromised by more toxicity. In contrast, treatment with EGFR inhibitors is better tolerated by the patients. These inhibitors are therefore suitable even for patients in poor conditions, who would not be eligible for chemotherapy. Another new drug target is the anaplastic lymphoma kinase (ALK), which is activated by chromosomal translocations in 3–5 % of all patients with adenocarcinoma of the lung. Patients respond to ALK inhibitors like crizotinib similar to how patients with EGFR mutations respond to EGFR inhibitors. Both inhibitors are commercially available. Many more drugs with different targets are tested in clinical trials (Buettner et al. 2013). Every patient with incurable lung cancer should therefore be evaluated for potential new drug targets, even if they are not curative and responses last only for about a year. Unfortunately, there has not been similar progress in SCLC.

In contrast to lung cancer, news about new drug targets in breast cancer is currently less prominent, since personalized therapy has been standard for many years. Compared with lung cancer, more women with breast cancer can be treated with targeted drugs. Estrogen deprivation is a very potent way of interfering with hormone-dependent (receptor positive) cancers. This well-established type of treatment is probably the most effective type of targeted therapy for patients with breast cancer. Three classes of agents, selective estrogen receptor modulators (SERM) such as tamoxifen, aromatase inhibitors such as anastrozole, and estrogen receptor antagonists such as fulvestrant, can be used sequentially. Many patients with low-risk, "luminal-type" breast cancer can successfully be treated for many months or years. Blocking of downstream-signaling pathways such as the mammalian target of rapamycin (mTOR) acts synergistically with hormonal and cytotoxic agents and is now a standard option at least for patients with receptor-positive tumors. Identification of agents that block signaling by the human epidermal growth factor receptor 2 (HER2 or HER2/neu) transformed a subgroup of breast cancer with poor prognosis into a highly treatable disease. By combining anti-HER2 agents with chemotherapy, remission rates of up to 80 % can be achieved in advanced breast cancer without compromising quality of life (Baselga et al. 2012). There are many more "druggable" targets in breast cancer, such as signal-transduction molecules,

DNA-repair enzymes, and receptors or soluble factors involved in angiogenesis. Biotechnology introduced highly effective new drug constructs, such as cytotoxic molecules linked to antibodies. They specifically deliver deadly loads of cytotoxic drugs to cancer cells while sparing normal cells. Even conventional cytotoxic drugs can now be used more efficiently, thanks to a better understanding of cancer cell response to DNA-damaging agents and better supportive care (el Saghir et al. 2011; Oostendorp et al. 2011). All this resulted in the transformation of metastatic breast cancer into a chronic relapsing and remitting disease, still incurable, but treatable in many patients. Median survival is still about 2 years, but the range is very wide (Cardoso et al. 2012a). The standstill of median survival for more than 20 years has been explained by balancing of more aggressive metastatic disease (after more effective primary treatment) by more effective treatment (Ufen et al. 2014).

The results of trials with molecular targeted drugs have to be put into perspective: most patients with lung cancer and many patients with breast cancer do not have molecular targets for this new class of drugs and have to rely on standard treatment options, which are improving at very low pace (Coleman et al. 2011; Owonikoko et al. 2013; Pitz et al. 2009). Patients usually ignore this fact and are misled by incomplete or wrong information in the lay media. One should also keep in mind that only about 3 % of adults with advanced cancer enroll on clinical trials. The numbers are higher in breast cancer and lower in lung cancer. Patients in clinical trials are typically highly selected to allow unbiased interpretation of the data. By this approach, results of these trials cannot be used for most patients walking through the door of an oncologist's office. "Real-life" patients are typically older and have more comorbidities. This applies more to patients with lung cancer than to patients with breast cancer (Townsley et al. 2005). In addition, clinical trials are more and more conducted only in high-volume and highly experienced centers to ensure rapid accrual of patients. Handling of adverse effects and access to subsequent treatment modalities are better in patients treated in these centers. Finally, patients with suitable targets can tremendously benefit from the new drugs regarding tumor shrinkage, symptom control, progression-free survival, and overall survival. But responses are mostly short-lived, and none of the currently available targeted drugs are curative for patients with metastatic lung and breast cancer (el Saghir et al. 2011; Ramalingam et al. 2011).

2.3 Symptoms and Palliative Needs of Patients with Lung Cancer and Breast Cancer

In *early stages*, cancer-associated symptoms differ fundamentally in patients with lung cancer and breast cancer. Breast cancer, limited to the breast or to regional lymph nodes, is mostly detected by the woman herself as a lump in her breast. Except for locally advanced or inflammatory breast cancer, it is asymptomatic. In contrast, even lung cancer confined to the chest is symptomatic in many patients. Lung parenchyma is not generously supplied with pain fibers. A neoplastic lesion can therefore reach considerable size without causing symptoms. If it does, patients have usually locally advanced, stage II–III disease. Patients may then suffer from pain due to invasion of the pleura, the ribs, the nerves, or other structures of the mediastinum. If the cancer grows into the bronchial tree, patients may experience cough or may develop pneumonia due to obstruction of the airways. Breathlessness and fear of suffocation is highly prevalent in these patients early on (Pass et al. 2010).

It is important to realize that many patients with lung cancer experience severe symptoms and a sense of threat to their life early in their disease trajectory. They need help with coping with the diagnosis of cancer like every patient with cancer, but even at early stages, many require more medical support for symptom control than women with early breast cancer.

In *late stages* of lung and breast cancer, symptoms and palliative needs gradually converge. They are driven by the sites of metastases and by systemic effects of uncontrolled disease such as fatigue or weight loss. However, patient- and disease-specific factors such as individual characteristics, adverse effects of treatment, comorbidities, and psychosocial factors differ in patients with lung cancer and with breast cancer and may modify the patients' performance and the course of the disease.

2.3.1 The Patient with Metastatic Lung Cancer

About 60 % of the patients with lung cancer present with metastatic cancer. Most patients are therefore faced with an incurable disease at the outset. This is in sharp contrast to breast cancer, where 95 % of the women present with localized and basically curable disease.

If metastasis is a secondary event after previous treatment of localized disease (30–40 % of all patients with metastatic NSCLC and 20–25 % of all patients with metastatic SCLC), the extent of metastatic spread may be limited. In this situation, symptoms are determined by the site of the metastases: pleural effusion or symptoms caused by compression of mediastinal structures due to thoracic metastases, skeletal pain due to bone metastases, abdominal pain or jaundice due to liver metastases, or headache, seizures, or other central nervous symptoms due to brain metastases (Pass et al. 2010).

Most patients who present with primary metastatic lung cancer have multiple metastatic sites. In a descending order, the bone, contralateral lung, brain, adrenal glands, pleura, liver, lymph nodes, skin, and abdominal viscera are involved. Patients may experience paraneoplastic syndromes, especially those with SCLC (Pass et al. 2010).

These patients face a wide spectrum of symptoms and problems (Table 2.2): physical symptoms (e.g., fatigue, loss of appetite, weight loss), psychological distress (e.g., worrying, nervousness, or anxiety), and disease-related symptoms at the site of the primary (e.g., cough, hemoptysis, shortness of breath, or chest pain) and at the sites of distant metastases (e.g., bone pain, abdominal pain, or headaches). Examples of treatment-related symptoms are peripheral neuropathy (e.g., caused by

Table 2.2 Specific (upper row of each parameter) and common (lower row, respectively) characteristics and symptoms of patients with metastatic lung cancer and breast cancer (for references, see Table 2.1 and text)

	Advanced lung cancer	Advanced breast cancer
Patient characteristics	Median age 70, men > women, metastasis as the presenting manifestation, smoker	Median age 61, women (99 %), metastasis as secondary event, nonsmoker
	Fear of facing a life-threatening disease, disability, loss of autonomy	
Tumor specific	Cough, breathlessness, hemoptysis	Inflammatory or ulcerating breast disease
Cancer associated	Fatigue, loss of appetite, weight loss, diarrhea, ascites, edema, pain, pathologic fracture, thromboembolic events, headache, confusion, seizures, palsies	
Treatment associated	Hearing impairment, renal disease, rash	Palmar-plantar erythrodysesthesia, myocardial disease
	Infection ("neutropenic fever"), bleeding, alopecia, nausea, vomiting, stomatitis, diarrhea, asthenia, fatigue, neuropathy, skin disorder, nail dystrophy, hypertension	
Psychosocial	Social network often less developed	Social network often well developed
	Difficulty sleeping, worrying, nervousness, anxiety, depression, cognitive impairment, decreased sexual interest, instability of partnership	

cisplatin), worsening of fatigue (e.g., caused by pemetrexed or gemcitabine), gastrointestinal symptoms (e.g., EGFR and ALK inhibitors), and rash, nail dystrophy, and paronychia (docetaxel, EGFR inhibitors). Patients rate 20–50 % of these symptoms as severe. The number and severity of symptoms increase toward the final phase of the disease (Alt-Epping et al. 2012; Gaertner et al. 2010, 2012; Hopwood and Stephens 1995; Koczywas et al. 2013; Lutz et al. 2001). Treatment recommendations are detailed in other chapters of this monograph.

Compared with patients with other cancers, symptoms of lung cancer patients are more severe, and many are difficult to treat. This applies first and foremost to dyspnea and pain (Alt-Epping et al. 2012; Vainio and Auvinen 1996). Considering older age and more smoking-associated diseases than women with breast cancer, patients with lung cancer have more comorbid conditions, such as obstructive lung disease and vascular disease. This leads to poorer tolerance of treatment and more complications.

Psychosocial distress is very common in patients with lung cancer. In a survey of 4,500 and 3,100 patients with different cancers, psychosocial distress was found to be highest in patients with lung cancer with a prevalence of 58 % and 43 %, respectively (Vainio and Auvinen 1996; Zabora et al. 2001). About a quarter of the patients report contact with the health-care system as causing them most distress at one or more time points close to the end of life, which is rarely detected by questionnaires (Tishelman et al. 2010). Distress is aggravated by the feeling of guilt, since the disease is so strongly associated with smoking. Patients are aware that their behavior contributed to their cancer and because of this are three times more likely to feel guilty than patients with breast and prostate cancer (LoConte et al. 2008). They also feel stigmatized or unjustly blamed if they stopped smoking many years ago (Chapple et al. 2004). This may cause isolation and unwillingness to seek help (Steele and Fitch 2008).

There are only a few data on spiritual needs in patients with lung cancer. Intuitively correct is the observation that patients who are open to spirituality and who see meaning in life feel better and have fewer distress symptoms (Meraviglia 2004; Murray et al. 2004). This is independent of religious beliefs and probably applies to all patients with advanced life-threatening disease.

2.3.2 The Woman with Metastatic Breast Cancer

Metastatic breast cancer is mostly a disease of women who relapsed after treatment of local breast cancer (Table 2.1). These women had experienced the existential threat of cancer before. Relapse may occur more than 10 years after the initial diagnosis. They had hoped to have overcome the disease, although they were always aware of the possibility of relapse.

Only 5 % of the women present with primary metastatic breast cancer at first diagnosis. Then, advanced metastatic disease and cancer-associated symptoms may be present, similar to patients suffering from lung cancer (Sect. 2.3.1, Table 2.2). However, chest symptoms do not usually dominate, as in lung cancer.

The most common metastatic sites in women presenting with metastatic breast cancer are the bone (40–75 %) followed by the lung (5–15 %), pleura (5–15 %), liver (3–10 %), and brain (5 %). At autopsy, the bone, lung, pleura, and liver are equally affected in about half of the patients. There is no organ that cannot be affected by breast cancer metastases. Five to 10 % of women who are treated for locoregional disease experience a relapse at the initial site, that is, in the remaining breast, the chest wall, or the regional lymph nodes (Harris et al. 2009).

Treatment of common symptoms of patients with systemic disease such as pain, fatigue, anxiety and depression, difficulty sleeping, lymphedema, dyspnea, and gastrointestinal symptoms is similar to patients with an according metastatic spread in lung cancer. Recommendations to control these symptoms are covered in other chapters of this monograph, and there is a good review of the current recommendations available from the Internet (Irvin et al. 2011).

Negative psychosocial consequences of metastatic breast cancer have been well described. Women complain that they cannot go on living a normal life. Quality of life decreases. They experience deterioration of physical and role functioning, especially within the family. Personal relationships may break, and they fear to be unable to care for themselves at the end of life (Kenne et al. 2007; Luoma and Hakamies-Blomqvist 2004; Mayer 2010). In one study in Australia, unmet needs were highest in the psychological and health information domains. Women asked for psychological support and counseling. They searched for information regarding things they could do to feel better, information on the status of their cancer, interpretation of test results, and risks and benefits of treatment (Aranda et al. 2005). One has to bear in mind that needs may be similar in different cultures, but priorities may be different (Lam et al. 2011).

Women with early metastatic breast cancer tend to have fewer cancer-related symptoms than patients with lung cancer (Sect. 2.3.1). The ability to control the disease with multiple lines of treatment (Mauri et al. 2008) may move the focus to treatment-related symptoms. Initially, metastatic breast cancer responds to "simple" treatment modalities such as anti-hormonal agents and well-tolerated, single cytotoxic drugs. With further lines of treatment and the development of drug resistance, less well-tolerated drugs and local treatment modalities such as surgery and radiation therapy have to be used. In conjunction with dwindling physical and emotional resources of the patients, the balance between antitumor effects and adverse effects tips at some point. In addition, prolonged control of the disease may select cancer cell clones with different biological characteristics and behavior. Patients experience more often brain metastases (Larsen et al. 2013) and metastases to otherwise unusual sites such as the skin, the spinal cord, the gut, or the heart. These events should urge to reconsider the benefit of anticancer treatment and discuss a change in goals and transition to palliative care.

2.3.3 Principles of Palliative Care

Professionals treating patients with metastatic lung cancer and breast cancer should keep in mind that the disease cannot be cured. The patient is the one setting therapeutic goals and deciding on how to reach these goals. Caregivers have the duty to inform her or him about what is possible from their point of view and what the consequences are of any decisions and actions taken.

Maintaining quality of life while optimizing disease control should be the mainstay of care (Irvin et al. 2011). Effects of antineoplastic, symptom-oriented, and supportive treatment should always be balanced against adverse effects of these modalities. One-sided and close-minded thinking should have no place in palliative care of patients at the end of life. Examples for unorthodox actions in the palliative setting include surgery and chemotherapy. Surgery is the most effective and most durable way of dealing with painful or infected tumor masses (Amann et al. 2013; Morrogh et al. 2010). Chemotherapy may be the best way to palliate symptoms such as breathlessness or cough due to effusions or to lymphangitic lung metastases, pain due to mass effects of metastases, paralysis or pain due to neoplastic meningitis, or constitutional symptoms caused by mediators released by cancer cells (Geels et al. 2000). Even minor effects of chemotherapy by standard oncologic evaluation criteria may result in symptomatic improvement (De Marinis et al. 2008; Geels et al. 2000). New drugs such as EGFR inhibitors in lung cancer or HER2 inhibitors in breast cancer require rethinking of the rules (Sect. 2.2.2). A classic "palliative" patient with known targets for drugs who never received these drugs should be informed about these treatment options. On the other hand, if palliative care without anticancer treatment options is the way to go, it should be palliative care and not leaving the patients alone (Lester et al. 2013).

Temel and colleagues demonstrated that palliative care in a broader sense has the capacity to improve the patients' well-being and survival that may rival oncologic approaches. They demonstrated that patients with metastatic lung cancer may live longer if they are accompanied by a dedicated team of palliative care specialists parallel to their oncologic treatment. Palliative care in this study included support to better understand the disease and its treatment, to optimize symptom management by systematically evaluating symptoms, to support decision-making, to help with coping, and to make sure that the patient adheres to the rules of treatment (Temel et al. 2010). A similar "early palliative care" approach has been demonstrated to improve the quality of life in patients with other solid tumors (Zimmermann et al. 2014). One may argue that this kind of support does not represent classical palliative care, but rather optimal oncological care. However, one has to acknowledge that accompanying a patient this way rarely succeeds in a busy oncological practice or hospital oncology ward. If the oncologist cannot do it, this support should be offered by someone who is trained to do it, for example, the palliative care specialist. He/she may be better prepared and may have more time to gather the patients' symptoms and needs (Okuyama et al. 2011). This topic is discussed in more detail in the chapter of Gaertner and colleagues.

Classical approaches to palliate specific symptoms and to palliative care in general are described in detail in this monograph and in recent guidelines or reviews (Ford et al. 2013; Irvin et al. 2011). They illustrate that care of patients with advanced cancer is a team approach. Knowledge and expertise of all team members is required to reach the optimal outcome for the patients.

2.4　Information Needs and Priorities of Patients with Incurable Cancer

Communicating with a patient with incurable cancer is challenging, and it does not always succeed. Women with breast cancer report unmet information needs relevant to health information, and many are dissatisfied with the information they receive from their providers. Information needs have been identified and programs aimed at specific patient groups have been described (Parker et al. 2009). However, they apply primarily to cancer prevention and treatment and not to patients in late stages of their disease. Research in this setting is more difficult due to the heterogeneity of the patients, and funding of palliative care research is difficult.

Recommendations on how to deal with the information needs of patients with lung cancer and breast cancer at the end of their life are mainly based on case series, qualitative research, expert opinion, and common sense. Only some research results applying to patients with lung cancer and breast cancer are discussed here.

Survival time is very important to many patients. Many palliative care professionals tend to generalize their view as healthy individuals of "adding life to days and not days to life." They may underestimate the importance of length of life for a patient with impending death. Many would be surprised by data demonstrating that many patients choose active and even aggressive treatment with the primary aim of prolonging life while accepting significant toxicity (Matsuyama et al. 2006).

However, most patients greatly overestimate the chance of prolongation of life in advanced stages of solid tumors, and many do not seem to fully understand their situation. Two out of three patients with advanced lung cancer do not understand that the treatment they receive is not curative (Weeks et al. 2012). An incorrect perception of the prognosis also applies to relatives of the patients. In a longitudinal study of patients with incurable cancer and their family caregivers, in 2/3 of the pairs, the patient, their caregiver, or both believed that the goal of treatment was curative or they stated that they did not know the aim of the treatment (Burns et al. 2007). The perception changed over time, but only as death approached did neither of the pair continued to believe that the treatment goal was cure. Unfortunately, if physicians are asked to estimate life expectancy, they also tend to overestimate survival, especially in patients near death (Gripp et al. 2007).

Physicians must realize that patients' preferences vary widely at one point in time and more so during the disease trajectory. Some patients faced with a life-threatening or terminal illness refuse any treatment, while others are willing to undergo almost any treatment for a small chance of benefit (Matsuyama et al. 2006). Elderly patients have accumulated a wealth of experience and knowledge and put other factors into decision-making than younger patients. Preferences are also influenced by social status, by having a partner or not, and by cultural and spiritual beliefs, to name only a few other parameters.

Physicians should honestly communicate options and outcomes to enable shared decision-making. They should realize that there are many misconceptions that may hinder adequate information (Mack and Smith 2012). Survival is best explained as worst-case, typical-case, and best-case scenarios (Kiely et al. 2011). Patients should be encouraged to express their preferences. Conjoint analysis – a widely used method in market research – is an interesting tool to better understand patients' reasoning and preferences (Bridges et al. 2012). Open communication about prognosis helps in the transition from active cancer treatment to palliative care (Grunfeld et al. 2006), and this kind of information is preferred by the patients if they are assured not to be abandoned (van Vliet et al. 2013).

2.5 Role of the Public

The team delivering palliative care to patients with advanced lung or breast cancer should realize that there are basic differences between these two patient groups beyond medical topics.

Breast cancer is a highly public disease. It is the most common cancer covered in the media (Stryker et al. 2007). There are hundreds of social groups for patients with breast cancer (De la Torre-Diez et al. 2012). Many celebrities do not hide their cancer but rather go public and share almost every detail of their disease. All this increases public awareness, facilitates funding of breast cancer research and support of women with breast cancer, and even influences legislation (Osuch et al. 2012).

In contrast, most people view lung cancer as the ugly disease of people who did not take care of themselves (Marlow et al. 2010). Patients with lung cancer tend to hide their disease, suffering from the stigma of a self-inflicted disease. There are only a few patient support groups compared to the amount of such groups for patients with breast cancer. Patients with lung cancer cannot nearly rely as much on support networks as patients with breast cancer. Funding of lung cancer research only got momentum when molecular targets for more effective treatment were discovered and chances of earning money with these expensive drugs increased dramatically.

Conclusions

Patients with lung cancer and breast cancer differ in several respects. They have different personal characteristics and social backgrounds, they present with different disease manifestations, and they rely on different treatment options. This accounts for different palliative care approaches. Due to the rapidly fatal course of advanced lung cancer, the full spectrum of palliative care should be offered to these patients as soon as a diagnosis of incurability is made. For women with breast cancer, offering palliative care for symptom control can often be delayed because these patients have more effective anticancer treatment options. However, because palliative care constitutes more than symptom control and women with breast cancer face similar complex psychological, social, and spiritual consequences of the disease and its treatment, contact with palliative care specialists should be offered as soon as the disease is considered incurable. Emphasis in the early phase of metastatic breast cancer should be put on counseling, help with coping, support with decision-making, and assistance with technical aspects of treatment. For both groups of patients, smoothly integrating palliative care into the oncology setting and continuing support throughout the course of the illness should be standard today (Peppercorn et al. 2011; Smith et al. 2012).

References

Aberle DR, Abtin F, Brown K (2013) Computed tomography screening for lung cancer: has it finally arrived? Implications of the national lung screening trial. J Clin Oncol 31:1002–1008

Aizer AA, Chen MH, McCarthy EP, Mendu ML, Koo S, Wilhite TJ, Graham PL, Choueiri TK, Hoffman KE, Martin NE, Hu JC, Nguyen PL (2013) Marital status and survival in patients with cancer. J Clin Oncol 31:3869–3876

Alt-Epping B, Staritz AE, Simon ST, Altfelder N, Hotz T, Lindena G, Nauck F (2012) What is special about patients with lung cancer and pulmonary metastases in palliative care? Results from a nationwide survey. J Palliat Med 15:971–977

Amann E, Huang DJ, Weber WP, Eppenberger-Castori S, Schmid SM, Hess TH, Guth U (2013) Disease-related surgery in patients with distant metastatic breast cancer. Eur J Surg Oncol 39:1192–1198

Aranda S, Schofield P, Weih L, Yates P, Milne D, Faulkner R, Voudouris N (2005) Mapping the quality of life and unmet needs of urban women with metastatic breast cancer. Eur J Cancer Care (Engl) 14:211–222

Arriagada R, Auperin A, Burdett S, Higgins JP, Johnson DH, Le CT, Le PC, Parmar MK, Pignon JP, Souhami RL, Stephens RJ, Stewart LA, Tierney JF, Tribodet H, van Meerbeeck J (2010) Adjuvant chemotherapy, with or without postoperative radiotherapy, in operable non-small-cell lung cancer: two meta-analyses of individual patient data. Lancet 375:1267–1277

Baselga J, Cortes J, Kim SB, Im SA, Hegg R, Im YH, Roman L, Pedrini JL, Pienkowski T, Knott A, Clark E, Benyunes MC, Ross G, Swain SM (2012) Pertuzumab plus trastuzumab plus docetaxel for metastatic breast cancer. N Engl J Med 366:109–119

Bridges JF, Mohamed AF, Finnern HW, Woehl A, Hauber AB (2012) Patients' preferences for treatment outcomes for advanced non-small cell lung cancer: a conjoint analysis. Lung Cancer 77:224–231

Buettner R, Wolf J, Thomas RK (2013) Lessons learned from lung cancer genomics: the emerging concept of individualized diagnostics and treatment. J Clin Oncol 31:1858–1865

Burns CM, Broom DH, Smith WT, Dear K, Craft PS (2007) Fluctuating awareness of treatment goals among patients and their caregivers: a longitudinal study of a dynamic process. Support Care Cancer 15:187–196

Cardoso F, Costa A, Norton L, Cameron D, Cufer T, Fallowfield L, Francis P, Gligorov J, Kyriakides S, Lin N, Pagani O, Senkus E, Thomssen C, Aapro M, Bergh J, Di LA, El SN, Ganz PA, Gelmon K, Goldhirsch A, Harbeck N, Houssami N, Hudis C, Kaufman B, Leadbeater M, Mayer M, Rodger A, Rugo H, Sacchini V, Sledge G, Van't Veer L, Viale G, Krop I, Winer E (2012a) 1st International consensus guidelines for advanced breast cancer (ABC 1). Breast 21:242–252

Cardoso F, Loibl S, Pagani O, Graziottin A, Panizza P, Martincich L, Gentilini O, Peccatori F, Fourquet A, Delaloge S, Marotti L, Perrault-Llorca F, Kotti-Kitromilidou AM, Rodger A, Harbeck N (2012b) The European Society of Breast Cancer Specialists recommendations for the management of young women with breast cancer. Eur J Cancer 48:3355–3377

Chapple A, Ziebland S, McPherson A (2004) Stigma, shame, and blame experienced by patients with lung cancer: qualitative study. BMJ 328:1470

Coleman MP, Forman D, Bryant H, Butler J, Rachet B, Maringe C, Nur U, Tracey E, Coory M, Hatcher J, McGahan CE, Turner D, Marrett L, Gjerstorff ML, Johannesen TB, Adolfsson J, Lambe M, Lawrence G, Meechan D, Morris EJ, Middleton R, Steward J, Richards MA (2011) Cancer survival in Australia, Canada, Denmark, Norway, Sweden, and the UK, 1995–2007 (the International Cancer Benchmarking Partnership): an analysis of population-based cancer registry data. Lancet 377:127–138

De Angelis R, Sant M, Coleman MP, Francisci S, Baili P, Pierannunzio D, Trama A, Visser O, Brenner H, Ardanaz E, Bielska-Lasota M, Engholm G, Nennecke A, Siesling S, Berrino F, Capocaccia R (2014) Cancer survival in Europe 1999–2007 by country and age: results of EUROCARE-5-a population-based study. Lancet Oncol 15:23–34

de Jong WK, ten Hacken NH, Groen HJ (2006) Third-line chemotherapy for small cell lung cancer. Lung Cancer 52:339–342

De la Torre-Diez I, Diaz-Pernas FJ, Anton-Rodriguez M (2012) A content analysis of chronic diseases social groups on Facebook and Twitter. Telemed J E Health 18:404–408

De Marinis F, Pereira JR, Fossella F, Perry MC, Reck M, Salzberg M, Jassem J, Peterson P, Liepa AM, Moore P, Gralla RJ (2008) Lung Cancer Symptom Scale outcomes in relation to standard efficacy measures: an analysis of the phase III study of pemetrexed versus docetaxel in advanced non-small cell lung cancer. J Thorac Oncol 3:30–36

Desantis C, Ma J, Bryan L, Jemal A (2014) Breast cancer statistics, 2013. CA Cancer J Clin 64:52–62

el Saghir NS, Tfayli A, Hatoum HA, Nachef Z, Dinh P, Awada A (2011) Treatment of metastatic breast cancer: state-of-the-art, subtypes and perspectives. Crit Rev Oncol Hematol 80:433–449

Ford DW, Koch KA, Ray DE, Selecky PA (2013) Palliative and end-of-life care in lung cancer: diagnosis and management of lung cancer, 3rd ed: American College of Chest Physicians evidence-based clinical practice guidelines. Chest 143:e498S–e512S

Gaertner J, Wolf J, Scheicht D, Frechen S, Klein U, Hellmich M, Ostgathe C, Hallek M, Voltz R (2010) Implementing WHO recommendations for palliative care into routine lung cancer therapy: a feasibility project. J Palliat Med 13:727–732

Gaertner J, Wolf J, Frechen S, Klein U, Scheicht D, Hellmich M, Toepelt K, Glossmann JP, Ostgathe C, Hallek M, Voltz R (2012) Recommending early integration of palliative care – does it work? Support Care Cancer 20:507–513

Geels P, Eisenhauer E, Bezjak A, Zee B, Day A (2000) Palliative effect of chemotherapy: objective tumor response is associated with symptom improvement in patients with metastatic breast cancer. J Clin Oncol 18:2395–2405

Goldhirsch A, Winer EP, Coates AS, Gelber RD, Piccart-Gebhart M, Thurlimann B, Senn HJ (2013) Personalizing the treatment of women with early breast cancer: highlights of the St Gallen International Expert Consensus on the Primary Therapy of Early Breast Cancer 2013. Ann Oncol 24:2206–2223

Goldstraw P, Crowley J, Chansky K, Giroux DJ, Groome PA, Rami-Porta R, Postmus PE, Rusch V, Sobin L (2007) The IASLC Lung Cancer Staging Project: proposals for the revision of the TNM stage groupings in the forthcoming (seventh) edition of the TNM Classification of malignant tumours. J Thorac Oncol 2:706–714

Greenberg PA, Hortobagyi GN, Smith TL, Ziegler LD, Frye DK, Buzdar AU (1996) Long-term follow-up of patients with complete remission following combination chemotherapy for metastatic breast cancer. J Clin Oncol 14:2197–2205

Gripp S, Moeller S, Bolke E, Schmitt G, Matuschek C, Asgari S, Asgharzadeh F, Roth S, Budach W, Franz M, Willers R (2007) Survival prediction in terminally ill cancer patients by clinical estimates, laboratory tests, and self-rated anxiety and depression. J Clin Oncol 25: 3313–3320

Grunfeld EA, Maher EJ, Browne S, Ward P, Young T, Vivat B, Walker G, Wilson C, Potts HW, Westcombe AM, Richards MA, Ramirez AJ (2006) Advanced breast cancer patients' perceptions of decision making for palliative chemotherapy. J Clin Oncol 24:1090–1098

Harris JR, Lippman ME, Osborne CK, Morrow M (2009) Diseases of the breast. Lippincott Williams & Wilkins, Philadelphia

Hoffe S, Balducci L (2012) Cancer and age: general considerations. Clin Geriatr Med 28:1–18

Hopwood P, Stephens RJ (1995) Symptoms at presentation for treatment in patients with lung cancer: implications for the evaluation of palliative treatment. The Medical Research Council (MRC) Lung Cancer Working Party. Br J Cancer 71:633–636

Ignatius Ou SH, Zell JA (2009) The applicability of the proposed IASLC staging revisions to small cell lung cancer (SCLC) with comparison to the current UICC 6th TNM Edition. J Thorac Oncol 4:300–310

Irvin W Jr, Muss HB, Mayer DK (2011) Symptom management in metastatic breast cancer. Oncologist 16:1203–1214

Kenne SE, Ohlen J, Jonsson T, Gaston-Johansson F (2007) Coping with recurrent breast cancer: predictors of distressing symptoms and health-related quality of life. J Pain Symptom Manage 34:24–39

Kenney LB, Yasui Y, Inskip PD, Hammond S, Neglia JP, Mertens AC, Meadows AT, Friedman D, Robison LL, Diller L (2004) Breast cancer after childhood cancer: a report from the Childhood Cancer Survivor Study. Ann Intern Med 141:590–597

Kiely BE, Soon YY, Tattersall MH, Stockler MR (2011) How long have I got? Estimating typical, best-case, and worst-case scenarios for patients starting first-line chemotherapy for metastatic breast cancer: a systematic review of recent randomized trials. J Clin Oncol 29:456–463

Koczywas M, Cristea M, Thomas J, McCarty C, Borneman T, Del FC, Sun V, Uman G, Ferrell B (2013) Interdisciplinary palliative care intervention in metastatic non-small-cell lung cancer. Clin Lung Cancer 14:736–744

Lam WW, Au AH, Wong JH, Lehmann C, Koch U, Fielding R, Mehnert A (2011) Unmet supportive care needs: a cross-cultural comparison between Hong Kong Chinese and German Caucasian women with breast cancer. Breast Cancer Res Treat 130:531–541

Larsen PB, Kumler I, Nielsen DL (2013) A systematic review of trastuzumab and lapatinib in the treatment of women with brain metastases from HER2-positive breast cancer. Cancer Treat Rev 39:720–727

Lester JF, Agulnik J, Akerborg O, Chouaid C, De GA, Finnern HW, Herder GJ, Lungershausen J, Mitchell PL, Vansteenkiste J, Ziske C, Goker E (2013) What constitutes best supportive care in the treatment of advanced non-small cell lung cancer patients?–results from the lung cancer economics and outcomes research (LUCEOR) study. Lung Cancer 82:128–135

LoConte NK, Else-Quest NM, Eickhoff J, Hyde J, Schiller JH (2008) Assessment of guilt and shame in patients with non-small-cell lung cancer compared with patients with breast and prostate cancer. Clin Lung Cancer 9:171–178

Luoma ML, Hakamies-Blomqvist L (2004) The meaning of quality of life in patients being treated for advanced breast cancer: a qualitative study. Psychooncology 13:729–739

Lutz S, Norrell R, Bertucio C, Kachnic L, Johnson C, Arthur D, Schwarz M, Palardy G (2001) Symptom frequency and severity in patients with metastatic or locally recurrent lung cancer: a prospective study using the Lung Cancer Symptom Scale in a community hospital. J Palliat Med 4:157–165

Mack JW, Smith TJ (2012) Reasons why physicians do not have discussions about poor prognosis, why it matters, and what can be improved. J Clin Oncol 30:2715–2717

Marlow LA, Waller J, Wardle J (2010) Variation in blame attributions across different cancer types. Cancer Epidemiol Biomarkers Prev 19:1799–1805

Massarelli E, Andre F, Liu DD, Lee JJ, Wolf M, Fandi A, Ochs J, le Chevalier T, Fossella F, Herbst RS (2003) A retrospective analysis of the outcome of patients who have received two prior chemotherapy regimens including platinum and docetaxel for recurrent non-small-cell lung cancer. Lung Cancer 39:55–61

Matsuyama R, Reddy S, Smith TJ (2006) Why do patients choose chemotherapy near the end of life? A review of the perspective of those facing death from cancer. J Clin Oncol 24:3490–3496

Mauri D, Polyzos NP, Salanti G, Pavlidis N, Icannidis JP (2008) Multiple-treatments meta-analysis of chemotherapy and targeted therapies in advanced breast cancer. J Natl Cancer Inst 100:1780–1791

Mavaddat N, Peock S, Frost D, Ellis S, Platte R, Fineberg E, Evans DG, Izatt L, Eeles RA, Adlard J, Davidson R, Eccles D, Cole T, Cook J, Brewer C, Tischkowitz M, Douglas F, Hodgson S, Walker L, Porteous ME, Morrison PJ, Side LE, Kennedy MJ, Houghton C, Donaldson A, Rogers MT, Dorkins H, Miedzybrodzka Z, Gregory H, Eason J, Barwell J, McCann E, Murray A, Antoniou AC, Easton DF (2013) Cancer risks for BRCA1 and BRCA2 mutation carriers: results from prospective analysis of EMBRACE. J Natl Cancer Inst 105:812–822

Mayer M (2010) Lessons learned from the metastatic breast cancer community. Semin Oncol Nurs 26:195–202

Meraviglia MG (2004) The effects of spirituality on well-being of people with lung cancer. Oncol Nurs Forum 31:89–94

Morrogh M, Miner TJ, Park A, Jenckes A, Gonen M, Seidman A, Morrow M, Jaques DP, King TA (2010) A prospective evaluation of the durability of palliative interventions for patients with metastatic breast cancer. Cancer 116:3338–3347

Murray SA, Kendall M, Boyd K, Worth A, Benton TF (2004) Exploring the spiritual needs of people dying of lung cancer or heart failure: a prospective qualitative interview study of patients and their carers. Palliat Med 18:39–45

Okuyama T, Akechi T, Yamashita H, Toyama T, Nakaguchi T, Uchida M, Furukawa TA (2011) Oncologists' recognition of supportive care needs and symptoms of their patients in a breast cancer outpatient consultation. Jpn J Clin Oncol 41:1251–1258

Oostendorp LJ, Stalmeier PF, Donders AR, van der Graaf WT, Ottevanger PB (2011) Efficacy and safety of palliative chemotherapy for patients with advanced breast cancer pretreated with anthracyclines and taxanes: a systematic review. Lancet Oncol 12:1053–1061

Osuch JR, Silk K, Price C, Barlow J, Miller K, Hernick A, Fonfa A (2012) A historical perspective on breast cancer activism in the United States: from education and support to partnership in scientific research. J Womens Health (Larchmt) 21:355–362

Ou SH, Ziogas A, Zell JA (2009) Prognostic factors for survival in extensive stage small cell lung cancer (ED-SCLC): the importance of smoking history, socioeconomic and marital statuses, and ethnicity. J Thorac Oncol 4:37–43

Owonikoko TK, Ragin C, Chen Z, Kim S, Behera M, Brandes JC, Saba NF, Pentz R, Ramalingam SS, Khuri FR (2013) Real-world effectiveness of systemic agents approved for advanced non-small cell lung cancer: a SEER-Medicare analysis. Oncologist 18:600–610

Pagani O, Senkus E, Wood W, Colleoni M, Cufer T, Kyriakides S, Costa A, Winer EP, Cardoso F (2010) International guidelines for management of metastatic breast cancer: can metastatic breast cancer be cured? J Natl Cancer Inst 102:456–463

Parker PA, Aaron J, Baile WF (2009) Breast cancer: unique communication challenges and strategies to address them. Breast J 15:69–75

Pass HI, Carbone DP, Johnson DH, Minna JD, Scagliotti GV, Turrisi AT (2010) Principles and practice of lung cancer. Lippincott Williams & Wilkins, Philadelphia

Patel JD, Krilov L, Adams S, Aghajanian C, Basch E, Brose MS, Carroll WL, De LM, Gilbert MR, Kris MG, Marshall JL, Masters GA, O'Day SJ, Polite B, Schwartz GK, Sharma S, Thompson I, Vogelzang NJ, Roth BJ (2014) Clinical cancer advances 2013: annual report on progress against cancer from the American society of clinical oncology. J Clin Oncol 32:129–160

Pentheroudakis G, Fountzilas G, Kalofonos HP, Golfinopoulos V, Aravantinos G, Bafaloukos D, Papakostas P, Pectasides D, Christodoulou C, Syrigos K, Economopoulos T, Pavlidis N (2008) Palliative chemotherapy in elderly patients with common metastatic malignancies: a Hellenic Cooperative Oncology Group registry analysis of management, outcome and clinical benefit predictors. Crit Rev Oncol Hematol 66:237–247

Peppercorn JM, Smith TJ, Helft PR, Debono DJ, Berry SR, Wollins DS, Hayes DM, Von Roenn JH, Schnipper LE (2011) American society of clinical oncology statement: toward individualized care for patients with advanced cancer. J Clin Oncol 29:755–760

Peto R, Darby S, Deo H, Silcocks P, Whitley E, Doll R (2000) Smoking, smoking cessation, and lung cancer in the UK since 1950. BMJ 321:323–329

Pirie K, Peto R, Reeves GK, Green J, Beral V (2013) The 21st century hazards of smoking and benefits of stopping: a prospective study of one million women in the UK. Lancet 381:133–141

Pitz MW, Musto G, Demers AA, Kliewer EV, Navaratnam S (2009) Survival and treatment pattern of non-small cell lung cancer over 20 years. J Thorac Oncol 4:492–498

Planchard D, Le PC (2011) Small cell lung cancer: new clinical recommendations and current status of biomarker assessment. Eur J Cancer 47(Suppl 3):S272–S283

Puts MTE, Tu HA, Tourangeau A, Howell D, Fitch M, Springall E, Alibhai SMH (2014) Factors influencing adherence to cancer treatment in older adults with cancer: a systematic review. Ann Oncol 25:564–577

Ramalingam SS, Owonikoko TK, Khuri FR (2011) Lung cancer: new biological insights and recent therapeutic advances. CA Cancer J Clin 61:91–112

SEER (2013) SEER Cancer Stat Fact Sheets, 2003–2009. National Cancer Institute. http://seer.cancer.gov/statfacts. Accessed 20 Dec 2013

Shepherd FA, Crowley J, Van HP, Postmus PE, Carney D, Chansky K, Shaikh Z, Goldstraw P (2007) The International Association for the Study of Lung Cancer lung cancer staging project: proposals regarding the clinical staging of small cell lung cancer in the forthcoming (seventh) edition of the tumor, node, metastasis classification for lung cancer. J Thorac Oncol 2:1067–1077

Slotman BJ, Mauer ME, Bottomley A, Faivre-Finn C, Kramer GW, Rankin EM, Snee M, Hatton M, Postmus PE, Collette L, Senan S (2008) Prophylactic cranial irradiation in extensive disease small-cell lung cancer: short-term health-related quality of life and patient reported symptoms–results of an international Phase III randomized controlled trial by the EORTC Radiation Oncology and Lung Cancer Groups. J Clin Oncol 22:3770–3776

Smith TJ, Temin S, Alesi ER, Abernethy AP, Balboni TA, Basch EM, Ferrell BR, Loscalzo M, Meier DE, Paice JA, Peppercorn JM, Somerfield M, Stovall E, Von Roenn JH (2012) American Society of Clinical Oncology provisional clinical opinion: the integration of palliative care into standard oncology care. J Clin Oncol 30:880–887

Steele R, Fitch MI (2008) Why patients with lung cancer do not want help with some needs. Support Care Cancer 16:251–259

Stryker JE, Emmons KM, Viswanath K (2007) Uncovering differences across the cancer control continuum: a comparison of ethnic and mainstream cancer newspaper stories. Prev Med 44:20–25

Temel JS, Greer JA, Muzikansky A, Gallagher ER, Admane S, Jackson VA, Dahlin CM, Blinderman CD, Jacobsen J, Pirl WF, Billings JA, Lynch TJ (2010) Early palliative care for patients with metastatic non-small-cell lung cancer. N Engl J Med 363:733–742

Tishelman C, Lovgren M, Broberger E, Hamberg K, Sprangers MA (2010) Are the most distressing concerns of patients with inoperable lung cancer adequately assessed? A mixed-methods analysis. J Clin Oncol 28:1942–1949

Townsley CA, Selby R, Siu LL (2005) Systematic review of barriers to the recruitment of older patients with cancer onto clinical trials. J Clin Oncol 23:3112–3124

Tumorregister München (2013) Basisstatistiken C50: Mammakarzinom (Frauen). http://www.tumorregister-muenchen.de. Accessed 22 Mar 2014

Ufen MP, Kohne CH, Wischneswky M, Wolters R, Novopashenny I, Fischer J, Constantinidou M, Possinger K, Regierer AC (2014) Metastatic breast cancer: are we treating the same patients as in the past? Ann Oncol 25:95–100

Vainio A, Auvinen A (1996) Prevalence of symptoms among patients with advanced cancer: an international collaborative study. Symptom Prevalence Group. J Pain Symptom Manage 12:3–10

van Vliet LM, van der Wall E, Plum NM, Bensing JM (2013) Explicit prognostic information and reassurance about nonabandonment when entering palliative breast cancer care: findings from a scripted video-vignette study. J Clin Oncol 31:3242–3249

Weeks JC, Catalano PJ, Cronin A, Finkelman MD, Mack JW, Keating NL, Schrag D (2012) Patients' expectations about effects of chemotherapy for advanced cancer. N Engl J Med 367:1616–1625

Zabora J, BrintzenhofeSzoc K, Curbow B, Hooker C, Piantadosi S (2001) The prevalence of psychological distress by cancer site. Psychooncology 10:19–28

Zhong C, Liu H, Jiang L, Zhang W, Yao F (2013) Chemotherapy plus best supportive care versus best supportive care in patients with non-small cell lung cancer: a meta-analysis of randomized controlled trials. PLoS One 8:e58466

Zimmermann C, Swami N, Krzyzanowska M, Hannon B, Leighl N, Oza A, Moore M, Rydall A, Rodin G, Tannock I, Donner A, Lo C (2014) Early palliative care for patients with advanced cancer: a cluster-randomised controlled trial. Lancet 383(9930):1721–1730

Palliative Care for Patients with Haematological Malignancies

3

Bernd Alt-Epping and Karin Hohloch

Contents

3.1 Introduction

Tremendous therapeutic advance has been made in treating patients with haematological disease during the past decades. Despite this, very many patients will eventually die from their disease, and another number of patients will die from complications and side effects of the therapeutic regimen itself. Given the burdensome and disease-specific course of most haematological malignancies, very little is known about the specific clinical, nursing and psychosocial needs of patients suffering from incurable and advanced haematological disease. Therefore, this chapter will on the one hand seek to provide haematologists with knowledge on the

B. Alt-Epping, MD (✉)
Department of Palliative Medicine, University Medical Center, Göttingen, Germany
e-mail: bernd.alt-epping@med.uni-goettingen.de

K. Hohloch, MD
Department of Haematology and Oncology, University Medical Center, Göttingen, Germany
e-mail: karin.hohloch@med.uni-goettingen.de

© Springer-Verlag Berlin Heidelberg 2015
B. Alt-Epping, F. Nauck (eds.), *Palliative Care in Oncology*,
DOI 10.1007/978-3-662-46202-7_3

assessment and multi-professional care of this particularly vulnerable group of patients and to demonstrate how palliative care structures may help in supporting the care for patients with incurable haematological disease. On the other hand, this chapter will provide palliative care physicians and teams with a basis of knowledge on the biology, the therapy and the prognostic trajectories of different haematological entities, enabling those of us who work in specialised palliative care to specifically support these patients and understand the complex clinical situations that differ markedly from those encountered in patients with solid tumour entities.

3.2   Clinical Implications of Haematological Malignancies

In Western societies, the most common malignancies are prostate cancer (26.1 %), lung cancer (13.9 %) and colorectal cancer (13.4 %) in men and breast cancer (31.3 %), colorectal cancer (12.7 %) and lung cancer (7.6 %) in women. In both genders, the prevalence of haematological malignancies (i.e. the group of the four most common haematological malignancies, which are non-Hodgkin's lymphoma, leukaemia, multiple myeloma and Hodgkin's disease) contributes to almost 7 % (Robert Koch Institute 2013). Of all haematological malignancies (ICD 10: C81–C95), 53.6 % of the patients will eventually die from their disease or its treatment in Germany (Husmann et al. 2010; Robert Koch Institute 2010).

The biology of haematological malignancies and its clinical and therapeutic implications differ from solid tumour entities in several respects. Some of these characteristics are reported here because they also have strong implications for the aims and adaptation of a focused palliative care concept:

- Haematological malignancies are a heterogeneous group of diseases, with different clinical presentations, outcomes and treatment strategies.
- For most patients the first symptoms are very shortly followed by diagnosis and treatment. Many haematological disease entities, for example, acute leukaemia, have the potential of both a rapid clinical decline and an ultimate improvement in a very short period of time (Epstein et al. 2012). This acuity may cause patients to slide from "daily routine" into a life-threatening situation within just a few days.
- Most often, urgent antineoplastic therapy is required immediately after diagnosis to reduce the risk of life-threatening complications. Recent medical progress has led to increasing remission rates, even to cure, or at least to long-term disease control (Manitta et al. 2010). For a number of haematological disease entities, the intensity of the antineoplastic therapies can be stratified and adapted to cytogenetic and molecular markers, and therefore, treatment can be applied in a more targeted way. But antineoplastic therapy is complicated by the nature of the haematological malignancies that infiltrate the bone marrow and may lead to pancytopenia and its respective complications, which aggravates the toxic effects of

chemotherapy on the bone marrow. Therefore, most patients will require red blood cell or platelet transfusions throughout the whole course of their disease, whereas in patients with solid tumours, transfusion dependence often implies an advanced stage of the disease. Bone marrow involvement may also lead to a high risk for viral, fungal or invasive bacterial infections or to (mucosal) bleeding complications.

– Treatment of acute haematological malignancies requires intensive and ongoing supportive care. Despite all efforts, a potentially life-saving treatment may itself cause lethal side effects or lead to profound and long-lasting morbidity. For instance, patients requiring autologous or allogeneic stem cell transplantation for an otherwise incurable and aggressive disease face a treatment-related mortality of up to 20–30 %, depending on disease-specific risk factors, on the chosen conditioning regimen, on the patient's comorbidities and on other factors (Sorror et al. 2007).

– Even in patients who are unable to undergo intensive treatment for acute haematological disease that aims at curing the disease, for instance, because of comorbidities or advanced age, "palliative" care concepts will include antiproliferative medication in order to limit the white blood cell count to maintain the best possible quality of life.

– In contrast to these acute scenarios, other haematological malignancies such as chronic myelogenous leukaemia (CML), B-cell chronic lymphocytic leukaemia (B-CLL) or indolent lymphoma are typically diagnosed as an incidental finding during a routine checkup, and patients may experience no or very mild symptoms for quite a long time during the course of their disease.

– The treatment of CML is considered a paradigmatic example for the development of new targeted therapies in haematology. As recently as two decades ago, CML treatment consisted of either cytotoxic (non-curative) chemotherapy with modest results or allogeneic stem cell (or bone marrow) transplantation, associated with the according treatment-related mortality, but also with a reasonable chance for cure. To date, though, the mainstay of CML treatment are oral tyrosine kinase inhibitors (TKI), taken once or twice daily, which in most cases leads to sustained cytogenetic remission of the disease. Since TKI are part of the treatment of CML, the patients' overall prognosis has improved significantly, with an almost normal life expectancy (Sacha 2014) and with tolerable side effects in general. Because of this, CML is now considered a chronic disease.

– Patients with B-CLL or indolent lymphoma (depending on stage, symptoms and other determining factors) may require no antineoplastic treatment at all for some time. Patients are followed up closely, or treatment may be installed intermittently over years. But still, even patients who experience a "chronic" course of their disease may be confronted with unforeseeable and life-threatening events such as septic infections that may require immediate and intensive support and particular expertise in the biological and immunological characteristics of the underlying disease. Therefore, difficulties in prognosticating the disease trajectory or the outcome of the respective treatment can be found not only in patients suffering from acute, but also from chronic haematological malignancies.

Considering these aspects, Manitta has stated in 2010:

The successful integration of palliative care into the care of hemato-oncological patients requires recognition by palliative care physicians of the particular issues encountered in care, namely, the difficulty in individual prognostication; ongoing therapeutic goals of curability or long term survival; the technical nature and complications of treatment; the speed of change to a terminal event; the need for pathology testing and transfusion of blood products as death approaches; the potentially reversible nature of intercurrent events such as infection; and the long relationships that develop between patients and their hematologists.

However, up to now, these disease-specific characteristics obviously contribute to the striking differences in end-of-life care of patients suffering from haematological malignancies compared with those with solid cancer entities. Hui et al. (2014) recently reported the following statistics for these differences: during the last 30 days of their life, patients suffering from haematological malignancies were more likely than patients with solid tumours to have emergency room visits (54 % vs. 43 %), hospital admissions (81 % vs. 47 %), ≥ 2 hospital admissions (23 % vs. 10 %), > 14 days of hospitalisation (38 % vs. 8 %), intensive care unit admissions (39 % vs. 8 %) and death (33 % vs. 4 %), chemotherapy use (43 % vs. 14 %) and targeted therapy use (34 % vs. 11 %).

3.3 Patients with Haematological Malignancies Between Intensive Care and Palliative Care

The clinical implications and complications described above, whether caused by the underlying disease or by the antineoplastic therapy, lead to a challenging and ambiguous relationship in haematology with regard to intensive care interventions: on the one hand, intensive care medicine is clearly indispensable for defending these complications. Gordon et al. (2005) found that 101 out of 1,437 patients (7 %) with underlying haematological malignancy required intensive care medicine even at first admission, and up to 40 % of all bone marrow transplant recipients will require intensive care at some point (Jackson et al. 1998).

On the other hand, the necessity for intensive care medicine predicts a grave outcome: the ICU-related mortality of patients suffering from acute leukaemia or other haematological disorders was found to be 42 % (Benoit et al. 2003), with great variability depending on the cause for ICU referral (like respiratory failure, sepsis or neurologic impairment) and the required ICU-specific actions, like ventilator support, vasopressors or renal replacement therapy (Roze des Ordons et al. 2010; Hampshire et al. 2009).

In the context of high-dose regimens and stem cell transplantation, especially from unrelated donors, the treatment-associated risk for (lethal) complications is even higher:

– The 1-year mortality in transplanted patients was found to be up to 94 % when haemodialysis had been required during an ICU stay (Scales et al. 2008). Mortality depends also in the post-transplantation setting on the underlying disease manifestations, its complications, additional comorbidities and related interventions

(invasive ventilation, renal replacement therapy, vasopressor therapy, progressive organ failure, APACHE score >45 and others; Jackson et al. 1998).
– A graft-versus-host reaction and a non-Hodgkin's lymphoma as underlying disease process were found to be associated with a better outcome (Agarwal et al. 2012).

Agarwal and colleagues (2012) also described an improvement of the ICU prognosis of patients after stem cell transplantation during the past two decades, with as many (or at least) 29 % and 24 % of all transplanted patients surviving for more than 6 and 12 months despite being treated on an ICU. The authors concluded that "HSCT patients should generally be favourably considered for ICU admission".

Therefore, it is mandatory in the care for patients with haematological malignancies to try to identify those patients whose conditions promise to be reversible. But often enough, especially in haematology, one cannot clearly predict whether a situation might be reversible, at which point on the haematological disease trajectory the patient is at the particular moment. or even whether a clinical situation in general is still curable in therapeutic intent or if it is already incurable. For a profoundly aplastic patient, for instance, who suffers from AML and is treated on ICU for septic complications, a sound prognostic assessment can be made at the earliest when the bone marrow is about to recover (physiologically or with blasts).

If conventional (dichotomous) prognostication cannot be applied, empirically validated risk scores may be useful (Krug et al. 2010; Scales et al. 2008; Gordon et al. 2005; Benoit et al. 2003; Jackson et al. 1998; Staudinger et al. 2000). But which statistical odds are deemed to justify initiating or maintaining intensive care? A 50 % chance for long-term survival? Or only a 10 % chance? And for how long should intensive care be maintained? This appraisal is a normative process where individual values of physicians, other team members, relatives and of course the patients need to be considered. For instance, patients have agreed to undergo toxic but possibly curative chemotherapy even when the chance for cure was only 1 % (Slevin et al. 1990) – this is obviously in conflict with the conventional values of health care professionals. Similarly, 58 % of patients with mostly incurable solid tumours who were treated on an oncology ward desired to be resuscitated in case of cardiocirculatory arrest (Ackroyd et al. 2007). These wishes of patients need to be balanced against the principle of non-maleficence (Beauchamp and Childress 2009) and require a thorough appraisal of what is medically indicated or what needs to be eschewed.

Therefore, there is need for studies and ethical reflection, despite the existing risk scores, to facilitate medical (and ethical) decision-making for or against the initiation and continuation of intensive care measures.

3.4 Symptoms and Needs of Patients Suffering from Haematological Malignancies

Despite the very intense medical attendance on patients suffering from haematological malignancies, very little is known about the symptoms and subjective needs of these patients, even from a palliative care perspective. Fadul et al. (2008) found an overall symptom severity similar to patients with solid tumour disease and increased occurrences of delirium and drowsiness. Like other studies that investigated symptom prevalences in patients with haematological malignancies (e.g. Corbett et al. 2013), symptom assessment was performed here at the time of referral to palliative care services; therefore, the overall symptom prevalences in haematology cannot be extrapolated from these data. Bonica (1980) found a prevalence of pain in only 5 % of leukaemic patients, for example, as opposed to 85 % in patients with selected solid tumour entities.

In a large, nationwide survey on all patients treated in palliative care and hospice institutions in Germany, pain was reported to be the most prevalent clinical problem with 81.7 % (Radbruch et al. 2003). In patients with haematological malignancies, the proportion of patients suffering from malignancy-associated pain (by compression, infiltration or displacement) is considered to be lower than in patients suffering from solid tumour disease (with the exception of bone pain in multiple myeloma; Niscola et al. 2010) – but the invasive and toxic character of haematological therapies and their side effects and complications might well be factors that predispose the patient to experience pain.

Dyspnoea, in particular, was reported to be extremely prevalent (80 %) in selected groups of haematology patients (Tendas et al. 2009). Fatigue seems to be even more prevalent (>90 %) in patients suffering from advanced haematological malignancies treated in either haematological or palliative care institutions (Alt-Epping et al. 2014). Moreover, fatigue seems to be particularly resistant to therapy; Alibhai et al. (2007) found prevalences of 98 % (baseline), 92 % (at one month after diagnosis), 97 % (at 4 months) and 93 % (at 6 months).

For patients undergoing bone marrow or allogeneic peripheral blood stem cell transplantation (BMT, allo-PBSCT), there have been no recent attempts to assess the according symptoms at all, according to Chung et al. (2009). Symptom management in haematology and BMT patients is described in terms of supportive care, addressing mucositis (Demarosi et al. 2004), therapy-induced nausea/vomiting, nutrition under antineoplastic therapy or GvHD care, but is not described in the context of palliative care.

The highly invasive therapies and their side effects, the uncertainty and hope for success as well as long-lasting hospital stays may lead to extraordinary psychical stress and psychosocial demands in patients and their relatives (Heinonen et al. 2005; Zabora et al. 2001) that need to be addressed in a comprehensive care model.

3.5 Implications for a Comprehensive Palliative Care of Patients Suffering from Haematological Disease

Palliative care aims at improving quality of life by early identification and treatment of symptoms and other complex needs of patients with advanced and progressive disease and comprises a multi-professional team approach for inpatient and outpatient settings and different levels of care intensity. This multi-professionality usually comprises medical, nursing, psychological, social and spiritual support.

During recent years, evidence has grown that patients with haematological malignancies are statistically underrepresented in specialised palliative care services (Maddocks et al. 1994; Hunt et al. 2002; McGrath 2002; Cheng et al. 2005; Joske and McGrath 2007; Fadul et al. 2007; Ansell et al. 2007; Manitta et al. 2010) compared with patients suffering from solid tumour disease. Hung et al. (2013) found that only 3.9 % of 3,156 patients who were treated in a specialised palliative care institution suffered from a haematological malignancy. At the MD Anderson Cancer Center (Houston, TX), patients with haematological malignancies were also significantly less likely to be admitted to palliative care units during the last 30 days of their life (8 % vs. 17 %; $p = 0.02$; Hui et al. 2014).

Similarly, in the German Hospice and Palliative Care Evaluation (HOPE, a large annual survey of patients requiring specialised palliative care support in palliative care units, hospices, oncology and outpatient settings), only 5.1 % of all documented patients (2002–2005) ($n = 5,684$) suffered from an underlying haematological disease (defined as ICD 10 C81–C96; unpublished data), whilst haematological disease contributes to age-adjusted cancer mortality in Germany by 7.1 % in male (16.0/100.000 out of 224.1/100.000) and by 7.7 % in female cancer patients (10.5/100.000 out of 136.8/100.000; RKI 2009).

In particular, the referral behaviour from haematology to palliative care has been criticised (McGrath 2001; Auret et al. 2003; Ibister 1992, Newton 2003). A study conducted by the MD Anderson Cancer Center found that patients with haematological malignancies had significantly later access to palliative care services, with only 13 days from the first palliative care consultation until death (as opposed to 46 days in patients suffering from solid cancer). There, 20 % of the patients suffering from haematological disease versus 44 % of patients suffering from solid tumour entities who died at this institution had been connected to specialised palliative care infrastructures (Fadul et al. 2007). These findings were recently confirmed by a large meta-analysis (Howell et al. 2011).

Numerous factors have been postulated as barriers for an appropriate timing for referral to/involvement of specialised palliative care structures (in part adapted from Howell et al. 2011):

– Treating focal symptoms such as pain is the traditional mainstay of palliative care. The described *lack of focal symptoms*, especially pain, in patients suffering from haematological malignancies might lead to a situation where palliative care services that are not experienced in the care of haematological patients might not be aware of the other particular needs and problems of this group of patients.
– The *difficulties in prognostication*, the likelihood for unexpected clinical developments and deterioration, and the related uncertainty about the proper time of transition to a palliative approach all may leave little time for a reasonable palliative care input. This is even more true if a model of palliative care is applied that relies more on prognosis than on current or future symptoms and demands.
– Often, *antiproliferative (chemotherapeutic) medication* is used rather continuously, for instance, to regulate the blood count and prevent the resulting symptoms

of leucocytosis. This demands ongoing care and management by the haematology team until the very final stages of the disease.

– Accordingly, *substitutive and supportive measures* (such as blood product substitution or anti-infective therapy) are pursued very continuously to prevent or control symptoms and to maintain physical autonomy as long as possible. For patients and relatives (and haematologists), blood product substitution denotes a self-evident therapeutic component throughout the whole disease process caused by disease- and treatment-related bone marrow failure and does not necessarily imply an advanced, near-death situation as in some solid tumour entities. Therefore, transfusion dependence and the reassessment of transfusion requirements with regard to altered treatment goals might lead to a major medical and ethical controversy. Not only medical values such as improved or prophylactic symptom control or a possible increase in end-of-life survival by maintaining transfusions (Brown and Bennett 2007) are affected, but normative values as well (Alt-Epping et al. 2010): the ethical considerations for an allocation of resources, the emotional aspects attributed to blood as a source of life (and bleeding as a sign that heralds death), and the common sense not to allow someone to bleed to death might influence the decision to proceed with or refrain from more transfusions and – implicitly – the decision of whether to involve palliative care structures.

– The *stem cell transplantation (SCT) scenario* might have several implications for palliative care involvement. In this group of haematology patients, huge efforts to cure an otherwise fatal disease are made, from which follows acceptance of a particularly high treatment-related morbidity and mortality. In this setting, haematological staff and their patients are strongly connected, which is a result from a long period of intense medical attendance. An understanding of palliative care that depends on a clearly incurable disease prognosis will exclude many patients who would benefit from better symptom control or profound psychosocial support. According to our experience, there are situations where patients might benefit from specialised palliative care even when the patient is formally in complete remission of his or her haematological disease: patients suffering from severe pulmonary or intestinal graft-versus-host disease, for instance, would profit from further expertise in symptom control and from other offers being made by specialised palliative care institutions.

– Especially (but not exclusively) in the SCT setting, it becomes obvious that there are numerous situations in medicine where a *dichotomous categorisation into curative or palliative care* does not reflect clinical reality, and therefore, the transition from curative intervention to a palliative care approach is considered to be especially difficult. Transplanters who are considering to seek support from palliative care services might wonder whether they had "given up too soon" or if they should better have "given up (their curative efforts) a long time ago" (Chung et al. 2009). Several observational studies with BMT patients showed that introducing a hospice team earlier in the disease process did not shorten survival or dismiss hope, but appeared to improve symptoms and allowed better planning (Chung et al. 2009).

– Until today, there is a persistent misunderstanding in haematology (and elsewhere) that *palliative care equates only to terminal care* (the concept of palliative care as the "death squad", Chung et al. 2009), and there is little awareness of the benefits of palliative care earlier in the illness trajectory (Manitta et al. 2010).

Both the statistical underrepresentation of patients in haematological disease in specialised palliative care structures and the described barriers to early palliative care access imply that traditional palliative care concepts (which have been clearly been proven on patients with solid tumour entities) cannot simply be imposed on patients suffering from haematological disease. Because palliative care originated in a tradition of postulating a "common pathway until death" for a majority of diseases (Solano et al. 2006), it has so far failed to provide a clear and flexible concept that is tailored to the specific disease characteristics and to the multi-faceted needs of patients with advanced haematological disease.

To define such a concept, a critical appraisal of the traditional practice in palliative care in defining the need for specialised palliative care involvement by prognostic parameters or scores is required. In a recent German study, a poor prognosis was associated with a low performance status, low platelet count, opioid-based pain therapy, high LDH and low albumin. The authors correctly concluded that "these parameters might help clinicians to estimate prognosis of remaining life-span and individualize treatment and/or end-of-life care options for patients" (Kripp et al. 2014). Nevertheless, such prognostic scores might not be appropriate to determine which patients in fact require additional palliative care expertise or can do without it.

In this respect, the conceptual considerations for patients suffering from haematological malignancies resemble modern palliative care concepts for patients with advanced non-malignant disease. These patients, who suffer from neurological disease, heart/lung/renal failure or other incurable progressive diseases, were found to have needs different from those of cancer patients, including more intense nursing demands, but had a lower incidence of focal symptoms that required specialist medical intervention (Ostgathe et al. 2011). For palliative care patients with non-malignant disease (as well as palliative care patients in intensive care units), an aligned concept has been proposed that adapts to the continuing treatment of the pretreating department (Lanken et al. 2008). In this model, a patient receives palliative care at the onset of symptoms from a progressive disease, concurrently with disease-specific therapy. The intensity of palliative care and of disease-specific interventions varies and thereby reflects the individual needs and preferences of patients and their families. This model is in contrast to the traditional, dichotomous palliative care models that are designed for patients with solid tumours, in which patients first receive disease-specific care until failure and then receive palliative care, or even the more recent concept of a linear increase in palliative care demands and a linear decrease in disease-specific therapy.

Table 3.1 Therapeutic elements of a multi-professional palliative care approach for patients suffering from haematological malignancies: institutional experience

Symptom control (counselling and pharmacotherapy for symptoms such as dyspnoea and fatigue)
Reassessment of therapeutic interventions such as blood product substitution, anti-infective therapy, antineoplastic therapy, wound care or nutrition and fluid intake tailored to their respective therapeutic goals
Psychological support, for example, providing coping strategies according to the uncertain disease trajectory and its prognostication difficulties
Advance care planning with precautionary and preparative measures for possible emergencies such as bleeding, dyspnoea, pain and other end-of-life crises
Facilitating an early interdisciplinary approach by consultative or outpatient palliative care or home care services (instead of inpatient treatment in a specialised PC unit)
Involvement of relatives, friends and other non-professionals such as community healthcare providers in home care

Adapted from Alt-Epping et al. (2011)

3.6 Own Experience

A case series of our own clinic demonstrated that the combination of inpatient, consultative and outpatient palliative care services provided multi-faceted and individually tailored support to stabilise the quality of life.

Here, the main therapeutic challenges were not necessarily refractory focal symptoms and end-of-life care alone, but instead social problems, mostly related to discharge planning and family support, organisational tasks or home care and to psychical problems that were in part related to alignments of therapeutic interventions with respect to the progressive underlying disease. Ethical advice, advance care planning and a 24-h response team to prevent emergency readmissions were additional facets of multi-professional treatment offers when taking care of patients with haematological malignancies (Table 3.1; Alt-Epping et al. 2011).

These palliative care offers can be combined into a conceptual framework that adjusts to the special requirements of haematology patients and their families at the end of life. Our experience demonstrates the necessity for a broad, comprehensive approach to patients with advanced and incurable haematological disease that is defined more by the underlying needs and symptoms than by prognosticative or infrastructural aspects.

Conclusions

Patients suffering from advanced and incurable haematological disease face numerous and complex clinical, ethical and psychosocial problems that can (and ought to) be addressed in a comprehensive, interdisciplinary and multi-professional approach.

So far, the discussion of when and why to "refer" patients to palliative care services is dominated and overlaid by prognostication queries and by a highly political discussion on care structures and facilities. More importantly for the care of these patients, though, we would like to propagate an integrative approach that defines palliative care as a support system (WHO definition of palliative care 2002) that addresses the needs and problems of particularly affected patients, in conjunction with disease-specific therapy, no matter how many days of life remain or who is going to provide this support – the haematologist, the palliative care specialist or the general practitioner.

References

Ackroyd R, Russon L, Newell R (2007) Views of oncology patients, their relatives and oncologists on cardiopulmonary resuscitation (CPR): questionnaire-based study. Palliat Med 21: 139–144

Agarwal S, O'Donoghue S, Gowardman J, Kennedy G, Bandeshe H, Boots R (2012) Intensive care unit experience of hematopoietic stem cell transplant patients. Intern Med J 42(7):748–754

Alibhai SMH, Leach M, Kowgier ME, Tomlinson GA, Brandwein JM, Minden MD (2007) Fatigue in older adults with acute myeloid leukaemia: predictors and associations with quality of life and functional status. Leukemia 21:845–848

Alt-Epping B, Simon A, Nauck F (2010) Blood product substitution in palliative care. Dtsch Med Wochenschr 135:2083–2087

Alt-Epping B, Wulf G, Nauck F (2011) Palliative care for patients with hematological malignancies – a case series. Letter to the editor. Ann Hematol 90:613–615

Alt-Epping B, Hinse P, Lindena G, Nauck F (2014) To treat or not to treat patients with hematological malignancies in specialized palliative care institutions – results from two prospective surveys. Abstract P298 EAPC Research Congress, Lleida (Spain), 5.-7.06.2014. Palliat Med 28(6):743–744

Ansell P, Howell D, Garry A, Kite S, Munro J, Roman E, Howard M (2007) What determines referral of UK patients with haematological malignancies to palliative care services? An exploratory study using hospital records. Palliat Med 21:487–492

Auret K, Bulsara C, Joske D (2003) Australasian haematologist referral patterns to palliative care: lack of consensus of when and why. Intern Med J 33:566–571

Beauchamp TL, Childress JF (2009) Principles of biomedical ethics, 6th edn. Oxford University Press, New York

Benoit DD, Vandewoude KH, Decruyenaere JM, Hoste EA, Colardyn FA (2003) Outcome and early prognostic indicators in patients with a hematologic malignancy admitted to the intensive care unit for a life-threatening complication. Crit Care Med 31(1):104–112

Bonica JJ (1980) Cancer pain. In: Bonica JJ (ed) Pain. Raven, New York, pp 335–362

Brown E, Bennett M (2007) Survey of blood transfusion practice for palliative care patients in Yorkshire: implications for clinical care. J Palliat Med 10:919–922

Cheng W, Willey J, Palmer JL, Zhang T, Bruera E (2005) Interval between palliative care referral and death among patients treated at a comprehensive cancer center. J Palliat Med 8:1025–1032

Chung HM, Lyckholm LJ, Smith TJ (2009) Palliative care in BMT. Bone Marrow Transplant 43:265–273

Corbett CL, Johnstone M, McCracken Trauer J, Spruyt O (2013) Palliative care and hematological malignancies: increased referrals at a comprehensive cancer centre. J Palliat Med 16(5): 537–541

Demarosi F et al (2004) Transdermal fentanyl in HSCT patients: an open trial using transdermal fentanyl for the treatment of oral mucositis pain. Bone Marrow Transplant 33(12):1247–1251

Epstein AS, Goldberg GR, Meier DE (2012) Palliative care and hematologic oncology: the promise of collaboration. Blood Rev 26:233–239

Fadul NA, Elsayem A, Palmer JL, Zhang T, Braiteh F, Bruera E (2007) Predictors of access to palliative care services among patients who died at a comprehensive cancer center. J Palliat Med 10(5):1146–1152

Fadul NA, El Osta B, Dalal S, Poulter VA, Bruera E (2008) Comparison of symptom burden among patients referred to palliative care with hematologic malignancies versus those with solid tumors. J Palliat Med 11(3):422–427

Gordon AC, Oakervee HE, Kaya B, Thomas JM, Barnett MJ, Rohatiner AZ et al (2005) Incidence and outcome of critical illness amongst hospitalized patients with haematological malignancy: a prospective observational study of ward and intensive care unit based care. Anaesthesia 60:340–347

Hampshire PA, Welch CA, McCrossan LA, Francis K, Harrison DA (2009) Admission factors associated with hospital mortality in patients with haematological malignancy admitted to UK adult, general critical care units: a secondary analysis of the ICNARC Case Mix Programme Database. Crit Care 13:R137

Heinonen H, Volin L, Zevon MA, Uutela A, Barrick C, Ruutu T (2005) Stress among allogeneic bone marrow transplantation patients. Patient Educ Couns 56:62–71

Howell D, Shellens R, Roman E, Garry A, Patmore R, Howard M (2011) Haematological malignancy: are patients appropriately referred for specialist palliative and hospice care? A systematic review and meta-analysis of published data. Palliat Med 25(6):630–641

Hui D, Didwaniya N, Vidal M, Shin SH, Chisholm G, Roquemore J, Bruera E (2014) Quality of end-of-life care in patients with hematologic malignancies: a retrospective cohort study. Cancer 15;120(10):1572–1578. doi:10.1002/cncr.28614. Epub 2014 Feb 18

Hung YS, Wu JH, Chang H, Wang PN, Kao CY, Wang HM, Liau CT, Chen JS, Lin YC, Su PJ, Hsieh CH, Chou WC (2013) Characteristics of patients with hematologic malignancies who received palliative care consultation services in a medical center. Am J Hosp Palliat Care 30:773–780

Hunt RW, Fazekas BS, Luke CG, Priest KR, Roder DM (2002) The coverage of cancer patients by designated palliative services: a population-based study, South Australia, 1999. Palliat Med 16:403–409

Husmann G, Kaatsch P, Katalinic A, Bertz J, Haberland J, Kraywinkel K, Wolf U (2010) Krebs in Deutschland 2005/2006. Häufigkeiten und Trends, 7th ed. http://www.rki.de/cln_226/nn_204124/DE/Content/GBE/DachdokKrebs/KID/kid__node.html?__nnn=true

Ibister J (1992) Palliative care: a clinical Haematologist's view. Coff's Harbour Palliative Care conference, Coff's Harbour

Jackson SR, Tweeddale MG, Barnett MJ, Spinelli JJ, Sutherland HJ, Reece DE, Klingemann HG, Nantel SH, Fung HC, Toze CL, Phillips GL, Shepherd JD (1998) Admission of bone marrow transplant recipients to the intensive care unit: outcome, survival and prognostic factors. Bone Marrow Transplant 21(7):697–704

Joske D, McGrath P (2007) Palliative care in haematology. Intern Med J 37:589–590

Kripp M, Willer A, Schmidt C, Pilz L, Gencer D, Buchheidt D, Hochhaus A, Hofmann WK, Hofheinz RD (2014) Patients with malignant hematological disorders treated on a palliative care unit: prognostic impact of clinical factors. Ann Hematol 93(2):317–325

Krug U, Röllig C, Koschmieder A, Heinecke A, Sauerland MC, Schaich M, Thiede C, Kramer C, Braess J, Spiekermann K, Haferlach T, Haferlach C, Koschmieder S, Rohde C, Serve H, Wörmann B, Hiddemann W, Ehninger G, Berdel WE, Büchner T, Müller-Tidow C (2010) Complete remission and early death after intensive chemotherapy in patients aged 60 years or older with acute myeloid leukaemia: a web-based application for prediction of outcomes. Lancet 376:2000–2008

Lanken PN, Terry PB, American Thoracic Society End-of Life Task Force et al (2008) Palliative care for patients with respiratory diseases and critical illnesses. Am J Respir Crit Care Med 177:912–927

Maddocks I, Bentley L, Sheedy J (1994) Quality of life issues in patients dying from haematological diseases. Ann Acad Med Singapore 23(2):244–248

Manitta V, Philip J, Cole-Sinclair MF (2010) Palliative care and the hemato-oncological patient: can we live together? A review of the literature. J Palliat Med 13(8):1021–1025

McGrath P (2001) Dying in the curative system: the haematology/oncology dilemma. Part 1. Aust J Holist Nurs 8:22–30

McGrath P (2002) Are we making progress? Not in haematology! Omega (Westport) 45(4):331–348

McGrath P, Joske D (2002) Palliative care and haematological malignancy: a case study. Aust Health Rev 25(3):60–66

Newton S (2003) Haematology and palliative care: blood, sweat and tears. Intern Med J 33(12):549–551

Niscola P, Scaramucci L, Romani C, Giovannini M, Tendas A, Brunetti G, Cartoni C, Palumbo R, Vischini G, Siniscalchi A et al (2010) Pain management in multiple myeloma. Expert Rev Anticancer Ther 10:415–425

Ostgathe C, Alt-Epping B, Golla H, Gaertner J, Lindena G, Radbruch L, Voltz R, Hospice and Palliative Care Evaluation (HOPE) Working Group in Germany (2011) Non-cancer patients in specialised palliative care in Germany: what are the problems? Palliat Med 25:148–152

Radbruch L, Nauck F, Ostgathe C, Elsner F, Bausewein C, Fuchs M, Lindena G, Neuwohner K, Schulenberg D (2003) What are the problems in palliative care? Results from a representative survey. Support Care Cancer 11:442–451

RKI, Robert Koch Institute (2013) Krebs in Deutschland. http://www.rki.de/Krebs/DE/Content/ Publikationen/Krebs_in_Deutschland/kid_2013/krebs_in_deutschland_2013.pdf?__ blob=publicationFile, Accessed 29.01.2015

Roze des Ordons AL, Chan K, Mirza I, Townsend DR, Bagshaw SM (2010) Clinical characteristics and outcomes of patients with acute myelogenous leukemia admitted to intensive care: a case-control study. BMC Cancer 10:516

Sacha T1 (2014). Imatinib in chronic myeloid leukemia: an overview. Mediterr J Hematol Infect Dis 6(1). doi: 10.4084/MJHID.2014.007

Scales DC, Thiruchelvam D, Kiss A, Sibbald WJ, Redelmeier DA (2008) Intensive care outcomes in bone marrow transplant recipients: a population-based cohort analysis. Crit Care 12:R77

Slevin ML, Stubbs L et al (1990) Attitudes to chemotherapy: comparing views of patients with cancer with those of doctors, nurses, and general public. BMJ 300(6737):1458–1460

Solano JP, Gomes B, Higginson IJ (2006) A comparison of symptom prevalence in far advanced cancer, AIDS, heart disease, chronic obstructive pulmonary disease and renal disease. J Pain Symptom Manage 31:58–69

Sorror ML, Sandmaier BM, Storer BE et al (2007) Comorbidity and disease status based risk stratification of outcomes among patients with acute myeloid leukemia or myelodysplasia receiving allogeneic hematopoietic cell transplantation. J Clin Oncol 25:4246–4254

Staudinger T, Stoiser B, Müllner M, Locker GJ, Laczika K, Knapp S, Burgmann H, Wilfing A, Kofler J, Thalhammer F, Frass M (2000) Outcome and prognostic factors in critically ill cancer patients admitted to the intensive care unit. Crit Care Med 28(5):1322–1328

Tendas A, Niscola P, Cupelli L et al (2009) Palliative sedation therapy in a bone marrow transplant unit. Support Care Cancer 17:107–108

World Health Organization (2002) WHO definition of palliative care. http://www.who.int/cancer/ palliative/definition/en/

Zabora J, BrintzenhofeSzoc K, Curbow B, Hooker C, Piantadosi S (2001) The prevalence of psychological distress by cancer site. Psychooncology 10:19–28

Part II

Symptom Control

Definition, Pathophysiology, and Assessment of Pain

4

Steffen Eychmüller

Contents

4.1 Multidimensional Pain Concept

This situation is typical for what we know about pathophysiology and the multidimensional character of pain in palliative care. Essential insights in this regard come from the basic knowledge of pain regulation in persistent pain (formerly: chronic pain). In addition to the so-called multidimensional pain concept (Ahles et al. 1983; Breitbart and Gibson 2007) with its four main sections of nociception, cognition, emotion, and social support, today we have other important insights that constitute the column on which modern understanding of pain is based on (Fig. 4.1).

S. Eychmüller, MD
Center for Palliative Care, University Hospital Inselspital, Bern, Switzerland
e-mail: steffen.eychmueller@insel.ch

© Springer-Verlag Berlin Heidelberg 2015
B. Alt-Epping, F. Nauck (eds.), *Palliative Care in Oncology*,
DOI 10.1007/978-3-662-46202-7_4

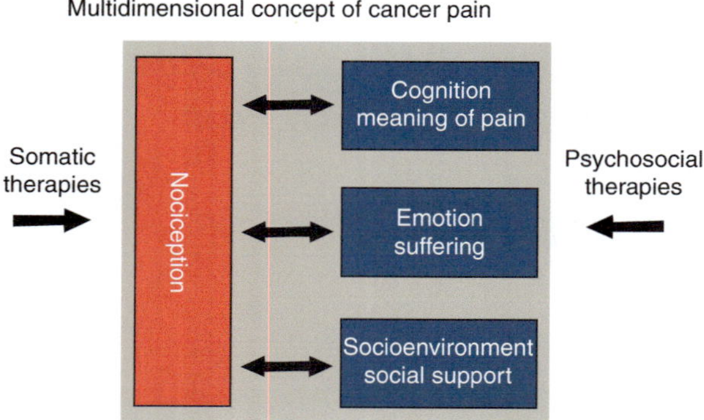

Fig. 4.1 Multidimensional concept of cancer pain (From Breitbart and Gibson 2007; http://primarypsychiatry.com/psychiatric-aspects-of-cancer-pain-management/. With permission of the publisher)

An essential column specifically in palliative care is the *role of fear and anxiety in pain perception*. In a seminal article in the journal *Pain*, Christopher Brown et al. (2008) found a clear correlation between fear and insecurity and, following from this, between uncertainty and intensity of pain. This corresponds very well with the common insight that fear cripples much more than the pain itself (Francis Keefe 2001: "fear is more disabling than pain"). The role and extent of fear needs to be particularly carefully taken into account in pain treatment in palliative care.

Apart from pain and fear, the clinical picture of *pain, depression, and insomnia* can be observed quite often. These fatal connections, which work like a "Bermuda triangle," of pain, are based on the essential insights of neuropsychology within the framework of the matrix of pain (Schadrack and Zieglgänsberger 2000).

4.2 Salutogenesis in Pain Treatment

Complementary to the deficit-oriented understanding of pain, in recent years more hopeful insights have been reported from the perspective of the salutogenetic model, in particular in managing pain. Our brain offers promising aspects within the framework of neuronal plasticity (Woolf 1983) to counter the "biologically meaningless" mechanisms of peripheral and central pain sensitization (these mechanisms may begin as early as a few hours after the first pain episode!). These mechanisms are propagated today with the buzzwords *neuroenhancement or relearning* and are based on excellent neuropsychological as well as neuroimaging results (e.g., Dodt et al. 2007). Neuroenhancement, or relearning, is an essential mechanism that points to the concept of *salutogenesis*: we can ourselves manipulate and reframe how we cope with pain, that is, how it affects our thinking, feeling, and acting.

Other essential impulses in the past years have come from complementary medicine. Awareness or, more to the point, the procedures of *mindfulness-based stress reduction (MBSR)* have developed into essential pillars of a self-directed pain management on the basis of neurophysiological results. In a broader context, these interventions are not only an indispensable part of multimodal pain programs, but may also inspire therapeutic strategies for acute and/or persistent pain in cancer.

These insights are crucial to understand all dimensions of assessment in pain. The following questions therefore belong to a proper multidimensional assessment of pain (Nicholas et al. 2013):

- Who is the person?
- What are her or his stressors/fears?
- How does the pain interact with her or his current lifestyle?
- Which are the main influencing factors?
- How can the person herself or himself influence the situation?
- What does she or he wish us to do or expect from us?

The importance of such patient-centered rather than diagnosis-oriented assessment is shown by surveys conducted to determine the effectiveness of pain therapy on severely ill or dying patients (e.g., Miettinen et al. 1998). The main factors for ineffectiveness were feelings of helplessness, insufficient self-management of the patient in the use of analgesics, insufficient information of relatives, little communication with the doctors and team, and unsatisfactory management of basic needs.

4.3 Persistent Pain and the Concept of "Total Pain"

In palliative care, the multidimensionality of pain is known as the so-called "total pain" concept, formulated by Dame C. Saunders to describe all dimensions of pain with its factors of physical, emotional, social, and spiritual suffering (Saunders 1970). This concept is complemented by another concept of C. Saunders, the "unit of care." Pain and its ramifications do not concern the patient alone, but also the relatives and the caregivers.

Distinctive features of "total pain," compared with persistent pain, are the following factors: in advanced illness, communication and cognitive function are altered with consecutive difficulty to express pain verbally; physical weakness as a main symptom hinders patients to cope actively; existential fears may dominate and create an atmosphere of helplessness and giving up; and finally the remaining life span may not allow to plan a long-term treatment. Thus, some strategies cannot be translated from one concept into the other without additional reflection and amendments.

Conclusion 1 Assessing the individual meaning of pain for the patient, including connected fears and expectations, is essential for determining the subsequent treatment and therapeutic possibilities in pain management in palliative care. The total pain concept is supported today by a wealth of new research results from neurophysiology and psychology in connection with persisting/chronic pain. The main pillars of treatment known from multimodal pain management can only be translated into palliative care with some modifications. Whenever possible it is indispensable to give the patient any available tools to manage difficult pain situations as autonomously as possible, including drug-based pain therapy.

4.4 Pain Definition and Pain Treatment

4.4.1 Pain Assessment

It has been proven effective to sort the pain according to the underlying pain diagnosis. The main distinction is made between nociceptive and neuropathic pain.

4.4.1.1 Nociceptive Pain
- Somatic
  - Continuous or intermittent
  - Often gnawing and piercing
  - Sometimes convulsive

Mechanism: nociceptive receptors are stimulated, for instance, by direct tissue damage (e.g., fracture, but also bone metastases).

- Visceral
  - Constant
  - Pressing and convulsive
  - In general not easily located, sometimes transferred (into the related dermatome) or radiating

Mechanism: nociceptive receptors are stimulated, for instance, by intra-abdominal masses or hepatic metastases.

4.4.1.2 Neuropathic Pain
- Dysesthetic pain (deafferentation), for instance, postherpetic neuralgia
  - Constant burning
  - Sometimes radiating
- Neuralgic pain, for example, trigeminal neuralgia and plexus infiltration by the tumor
  - Suddenly electrifying burning pain
  - Sharply thrusting pain

These distinctions can help to define the stratification of the initial pharmaceutical measures, and it is evident that neuropathic pain in particular is difficult to treat with pharmaceutical measures alone. The underlying pathophysiological mechanisms are complex and therefore difficult to treat with a single modality therapy.

Note that in palliative care, particularly in patients suffering from advanced cancer, one often finds a mix of nociceptive and neuropathic pain components (a typical example is bone pain in conjunction with plexus infiltration). In consequence, a mix of therapeutic strategies including administration of multiple classes of drugs may be needed.

4.4.2   Systematics of Pain Assessment: The Seven Dimensions

The components in the patient history include the temporal sequence, localization, pain quality, intensity, triggering events for secondary signals (in particular influence by activity or rest), and intensifying and mitigating factors.

Additional diagnostic measure may be necessary or helpful:

- Radiological imaging (often MRI, especially for assessing soft tissue components including neuronal compression)
- Fears connected with the use of strong analgesics ("morphine myth")
- Possible cultural particularities (meaning of pain)
- Spiritual aspects (stressors, but possibly also resources)
- Existing self-help strategies

4.4.2.1 Assessing Pain Intensity

The most important source for pain assessment is the information provided by the patient. Most often a visual analogue scale (VAS) is used. Numerical scales (mostly 11-step Likert scales ranging from 0 = no pain to 11 = strongest pain imaginable) and descriptions in words are useful as well. Likewise, words, fingers, and other figures such as smiling or sad faces can be used to assess pain intensity.

Long-lasting pain often causes a shift in the perception of pain intensity that is being reflected by the measurements: on the VAS, for instance, a lack of intensities below 5 indicates the extent of the sensitization of pain in the context of neuronal plasticity. It is therefore not useful to evaluate pain intensity in these patients. Instead, acceptable level of pain and most of all function, such as sleep, mood, or number of social contacts, should be measured.

In cognitively disabled patients, observation by professionals turns out to be the only way to "assess" pain. A validated measurement tool for this situation is ECPA (Echelle comportementale de la douleur pour personnes âgées non communicates), an observational tool defined by nurses, similar to DOLOPLUS 2 © (Zwakhalen et al. 2006).

4.4.3   Recording Pain Effects

The effects of pain on muscle activity and tension are underestimated and need to be specifically investigated: changes in motions, sleeping position, postures assumed to avoid pain, shortened muscles, asymmetry, and atrophy are relevant factors for completing the clinical picture of pain.

Particular attention is recommended in these cases to ameliorate muscular tone, for instance, with local actions (warmth, massages, anesthesia) including general muscle relaxation (e.g., according to Jacobson), but also acupuncture, body packs, or other relaxing measures (including hypnosis, etc.).

4.4.4 Assessing Expectations

It is essential in diagnosing the actual pain situation to accurately *assess the expectations* of the patients and their social surrounding. This is particularly true for expectations of drug therapy, which are often far too high. To establish an effective pain therapy, it is recommended to define and later evaluate three steps of analgesic effectiveness before the actual treatment:

1. Pain reduction during the night/while sleeping
2. Pain reduction while at rest during the day
3. Pain reduction while moving/during certain everyday movements

4.4.5 Assessing Possible Relevant Side Effects and Drug Interactions

Before beginning an analgesic therapy, one needs to determine possible comorbidities such as gastric ulcers, already existing tendencies for obstipation, diverticulosis, renal insufficiency, addiction (see below), and a tendency for nausea in connection with medication. While adding a new drug a check for pharmacological interaction may be needed, especially in multiple organ insufficiency (see Chap. 10) medication needs to be checked for potential pharmacological interactions.

4.4.6 Breakthrough Pain

Despite the best possible pain treatment, breakthrough pain may occur, particularly in connection with movement, and is most frequent in cachectic patients. The phenomenon of breakthrough pain has been widely studied. A definition is given as "a transient increase in pain intensity that occurs in patients with stable, baseline persistent pain" (Medical dictionary). Therapeutic strategies, however, are unfortunately very heterogeneous (Mishra et al. 2009). According to this general overview, the incidence of breakthrough pain in cancer patients is very high (40–86 %). Most often we see nociceptive pain in connection with bone or joint instabilities (for instance, bone metastases), but neuropathic pain also occurs in connection with neural compression. Because this is such a frequent pattern of pain, the following points are essential:

1. Capacity building
   In the first step, the aim is to enable patients and their relatives to react to pain exacerbation autonomously. Training and monitoring of pain and basic

understanding of pain treatment (including essentials about pain medication) is a mandatory part of patient education. This helps to reduce the fear of being helpless but also unrealistic expectations of the medication effectiveness.

2. Medication according to the basis–bolus principle
   Similar to, insulin therapy, patients (and their relatives!) need to be instructed in the use of a basis–bolus strategy of pain medication in order to control basic pain levels as well as breakthrough pain. As an example, patient instructions may include the self-administration of preventive pain medication BEFORE a movement short acting is planned that in the past has triggered breakthrough pain (comparable to taking insulin before a meal).

3. Sufficient on-demand medication and frequency of repetition
   A frequent reason for insufficient treatment of breakthrough pain is a too low PRN (on-demand) dose in relation to the daily dose of the analgesics. Usually, strong opioids are used, and then the on-demand dose is recommended to be 10–16 % (the four-hourly dose) of the total daily opioid dose. A too long interval between two PRN doses is another factor: as a rule, opioids should be applied again – except for renal insufficiency – after only 60 min if the analgesic effect is insufficient. This also applies to treatments at home.

4.4.7 Follow-Up Evaluation

It is essential for a follow-up evaluation to determine

- The onset of effect and duration of pain reduction when taking regular dose and on-demand medication
- The pain quality and localization that do not respond to the medical treatment (additional diagnosis and assessment of other factors such as nerve compression or undetected fears may be needed)
- The incidence of new pain spots or pain qualities

4.4.8 Pain Therapy in Palliative Care and Addiction

Fear of addiction when using opioids is often a reason for caution and reluctance by patients and doctors alike when these drugs are prescribed, even in far-advanced disease. Addiction is rare in patients suffering from progressive (tumor) pain; this is also true for end-stage neurodegenerative pain. On the other hand, preexisting addiction of drugs and alcohol and drug dependence are unfavorable prognostic factors for immediate acting drug-based pain management, and one needs to actively investigate whether this is the case (see modified CAGE test for all addictions, Kwon et al. 2013). Nonetheless, the limited lifetime of patients in palliative care makes addiction a minor concern compared with potentially addiction-related medication while treating persistent pain. "A little euphoria should be allowed" may be a reasonable point of view in this situation.

Conclusion

The distinction of nociceptive and neuropathic pain mechanism (pain diagnosis) is of clinical relevance. Neuropathic components of pain are frequent in oncology and especially in advanced cancer and difficult to treat with medication alone. Specific challenges in pain management of patients with advanced cancer are empowerment of patients and family in self-administration of PRN pain medication for breakthrough pain, evaluation of expectations in regard of analgesic drugs in order to avoid overoptimism and frustration, pain assessment in cognitively impaired patients (frequently requires the use of observational measurement tools), and specific attention to muscular response to pain which may not be responsive to analgesic drug use alone. Addiction is not a frequent clinical challenge in palliative care.

References

Ahles TA, Blanchard EB, Ruckdeschel JC (1983) The multidimensional nature of cancer-related pain. Pain 17:277–288

Breitbart W, Gibson CA (2007) Psychiatric aspects of cancer pain management. Primary Psychiatry 14(9):81–91

Brown CA, Seymour B, Boyle Y, El-Deredy W, Jones AK (2008) Modulation of pain ratings by expectation and uncertainty: behavioral characteristics and anticipatory neural correlates. Pain 135(3):240–250

Dodt HU, Leischner U, Schierloh A, Jährling N, Mauch CP et al (2007) Ultramicroscopy: three-dimensional visualization of neuronal networks in the whole mouse brain. Nat Methods 4:331–336

Kwon JH et al (2013) Predictors of long-term opioid treatment among patients who receive chemo-radiation for head and neck cancer. Oncologist 18(6):768–774

Miettinen TT et al (1998) Why is the pain relief of dying patients often unsuccessful? The relatives' perspectives. Palliat Med 12(6):429–435

Mishra S, Bhatnagar S, Chaudhary P, Rana SP (2009) Breakthrough cancer pain: review of prevalence, characteristics and management. Indian J Palliat Care 15(1):14–18

Nicholas M, Molloy A, Tonkin L, Beeston L (2013) Manage your pain, 3rd edn. ABC Books, Sydney, Australia

Saunders C (1970) Nature and management of terminal pain. In: Shotter EF (ed) Matters of life and death. Dartman, Longman, and Todd, London, pp 15–26

Schadrack J, Zieglgänsberger W (2000) Activity- dependent changes in the pain matrix. Scand J Rheumatol Suppl 113:19–23

Sullivan MJL, Thorn B, Haythornthwaite JA, Keefe FJ (2001) Theoretical perspectives on the relation between catastrophizing and pain. Clin J Pain 17:52–64

Woolf CJ (1983) Evidence for a central component of post-injury pain hypersensitivity. Nature 306:686–688

Zwakhalen SM, Hamers JP, Abu-Saad HH, Berger MP (2006) Pain in elderly people with severe dementia: a systematic review of behavioural pain assessment tools. BMC Geriatr 6:3

Therapy of Cancer-Related Pain and Cancer Therapy-Related Pain

5

Christoph Ostgathe and Bernd-Oliver Maier

Contents

C. Ostgathe, MD (⊠)
Department of Palliative Medicine, University Hospital,
Krankenhausstrasse 12, 91054 Erlangen, Germany
e-mail: christoph.ostgathe@uk-erlangen.de

B.-O. Maier, MD, MSc
St. Joseph's Hospital, Wiesbaden, Germany
e-mail: bomaier@joho.de

© Springer-Verlag Berlin Heidelberg 2015
B. Alt-Epping, F. Nauck (eds.), *Palliative Care in Oncology*,
DOI 10.1007/978-3-662-46202-7_5

5.1 Introduction

One third of all patients receiving active anticancer therapy and two thirds of patients with advanced cancer experience pain related to cancer or to anticancer therapy that requires treatment (Foley 2011). In 70–90 % of these patients, adequate pain control can be achieved. Although evidence has been accumulated over the past decades and many national and international recommendations are available, still about 50 % of patients are undertreated (Deandrea et al. 2008). An exact pain diagnosis is essential for successful management of pain in cancer patients. A sound medical history and physical examination need to be performed to determine pain type, localization, intensity, and factors that affect occurrence and intensity.

The main backbone of managing pain in cancer patients is drug therapy. Within a short period of time, adequate pain reduction is achievable in many patients. In particular in oncological patients, new pain or pain exacerbations may be interpreted as signs of disease progression. Therefore, anxiety is often a coexisting symptom, which may even aggravate pain perception. Together with adequate symptom-oriented treatment, it is crucial to identify treatable causes for the pain. Additional non-pharmacological measures can play an important role in the comprehensive management of cancer pain.

5.2 Basic Treatment Algorithm for Cancer Pain

The WHO guideline for cancer pain therapy is widely accepted (WHO 1998). It offers an easy-to-use stepwise approach. Essential principles of drug-focused pain management are to keep administration as simple as possible ("by the mouth," transdermal) (WHO 1998; Caraceni et al. 2012) and to choose the application interval according to the duration of drug action ("by the clock") (WHO 1998). The major benefit of the WHO guideline is that it is based upon pain intensity and opioid strength and outlines the idea of combining opioids and non-opioids. Despite or maybe because of this wide acceptance, the guideline has never been formally evaluated or validated. Important issues for treatment decision such as the underlying mechanisms of pain are not taken into account. This shortcoming has recently been criticized (Raphael et al. 2010). On the basis of the WHO ladder, we prefer a combination of the didactic advantages of a simple scheme (Mercadante 2010) and an approach based on the respective mechanism.

5.2.1 WHO Step I

Following the WHO guideline (Fig. 5.1), non-opioids may be prescribed for mild pain. The suspected pain mechanism is supposed to lead the decision about which substance to prescribe. The majority of patients can easily localize their pain, and it is often described as "bright and stabbing." NSAIDs such as ibuprofen or celecoxib

Step 3: strong opioids (e.g. morphine, hydromorphone, fentanyl, buprenorphine, oxycodone, (levo-) methadone) ± non-opioids ± co-analgetics

Step 2: weak-to-moderate opioids (e.g. tramadol, dihydrocodein, low-dose step 3 opioids) ± non-opioids ± co-analgetics

Step 1: non-opioids (e.g. ibuprofen, paracetamol, celecoxib, dipyrone) ± co-analgetics

Fig. 5.1 WHO guidelines for cancer pain management (WHO 1998)

Table 5.1 Common non-opioids for treating cancer pain

Drug	Single dose [mg]	Interval [h]	Comments/side effects
Dipyrone	500–1,000	4	Potent non-opioid
			Not available in all countries
			Very rarely agranulocytosis
Paracetamol	500–1,000	4	No gastrointestinal side effects
			Daily dose <6 g
Ibuprofen	400–800	4–8	Gastrointestinal side effects
			Combination with PPI recommended
Celecoxib	100–200	12	Less gastrointestinal toxicity
			Rarely edema, hypertension
Naproxen	200	8–12	Fewer side effects in patients at cardiovascular risk
			Dose reduction in renal and/or liver impairment

are effective when musculoskeletal nociceptive pain is predominant (Table 5.1). Pain caused by bone metastases, for example, may benefit from NSAIDs because of the anti-inflammatory effect of these substances. The risk of side effects or adverse events such as edema, confusion, or in particular gastrointestinal bleeding has to be taken into account and needs to be weighed against the benefits individually. The overall risk of bleeding is described to be somewhat lower for selective COX-2 inhibitors (Buvanendran et al. 2003). But for a moderately increased risk for gastrointestinal bleeding, nonselective NSAIDs in combination with proton pump inhibitors (PPI) are equal to selective COX-2 inhibitors (Brooks et al. 2013). In patients with a history of previous ulcer or hemorrhage and thus a high risk for bleeding, it is preferable to combine a COX-2 inhibitor with a PPI to reduce the risk of gastrointestinal events (Brooks et al. 2013). Patients at high cardiovascular risk are expected to benefit most from naproxen (Bhala et al. 2013).

Affection of the intestines, hollow organs, or pleura may lead to visceral nociceptive pain. This is often described as "crampy," and many patients have trouble to localize the pain. Dipyrone (metamizole) is a non-opioid with good analgesic properties (Edwards et al. 2010) and is a good choice for visceral pain because of its additional spasmolytic properties. It is widely used in many countries (e.g., Germany, France, Latin America, India), but has been withdrawn from the market in some countries (e.g., Sweden, UK) because of possible agranulocytosis (Edwards and McQuay 2002). The different non-opioids should in general not be combined, but in selected cases, the clinical impression is that a combination of NSAIDs with dipyrone or paracetamol may be beneficial.

5.2.2 WHO Step II/Step III

The step I drugs are to be chosen in case of mild pain. Nevertheless, many cancer patients need additional analgesics, in particular when the disease progresses. In case of moderate pain, weak opioids (codeine, hydrocodone, tramadol, or tilidine (only available in some countries)) or, following the new recommendations of the EAPC, strong opioids in lower doses (morphine ≤ 30 mg, oxycodone ≤ 20 mg or hydromorphone ≤ 4 mg ad day) (Caraceni et al. 2012) are combined in step II with the non-opioids. In patients with severe pain, step III strong opioids are recommended to replace the weak opioid.

5.3 Strong Opioids

Opioids are essential in treating cancer pain. For many years, morphine was the gold standard (Hanks et al. 2001). Evidence on and use of other opioids have evolved over the past decade, and now morphine, oxycodone, and hydromorphone given by the oral route can be used as the first choice for moderate to severe cancer pain (Caraceni et al. 2012). Alternatives to oral opioids are transdermal fentanyl and buprenorphine. Both drugs may be the preferred step III opioid for some patients, in particular if patients are unable to swallow (Caraceni et al. 2012).

5.3.1 Morphine

Morphine is widely used for cancer pain (Nauck et al. 2004). All other strong opioids are related to morphine concerning their effects, side effects, and costs. Morphine is a mere μ-receptor-agonist with an oral bioavailability of 35 %. It is metabolized in morphin-3-glucuronide (no analgesic effect) and morphin-6-glucuronide (stronger effect than morphine). In case of renal insufficiency, the metabolites of morphine may accumulate and provoke pronounced side effects such as sedation or myoclonus. Liver disease has no negative impact on treating patients with morphine.

5.3.2 Hydromorphone

Hydromorphone is another mere μ-receptor-agonist with an oral bioavailability of 50 %. Compared with morphine, clinical data suggest some advantage of hydromorphone concerning side effects (Lussier et al. 2010). This may be because hydromorphone seems to have no clinically relevant metabolites. The importance of hydromorphone-3-glucoronide is not clear yet (McCann et al. 2010). In addition, the low plasma protein binding (14 %) (Saari et al. 2012) is discussed to be favorable in case of renal insufficiency.

5.3.3 Oxycodone

Oxycodone – and in particular the active metabolite oxymorphone – is effective as an agonist at the μ-receptor. In addition, it has been discussed that the intrinsic anti-nociceptive effects are mediated by κ-opioid receptors (Ross and Smith 1997). The oral bioavailability is >60 % (Kalso 2005). In cases of liver and renal dysfunction, plasma concentrations may be elevated by 50 %; therefore, a dose reduction may be necessary. There is growing evidence that in cancer patients, a fixed combination of oxycodone with naloxone – both sustained released – is associated with a better bowel function and less additional laxative intake (Ahmedzai et al. 2012).

5.3.4 Fentanyl

The μ-receptor agonist fentanyl is highly lipophilic. Thus, it is well absorbed and can be administered transdermal and transmucosal. Using a patch, the strongest effect will occur with a delay of 12–24 h and mostly lasts for about 72 h. When removed because of complications or side effects, the half-life is 16 h, so that monitoring may be required. Buccal or nasal administration leads to rapid onset and short duration of action. In some cases of breakthrough or incident pain, buccal or nasal fentanyl may therefore be preferable to immediate-release oral opioids (Caraceni et al. 2012). In patients with reduced liver function or renal impairment, a moderate dose reduction is recommended (Pergolizzi et al. 2008).

5.3.5 Buprenorphine

Buprenorphine is a μ-agonist and κ-antagonist with a high receptor affinity. Onset of action is slow. It causes partial antagonism; therefore, ceiling effects have been discussed. Recent data show that titrating to higher doses can lead to adequate pain reduction, which contradicts a ceiling effect on analgesia (Clement et al. 2013). For respiratory depression, however, a ceiling effect has been described (Davis 2005). Apart from this, constipation (Likar et al. 2006) and cognitive dysfunction (Davis 2005) seem to be less common than for other opioids. In renal impairment or failure as well as in dialysis, it is safe and effective (Filitz et al. 2006) because elimination occurs mainly via the gastrointestinal tract. Because of its pharmacokinetic properties, buprenorphine can also be administered via the transdermal and transmucosal route. The sublingual bioavailability is 30–50 % (Davis 2005). The galenic formulation of selected patches allows 7-day changing intervals.

5.3.6 Tapentadol

The only new synthetic opioid developed in the past decade is tapentadol. It is a dual-action molecule due to the μ-agonism and the norepinephrine reuptake inhibition. This dual action may be beneficial in case of neuropathic pain. However, up to now, the role of this new central-acting analgesic has not been defined. The analgesic effect was shown in acute postoperative (Daniels et al. 2009) and chronic non-cancer (Buynak et al. 2010) pain. A better tolerability than for other strong opioids has been reported (Hale et al. 2009; Daniels et al. 2009). In patients suffering from renal or liver impairment, the dose does not have to be adjusted. Results of clinical trials for usage of tapentadol in the context of palliative care are pending (Klein et al. 2011). To date, no immediate release formulation is available, which may hamper its use in cancer pain management.

5.3.7 Methadone/Levo-Methadone

Owing to its complex pharmacokinetic profile, the use of methadone and levo-methadone in cancer pain management is rather limited (Klepstad et al. 2005; Nauck et al. 2004). However, it is recommended as a second-line opioid in cases of complex or neuropathic pain or opioid tolerance (Caraceni et al. 2012). In addition to the effects on the opioid receptor, analgesic properties are enhanced by presynaptic reuptake inhibition of serotonin and an additional antagonism at the NMDA receptor. It is lipophilic and has a high oral bioavailability of 85 % (Inturrisi 2002). In Germany, the racemic methadone and the isolated isomer levo-methadone are both available. When used in cancer pain management, the substance of choice is levo-methadone (Ostgathe et al. 2012) because necessary doses are lower because it is twice as potent as methadone and is preferable with respect to cardiac side effects (Ansermot et al. 2010). Due to the high protein-binding proportion (60–90 %) and a variable plasma half-life (8–75 h), the risk of accumulation in case of repetitive doses is higher than for other opioids. Therefore, specific conversion and titration schemes for methadone (Morley and Makin 1998; Ripamonti et al. 1998) and levo-methadone (Nauck et al. 2001; Ostgathe et al. 2012) have been developed.

5.3.8 Side Effects of Opioids

Most commonly, patients treated with opioids complain of nausea, vomiting, and constipation. Furthermore, opioids can cause sedation, dry mouth, confusion, hallucinations, nightmares, itching, sweating, urinary retention, or myoclonus. Most side effects occur especially in the initial treatment setting and after dose increases. Co-medication as prophylaxis or treatment is often necessary on a temporary or continuous basis.

5.3.9 Practical Proceeding in Cancer Pain Management

If pain is insufficiently controlled with step I/II or patients are in strong pain, a therapy with strong opioids needs to be initiated. In naïve patients, a dose titration phase is beneficial. Therefore, immediate-release preparations of all three first-line opioids (morphine, hydromorphone, oxycodone) (Caraceni et al. 2012) are recommended. The decision of which opioid to use should be based on organ function, availability, and preferred route of administration. In many situations, the oral route is feasible. In particular in patients that are unable to swallow and/or in the dying phase, the subcutaneous administration of drugs is a flexible, feasible, safe, and non-burdening method (Bartz et al. 2013).

A titration strategy – to start with low-dose immediate-release opioid given every 4 h (parenteral 2.5 mg or oral 5 mg morphine, hydromorphone 0.5–1 mg or oxycodone 1–2 mg) individualized by dose adjustment until sufficient pain relief is achieved – is widely used and well described; however, it is not based on controlled clinical studies but on pharmacological properties (Caraceni et al. 2012). Dose escalation of step III opioids is only limited by side effects. If no sufficient pain reduction is achieved or intolerable side effects occur, rotation to another opioid or other measures should be considered (Fine and Portenoy 2009; Cherny et al. 2001). Strong opioids may also be initiated in the outpatient setting. It is recommended to start with the oral administration of a low dose of a slow-acting opioid.

For acute pain exacerbations, 1/6th (individual range 1/12th–1/3rd) of the regular opioid daily dose should be prescribed as an immediate-release solution. This on-demand medication should be administered with a minimum interval of 45 min between two doses. If the patient requires the additional rapid-acting opioid more than 3–5 times a day, the regular dose should be increased accordingly. Patients can be educated that in case of predictable pain exacerbations, for instance, on movement, this additional medication should be given 30–45 min prior to the anticipated painful stimulus. Rapid-acting fentanyl preparations are an option for on-demand medication in case of transient severe pain crises (breakthrough pain) while background pain is otherwise generally well controlled. It has a fast onset (between 5 and 15 min) and short duration of action. Xerostomia sometimes makes dissolution of the buccal tablets difficult, and some patients dislike the perception of dizziness that is provoked by the rapid absorption of the opioid. In fast-acting fentanyl preparations, dose titration should start at the lowest dose; unlike with other opioids, it is not possible to calculate the dose necessary for breakthrough pain control according to the regular total daily opioid dose. To prevent disappointment, dose titration should be performed with the first pain crisis.

Table 5.2 Evidence-based relative analgesic ratios for opioid switching

	Relative analgesic ratio	Strength of the recommendation for use (GRADE)
Oral morphine to oral oxycodone	1.5:1	Strong
Oral oxycodone to oral hydromorphone	4:1	Strong
Oral morphine to oral hydromorphone	5:1	Weak
Oral morphine to TD buprenorphine	75:1	Weak
Oral morphine to TD fentanyl	100:1	Weak

Modified after Caraceni et al. (2012)

TD transdermal

5.3.10 Opioid Rotation

The first step when rotation is considered is to calculate the equianalgesic dose of the new drug according to its relative analgesic potency (Table 5.2). Because of incomplete tolerance between different opioids, it is advisable to reduce the starting dose of the new opioid at least by one third (Vadalouca et al. 2008).

5.3.11 Management of Opioid-Induced Side Effects

Potential side effects need to be discussed with the patients because they should be aware that side effects may persist, and some may appear transient during opioid application. For most patients, opioid-induced constipation is a persistent phenomenon and needs to be treated. For some patients, distress induced by constipation can be worse than pain, and some even refuse to continue the opioid (Hurdon et al. 2000). Evidence on the treatment of constipation is inadequate (Miles et al. 2006). The European Consensus Group on Constipation therefore published consensus-based recommendations on a stepwise approach to treat constipation (Larkin et al. 2008). As rescue medication, or if enteral administration of a laxative is not achievable, the opioid antagonist methylnaltrexone can be administered for opioid-induced constipation (Candy et al. 2011). In the beginning of an opioid medication or when the dose is adapted, mild sedation can occur. Patients can be reassured with the information that sedation will commonly disappear within a few days up to a week after onset of opioid medication. Nausea and emesis do occur with an incidence of 25–35 % and may have a negative impact on the patient's quality of life (Aparasu et al. 1999). For 7–10 days, antiemetic drugs should be prescribed prophylactically parallel to the onset of the opioid medication. Drugs with antidopaminergic action such as haloperidol or metoclopramide are recommended to be used prophylactically and in case of opioid-induced nausea and emesis (Caraceni et al. 2012). Rare side effects are confusion, nightmares, itching, sweating, myoclonus, urinary retention, or loss of sexual interest (Table 5.3). In case of distress caused by any side effect not sufficiently manageable by other measures, the opioid dose should be reduced or an opioid rotation considered (Caraceni et al. 2012).

Table 5.3 Rare side effects of opioids and possible measures

Side effect	Remarks	Possible measures
Confusion, hallucination	Often multiple causes, DD: paraneoplastic	Dose reduction
		Opioid rotation
		Neuroleptic drugs
Sweating	Often in patients with liver metastases	Anticholinergic drugs
		Salvia
		Washing the whole body
		Opioid rotation
Itching	Intradermal histamine deliberation and alteration of the sensory modulation in the medullary dorsal horn	Antihistaminic drugs
		Skin care
		Washing the whole body with diluted vinegar
		Antidepressant
		5-HT3-antagonist
		Opioid rotation
Urinary retention	Opioids can increase tonus of smooth muscles (higher tonus of the sphincter, lower tonus of the detrusor)	If possible, reduction of medication that has similar effects on smooth muscle (e.g., tricyclic antidepressants)
		Parasympathomimetics
		Dose reduction
		Opioid rotation
Myoclonus	Possible sign for intoxication, accumulation in case of renal dysfunction	Dose reduction
		Opioid rotation
		Antiepileptic drugs (e.g., clonazepam)
		Baclofen
Loss of sexual interest	Opioid-induced hypogonadism	If possible, reduction of medication that has similar effects (e.g., SSRI, tricyclic antidepressants)
		Dose reduction

Sometimes patients as well as professionals are concerned about problems like respiratory depression or that starting with an opioid may be "the beginning of the end." Here, good communication is necessary because there is no reason for such concerns when the principles mentioned above are followed. Respiratory depression, for example, does not occur as long as pain reduction guides the dose titration of the opioid. Pain is the physiological antagonist of an opioid-induced respiratory depression. Moreover, when the general principles are followed, opioids can be administered over long periods.

5.4 Neuropathic Pain

Cancer-related neuropathic pain is a common and severe symptom (Rodriguez et al. 2013; Rayment et al. 2013). Its origin is to be found either in the disease itself (cancer-related neuropathic pain), as a side effect of neurotoxic therapy (chemotherapy-induced neuropathic pain – CINP), or in preexisting health conditions that are not related to cancer, but contribute to the development of neuropathic pain, such as diabetes mellitus or postherpetic neuralgia (cancer-associated pain) (Fallon 2013). Neuropathic pain is defined as "pain arising as direct consequence of a lesion of disease affecting the somatosensory system" (Treede et al. 2008), and in the context of cancer, this lesion may derive from a wide variety of reasons. These reasons have to be explored carefully before treatment starts so that one can find the treatment options that promise to be the most effective.

5.4.1   Basic Treatment Algorithm for Neuropathic Cancer Pain

The foundation for a reflected treatment decision is based on many factors. These begin with a thorough and comprehensive examination and documentation of neuropathological clinical features; general medical and oncological medical history including current spread of disease, previous treatment regimens, and cumulative drug dosages; and also include concurrent medication and coexisting non-neuropathic pain syndromes (Laird et al. 2008).

The basic question is whether the neuropathic cancer pain results from cancer growth and progressive disease, which urges for causative treatment, if available. If local irritation or invasion of neural tissue is diagnosed to cause the neuropathic cancer pain, effective local treatment measures such as surgery, radiotherapy, or – in rare circumstances – neural ablation should be considered (Cleeland et al. 2010). In some cancers, for instance, in multiple myeloma or small cell cancer of the lung, neuropathy may be a sign of metabolic tumor activity. Decision is needed whether systemic anticancer treatment might improve the symptomatic neuropathy itself if the tumor responds or even without objective response (Richardson et al. 2006; van Oosterhout et al. 1996; Vedeler et al. 2006). In addition to causative treatment options, pharmacological treatment is the mainstay in addressing neuropathic cancer pain.

Despite the clear notion that neuropathic cancer pain might be more complex to treat than pain syndromes without a neuropathic component, the WHO ladder is strongly recommended as a basis for neuropathic cancer pain management (Foley 2003). However, there are contradictory data and recommendations for whether the combination of analgesics and adjuvants should be the first-line treatment, or whether one class of drugs should be titrated properly before introducing a second one (Raptis et al. 2014; Paice 2003).

5.4.2   Neuropathic Pain in Cancer and Non-cancer Patients

General differences in the therapeutic approach to cancer-related and non-cancer pain are reflected in differences in recommendations: on the one hand, underlying neuropathophysiological pathways show many similarities, which leads to similar recommendations for both types of pain. However, the overall clinical conditions can vary greatly between patients suffering from nonmalignant neuropathic pain syndromes and patients suffering from neuropathic cancer pain. Therefore, recommendations for treatment of neuropathic cancer pain often differ for practical reasons from those for non-cancer neuropathic pain despite their similarities. A prevalence of

19–39% of neuropathic pain (including mixed pain) in cancer patients is remarkably high, which calls for specific treatment. But the majority of cancer patients suffer from at least two and more pain types at the same time. This leads to a different practical approach, emphasizing drugs with a high analgesic potential for all pain types, such as opioids (Bennett et al. 2012; Banning et al. 1991). To avoid polypharmacy, first-line medication then often pragmatically covers the whole picture of a mixed-pain syndrome such as that frequently found in cancer patients. The most important drug classes used specifically to treat neuropathic cancer pain are also the substances featured in the WHO analgesic ladder; they are mainly antidepressants, anticonvulsants, steroids, NMDA antagonists, cannabinoids, and topicals.

5.4.3 Drugs for Managing Neuropathic Cancer Pain

5.4.3.1 Opioids

The role of opioids is still debated. The last update of a Cochrane review (2013) on this question showed a benefit for opioids over placebo only in intermediate-term studies, with strong hints for significant bias in the overall results (McNicol et al. 2013). This means that supporting evidence remains weak for opioids in the treatment of neuropathic pain, at least if etiological reasons are not differentiated. Specifically, studies that focused on neuropathic cancer pain reported that there is evidence for a useful role of opioids according to some small interventional studies, but again the wider picture remains unclear (Jongen et al. 2013). There are different reasons for that: by now oxycodone is the only opioid studied regarding its efficiency in neuropathic cancer pain. Due to the existing lack of common definitions, criteria for diagnosis and assessment results are difficult to compare (Cartoni et al. 2012; Garassino et al. 2013). It is already considered to be good clinical standard to actually apply the principles of the WHO analgesic ladder in cancer pain patients, including patients suffering from neuropathic pain. Consequently, in studies that examine the efficiency of co-analgesics head-to-head including a placebo arm, opioids are referred to as effective rescue medication, underlining the clinical relevance of opioids despite the comparably weak evidence (Mishra et al. 2012).

Moreover, the choice of analgesics is significantly influenced by the overall symptom burden, existing comorbidities, and co-medication. Therefore, opioids do play an important practical role in the treatment of neuropathic cancer pain, especially in the context of palliative care. All in all, there is no evidence supporting the superiority of one opioid to another.

5.4.3.2 Antidepressants

Antidepressants have been known to be effective in neuropathic pain for many years. Published data specifically on neuropathic cancer pain suggest a superiority over placebo for amitriptyline (Mishra et al. 2012), duloxetine (Smith et al. 2013), and venlafaxine (Durand et al. 2012). Each of these positive studies examined special aspects of neuropathic cancer pain. Mainly focusing on chemotherapy-induced peripheral neuropathy, they do not allow general conclusions for all types of neuropathic pain.

A Cochrane review on the effect of amitriptyline in general neuropathic pain did not find enough evidence to actually support the use of amitriptyline (Moore et al.

2012), nor did some specifically designed studies on neuropathic cancer pain (Mercadante et al. 2002). More recently, preventing chemotherapy-induced neuropathic symptoms was the aim of studies with upfront administration of amitriptyline up to 100 mg/daily against placebo in asymptomatic chemotherapy patients who received vinca alkaloids, platina derivates, or taxanes. These studies showed no difference of amitriptyline against placebo (Kautio et al. 2009). Despite the lack of evidence, amitriptyline is still often considered to be helpful, and the clinical experience should not be neglected when one evaluates its role.

Duloxetine and venlafaxine have recently been shown to be efficient (Smith et al. 2013; Durand et al. 2012) in neuropathic cancer pain, especially in chemotherapy-induced peripheral neuropathy. These drugs should be considered among the first-line options in addition to pain treatment according to the WHO ladder. Venlafaxine even showed some efficiency in preventing CIPN.

Almost every newer antidepressant is said to be somewhat effective on an anecdotal basis, but judging from hard data alone, none of them can be regularly recommended (Bennett 2011).

In summary, evidence for the use of antidepressants is present with no real first-line medication. According to the data, amitriptyline is not considered to be as effective as its wide acceptance for treatment would suggest. Duloxetine and venlafaxine are promising alternatives, but their real value still has to be proven.

5.4.3.3 Anticonvulsants

Gabapentin and pregabalin are widely used as alternatives to or in combination with other drugs in the treatment of neuropathic cancer pain; lamotrigine is another often-discussed option. Evidence especially supports the use of gabapentin (Caraceni et al. 1999; Yan et al. 2013). A Cochrane review on a mixed population including cancer patients resulted in a significant reduction of neuropathic pain in one third of the patients taking gabapentin for this reason (Moore et al. 2011). In addition, the combination with opioids is specifically backed by evidence (Caraceni et al. 2004). Pregabalin is often used, but its use lacks comparable evidence (Bennett et al. 2013). It became very popular because it is considered to be faster in onset. Hard data supporting this are still lacking. Evidence for its activity against neuropathic cancer measured as an opioid-sparing effect is found in the literature (Raptis et al. 2014).

Lamotrigine is neither effective nor safe enough to be recommended for the treatment of neuropathic cancer pain (Wiffen et al. 2013; Rao et al. 2008).

Anecdotal evidence only exists for the use of valproic acid, topiramate, phenytoin, and carbamazepine for the specific use in neuropathic cancer pain. With existing alternatives available, their use can therefore not be recommended (Bendaly et al. 2007; Hardy et al. 2001).

Recent literature suggests gabapentin as the drug of choice when anticonvulsants are considered for treatment of neuropathic cancer pain.

5.4.3.4 Steroids

Despite its wide use, there is only little evidence for the role of steroids in the treatment of neuropathic cancer pain. The use of corticosteroids in spinal cord compression, superior vena cava obstruction, raised intracranial pressure, and bowel obstruction is better established than in other nonspecific pain indications. Recommendations for dosage and drug of choice vary. However, dexamethasone is most often prescribed for pain treatment. An advantage of long-acting dexamethasone is the comparably less fluid retention due to less mineralocorticoid action than in other steroids (Leppert and Buss 2012).

5.4.3.5 NMDA Antagonists

NMDA antagonists such as ketamine, memantine, and dextromethorphan are used in complicated pain syndromes with the aim to resensitize the opioid receptors for μ-agonist activity. Clinical evaluation remains limited. Efficiency is described on a rather anecdotal level in the form of small case studies and case reports (Grande et al. 2008). Systematic evaluation is rare and leads to a complicated picture: the use of NMDA antagonists is limited by severe side central nervous effects if given in the so-considered appropriate dose (Mercadante et al. 2000). At the same time, low-dose application does not show any reliable effects (Mercadante et al. 1998). If an opioid is needed and the standard options have failed, (levo-) methadone can be used. It is – in addition to its opioid properties – a potent antagonist to the NMDA receptor (Caraceni et al. 2012). The positive effects in neuropathic cancer pain are enhanced by a presynaptic reuptake inhibition of serotonin.

Reasons for the limited data are surely to be found in the methodological difficulties of conducting proper studies on the issue, but currently, NMDA antagonists are not generally recommended and should be only considered when other options fail.

5.4.3.6 Cannabinoids

For years, cannabinoids have been attributed with anti-neuropathic capacity. Here also, evidence on the subject remains limited, especially for neuropathic cancer pain. Small studies describe the feasibility and moderate efficiency of cannabinoids (Lynch et al. 2013). An overall modest effect is confirmed for the efficiency of cannabinoids in non-cancer pain (Lynch and Campbell 2011). These data clearly suggest that cannabinoids are not to be recommended as first-line therapy, neither as monotherapy, nor as first-line adjuvant. But cannabinoids can be an interesting effort in subduing refractory pain syndromes.

5.4.3.7 Topicals

Topicals such as lidocaine 5 % and capsaicin 8 % patches have been widely studied in non-cancer neuropathic pain and have been shown to be an effective measure there (Sawynok 2013). Only very few data on patients suffering from specific types of cancer or patients treated in the oncological setting are available (Lopez Ramirez 2013; Fleming and O'Connor 2009). An explanation might be that topical treatment is not considered to be as different in cancer and non-cancer patients, and therefore results of non-cancer patients are more easily accepted for their applicability in cancer patients. With limited data on patients in the oncology setting, topical treatment can be considered an option in individual cases but needs to be explored in more detail. Procedural management of the capsaicin patch does require great care and special skills, which limits its use in a generalist setting.

5.4.3.8 Others

Complementary psychological and physiotherapeutic approaches may enhance efficacy of treatment and improve the patient's quality of life when they suffer from neuropathic cancer pain (Cassileth and Keefe 2010). These strategies are embedded in a holistic multidisciplinary framework of care. It is difficult to assess whether there is a specific influence on neuropathic pain as such, but without doubt the quality of holistic care is helpful for the development of good coping strategies for the patients.

5.4.3.9 A Pragmatic Approach to Managing Neuropathic Cancer Pain

There is no gold standard available for the treatment of neuropathic cancer pain, and there is little evidence compared with the treatment on non-cancer neuropathic pain. One might question whether this actually is of any therapeutic relevance because the neural pathways, ion channels, receptors, and neurotransmitters affected are the same in both types of neuropathies. However, the mode of damage to the nerves together with the coexistence of noncancerous factors leads to a physiologically different constellation of receptor transmission in the context of cancer pain (Urch and Dickenson 2008). In addition, the clinical features of neuropathic cancer pain are frequently found in combination with other severe symptoms, which urges for an appropriate simultaneous treatment (Stute et al. 2003). This influences the choice of drugs, because drugs with a known activity for neuropathic pain and other symptoms are certainly preferable to those with neuropathic pain activity alone.

From a pragmatic side, the following guidance for treatment of neuropathic cancer pain is therefore recommended:

> Step1: Treatment according to the WHO ladder, including appropriate titration of opioids
> If the result is good, the treatment can be continued, otherwise proceed to step 2.
> Step 2: Additional use of either an antidepressant (duloxetine/venlafaxine) or an anticonvulsant (gabapentin), including appropriate titration of the drug chosen
> If the result is good, the treatment can be continued, otherwise proceed to step 3.
> Step 3: Additional use of the class of drugs that is not being used in step 2, including appropriate titration of the drug chosen
> If the result is good, the treatment can be continued, otherwise proceed to step 4.
> Step 4: Additional use or replacement of co-analgesics with drugs of anecdotal evidence such as cannabinoids and NMDA antagonists

Basics throughout the treatment process:

> Evaluate causative options.
> Make use of integrative approaches.

5.4.3.10 Cancer Therapy-Related Pain

Pain related to anticancer therapy needs to be treated adequately and in accordance with the existing guidelines for acute and chronic pain syndromes. However, it is important to reflect on some special aspects of therapy-related pain in comparison with other pain syndromes.

Pain related to anticancer therapy is very troublesome to patients because for the majority of patients the pain is a constant reminder of the disease itself. Increasing pain intensity becomes emotionally associated with tumor progression (Portenoy and Hagen 1990; Zeppetella et al. 2000). Explaining therapy-related pain syndromes and patient education is therefore crucial in helping patients set the pain they experience into perspective.

The most important therapy-related pain syndrome for cancer patients is chemotherapy-induced neuropathic pain (CINP).

As outlined above, pharmacological treatment options are variable and have to be seen as one part of a wider picture.

Chemotherapeutic agents with a high likelihood of causing peripheral neuropathy are platinum drugs (cisplatin, carboplatin, oxaliplatin), plant alkaloids (vincristine, vindesine, vinblastine, vinorelbine, etoposide), taxanes (paclitaxel, docetaxel, cabazitaxel), epothilones (ixapebilone), bortezomib, carfilzomib, eribulin, and thalidomide/lenalidomide. Some of these drugs (like bortezomib, lenalidomide, and thalidomide in multiple myeloma) are actually used to prevent neuropathic cancer pain despite their potential side effects. As they are well capable of treating the underlying disease, they can improve and alleviate the symptom of neuropathic pain, if this is the main reason.

Pharmacological prevention of CIPN was studied intensely especially for oxaliplatin because one was apprehensive of its acute neurosensory toxicity. Up to now, little support or conflicting results regarding the upfront administration of drugs to asymptomatic patients can be stated. Despite reports on some activity of neuromodulatory agents such as calcium-magnesium infusions, glutathione, antiepileptic drugs such as carbamazepine and gabapentin, and a-lipoic acid, none of them proved to be effective in proper phase II or III trials (Grothey 2005). Even the previously highly ranked calcium-magnesium infusion regimen was shown to be ineffective in a phase III trial (Gamelin et al. 2004; Loprinzi et al. 2013; Kautio et al. 2009). The only drug with a positive phase III trial at the moment is venlafaxine 50 mg prior to infusion and 37.5 mg twice daily for the following 10 days. In comparison with placebo, venlafaxine showed a higher clinical activity against oxaliplatin-induced acute neurosensory toxicity (Durand et al. 2012).

Other aspects of therapy-related pain such as painful mucositis or bone pain in hematological recovery after chemotherapy nadir need to be treated cautiously according to guidelines on acute pain management and need to be embedded in a counseling and educational process.

References

Ahmedzai SH, Nauck F, Bar-Sela G, Bosse B, Leyendecker P, Hopp M (2012) A randomized, double-blind, active-controlled, double-dummy, parallel-group study to determine the safety and efficacy of oxycodone/naloxone prolonged-release tablets in patients with moderate/severe, chronic cancer pain. Palliat Med 26:50–60

Ansermot N, Albayrak O, Schlapfer J, Crettol S, Croquette-Krokar M, Bourquin M, Deglon JJ, Faouzi M, Scherbaum N, Eap CB (2010) Substitution of (R, S)-methadone by (R)-methadone: Impact on QTc interval. Arch Intern Med 170:529–536

Aparasu R, McCoy RA, Weber C, Mair D, Parasuraman TV (1999) Opioid-induced emesis among hospitalized nonsurgical patients: effect on pain and quality of life. J Pain Symptom Manage 18:280–288

Banning A, Sjogren P, Henriksen H (1991) Pain causes in 200 patients referred to a multidisciplinary cancer pain clinic. Pain 45:45–48

Bartz L, Klein C, Seifert A, Herget I, Ostgathe C, Stiel S (2013) Subcutaneous administration of drugs in palliative care – results of a systematic observational study. J Pain Symptom Manage 48(4):540–547

Bendaly EA, Jordan CA, Staehler SS, Rushing DA (2007) Topiramate in the treatment of neuropathic pain in patients with cancer. Support Cancer Ther 4:241–246

Bennett MI (2011) Effectiveness of antiepileptic or antidepressant drugs when added to opioids for cancer pain: systematic review. Palliat Med 25:553–559

Bennett MI, Rayment C, Hjermstad M, Aass N, Caraceni A, Kaasa S (2012) Prevalence and aetiology of neuropathic pain in cancer patients: a systematic review. Pain 153:359–365

Bennett MI, Laird B, van Litsenburg C, Nimour M (2013) Pregabalin for the management of neuropathic pain in adults with cancer: a systematic review of the literature. Pain Med 14:1681–1688

Bhala N, Emberson J, Merhi A, Abramson S, Arber N, Baron JA, Bombardier C, Cannon C, Farkouh ME, Fitzgerald GA, Goss P, Halls H, Hawk E, Hawkey C, Hennekens C, Hochberg M, Holland LE, Kearney PM, Laine L, Lanas A, Lance P, Laupacis A, Oates J, Patrono C, Schnitzer TJ, Solomon S, Tugwell P, Wilson K, Wittes J, Baigent C (2013) Vascular and upper gastrointestinal effects of non-steroidal anti-inflammatory drugs: meta-analyses of individual participant data from randomised trials. Lancet 382:769–779

Brooks J, Warburton R, Beales IL (2013) Prevention of upper gastrointestinal haemorrhage: current controversies and clinical guidance. Ther Adv Chronic Dis 4:206–222

Buvanendran A, Kroin JS, Tuman KJ, Lubenow TR, Elmofty D, Moric M, Rosenberg AG (2003) Effects of perioperative administration of a selective cyclooxygenase 2 inhibitor on pain management and recovery of function after knee replacement: a randomized controlled trial. JAMA 290:2411–2418

Buynak R, Shapiro DY, Okamoto A, Van Hove I, Rauschkolb C, Steup A, Lange B, Lange C, Etropolski M (2010) Efficacy and safety of tapentadol extended release for the management of chronic low back pain: results of a prospective, randomized, double-blind, placebo- and active-controlled Phase III study. Expert Opin Pharmacother 11:1787–1804

Candy B, Jones L, Goodman ML, Drake R, Tookman A (2011) Laxatives or methylnaltrexone for the management of constipation in palliative care patients. Cochrane Database Syst Rev (1):CD003448

Caraceni A, Zecca E, Martini C, De Conno F (1999) Gabapentin as an adjuvant to opioid analgesia for neuropathic cancer pain. J Pain Symptom Manage 17:441–445

Caraceni A, Zecca E, Bonezzi C, Arcuri E, Tur RY, Maltoni M, Visentin M, Gorni G, Martini C, Tirelli W, Barbieri M, De Conno F (2004) Gabapentin for neuropathic cancer pain: a randomized controlled trial from the Gabapentin Cancer Pain Study Group. J Clin Oncol 22:2909–2917

Caraceni A, Hanks G, Kaasa S, Bennett MI, Brunelli C, Cherny N, Dale O, De Conno F, Fallon M, Hanna M, Haugen DF, Juhl G, King S, Klepstad P, Laugsand EA, Maltoni M, Mercadante S, Nabal M, Pigni A, Radbruch L, Reid C, Sjogren P, Stone PC, Tassinari D, Zeppetella G (2012) Use of opioid analgesics in the treatment of cancer pain: evidence-based recommendations from the EAPC. Lancet Oncol 13:e58–e68

Cartoni C, Brunetti GA, Federico V, Efficace F, Grammatico S, Tendas A, Scaramucci L, Cupelli L, D'Elia GM, Truini A, Niscola P, Petrucci MT (2012) Controlled-release oxycodone for the treatment of bortezomib-induced neuropathic pain in patients with multiple myeloma. Support Care Cancer 20:2621–2626

Cassileth BR, Keefe FJ (2010) Integrative and behavioral approaches to the treatment of cancer-related neuropathic pain. Oncologist 15(Suppl 2):19–23

Cherny N, Ripamonti C, Pereira J, Davis C, Fallon M, McQuay H, Mercadante S, Pasternak G, Ventafridda V (2001) Strategies to manage the adverse effects of oral morphine: an evidence-based report. J Clin Oncol 19:2542–2554

Cleeland CS, Farrar JT, Hausheer FH (2010) Assessment of cancer-related neuropathy and neuropathic pain. Oncologist 15(Suppl 2):13–18

Clement PM, Beuselinck B, Mertens PG, Cornelissen P, Menten J (2013) Pain management in palliative cancer patients: a prospective observational study on the use of high dosages of transdermal buprenorphine. Acta Clin Belg 68:37–91

Daniels SE, Upmalis D, Okamoto A, Lange C, Haeussler J (2009) A randomized, double-blind, phase III study comparing multiple doses of tapentadol IR, oxycodone IR, and placebo for postoperative (bunionectomy) pain. Curr Med Res Opin 25:765–776

Davis MP (2005) Buprenorphine in cancer pain. Support Care Cancer 13(11):878–887

Deandrea S, Montanari M, Moja L, Apolone G (2008) Prevalence of undertreatment in cancer pain. A review of published literature. Ann Oncol 19:1985–1991

Durand JP, Deplanque G, Montheil V, Gornet JM, Scotte F, Mir O, Cessot A, Coriat R, Raymond E, Mitry E, Herait P, Yataghene Y, Goldwasser F (2012) Efficacy of venlafaxine for the prevention and relief of oxaliplatin-induced acute neurotoxicity: results of EFFOX, a randomized, double-blind, placebo-controlled phase III trial. Ann Oncol 23:200–205

Edwards JE, McQuay HJ (2002) Dipyrone and agranulocytosis: what is the risk? Lancet 360:1438

Edwards J, Meseguer F, Faura C, Moore RA, McQuay HJ, Derry S (2010) Single dose dipyrone for acute postoperative pain. Cochrane Database Syst Rev (3):CD003227

Fallon MT (2013) Neuropathic pain in cancer. Br J Anaesth 111:105–111

Filitz J, Griessinger N, Sittl R, Likar R, Schuttler J, Koppert W (2006) Effects of intermittent hemodialysis on buprenorphine and norbuprenorphine plasma concentrations in chronic pain patients treated with transdermal buprenorphine. Eur J Pain 10:743–748

Fine PG, Portenoy RK (2009) Establishing "best practices" for opioid rotation: conclusions of an expert panel. J Pain Symptom Manage 38:418–425

Fleming JA, O'Connor BD (2009) Use of lidocaine patches for neuropathic pain in a comprehensive cancer centre. Pain Res Manag 14:381–388

Foley KM (2003) Opioids and chronic neuropathic pain. N Engl J Med 348:1279–1281

Foley KM (2011) How well is cancer pain treated? Palliat Med 25:398–401

Gamelin L, Boisdron-Celle M, Delva R, Guerin-Meyer V, Ifrah N, Morel A, Gamelin E (2004) Prevention of oxaliplatin-related neurotoxicity by calcium and magnesium infusions: a retrospective study of 161 patients receiving oxaliplatin combined with 5-Fluorouracil and leucovorin for advanced colorectal cancer. Clin Cancer Res 10:4055–4061

Garassino MC, Piva S, La Verde N, Spagnoletti I, Iorno V, Carbone C, Febbraro A, Bianchi A, Bramati A, Moretti A, Ganzinelli M, Marabese M, Gentili M, Torri V, Farina G (2013) Randomised phase II trial (NCT00637975) evaluating activity and toxicity of two different escalating strategies for pregabalin and oxycodone combination therapy for neuropathic pain in cancer patients. PLoS One 8:e59981

Grande LA, O'Donnell BR, Fitzgibbon DR, Terman GW (2008) Ultra-low dose ketamine and memantine treatment for pain in an opioid-tolerant oncology patient. Anesth Analg 107:1380–1383

Grothey A (2005) Clinical management of oxaliplatin-associated neurotoxicity. Clin Colorectal Cancer 5(Suppl 1):S38–S46

Hale M, Upmalis D, Okamoto A, Lange C, Rauschkolb C (2009) Tolerability of tapentadol immediate release in patients with lower back pain or osteoarthritis of the hip or knee over 90 days: a randomized, double-blind study. Curr Med Res Opin 25:1095–1104

Hanks GW, Deconno F, Cherny N, Hanna M, Kalso E, McQuay H, Mercadante S, Meynardier J, Poulin P, Ripamonti C, Radbruch L, Casas JR, Sawe J, Twycross RG, Ventafridda V (2001) Morphine and alternative opioids in cancer pain: the EAPC recommendations. Br J Cancer 84:587–593

Hardy JR, Rees EA, Gwilliam B, Ling J, Broadley K, A'Hern R (2001) A phase II study to establish the efficacy and toxicity of sodium valproate in patients with cancer-related neuropathic pain. J Pain Symptom Manage 21:204–209

Hurdon V, Viola R, Schroder C (2000) How useful is docusate in patients at risk for constipation? A systematic review of the evidence in the chronically ill. J Pain Symptom Manage 19:130–136

Inturrisi CE (2002) Clinical pharmacology of opioids for pain. Clin J Pain 18:S3–S13

Jongen JL, Hans G, Benzon HT, Huygen F, Hartrick CT (2013) Neuropathic pain and pharmacological treatment. Pain Pract 14(3):283–295

Kalso E (2005) Oxycodone. J Pain Symptom Manage 29:47–56

Kautio AL, Haanpaa M, Leminen A, Kalso E, Kautiainen H, Saarto T (2009) Amitriptyline in the prevention of chemotherapy-induced neuropathic symptoms. Anticancer Res 29:2601–2606

Klein C, Lang U, Bukki J, Sittl R, Ostgathe C (2011) Pain management and symptom-oriented drug therapy in palliative care. Breast Care (Basel) 6:27–34

Klepstad P, Kaasa S, Cherny N, Hanks G, De Conno F, Eapc RSC (2005) Pain and pain treatments in European palliative care units. A cross sectional survey from the European Association for Palliative Care Research Network. Palliat Med 19:477–484

Laird B, Colvin L, Fallon M (2008) Management of cancer pain: basic principles and neuropathic cancer pain. Eur J Cancer 44:1078–1082

Larkin PJ, Sykes NP, Centeno C, Ellershaw JE, Elsner F, Eugene B, Gootjes JR, Nabal M, Noguera A, Ripamonti C, Zucco F, Zuurmond WW (2008) The management of constipation in palliative care: clinical practice recommendations. Palliat Med 22:796–807

Leppert W, Buss T (2012) The role of corticosteroids in the treatment of pain in cancer patients. Curr Pain Headache Rep 16:307–313

Likar R, Kayser H, Sittl R (2006) Long-term management of chronic pain with transdermal buprenorphine: a multicenter, open-label, follow-up study in patients from three short-term clinical trials. Clin Ther 28:943–952

Lopez Ramirez E (2013) Treatment of acute and chronic focal neuropathic pain in cancer patients with lidocaine 5% patches. A radiation and oncology department experience. Support Care Cancer 21:1329–1334

Loprinzi CL, Qin R, Dakhil SR, Fehrenbacher L, Flynn KA, Atherton P, Seisler D, Qamar R, Lewis GC, Grothey A (2013) Phase III randomized, placebo-controlled, double-blind study of intravenous calcium and magnesium to prevent oxaliplatin-induced sensory neurotoxicity (N08CB/Alliance). J Clin Oncol 32(10):997–1005

Lussier D, Richarz U, Finco G (2010) Use of hydromorphone, with particular reference to the OROS formulation, in the elderly. Drugs Aging 27:327–335

Lynch ME, Campbell F (2011) Cannabinoids for treatment of chronic non-cancer pain; a systematic review of randomized trials. Br J Clin Pharmacol 72(5):735–744

Lynch ME, Cesar-Rittenberg P, Hohmann AG (2013) A double-blind, placebo-controlled, crossover pilot trial with extension using an oral mucosal cannabinoid extract for treatment of chemotherapy-induced neuropathic pain. J Pain Symptom Manage 47(1):166–173

McCann S, Yaksh TL, von Gunten CF (2010) Correlation between myoclonus and the 3-glucuronide metabolites in patients treated with morphine or hydromorphone: a pilot study. J Opioid Manag 6:87–94

McNicol ED, Midbari A, Eisenberg E (2013) Opioids for neuropathic pain. Cochrane Database Syst Rev (8):CD006146

Mercadante S (2010) Management of cancer pain. Intern Emerg Med 5(Suppl 1):S31–S35

Mercadante S, Casuccio A, Genovese G (1998) Ineffectiveness of dextromethorphan in cancer pain. J Pain Symptom Manage 16:317–322

Mercadante S, Arcuri E, Tirelli W, Casuccio A (2000) Analgesic effect of intravenous ketamine in cancer patients on morphine therapy: a randomized, controlled, double-blind, crossover, double-dose study. J Pain Symptom Manage 20:246–252

Mercadante S, Arcuri E, Tirelli W, Villari P, Casuccio A (2002) Amitriptyline in neuropathic cancer pain in patients on morphine therapy: a randomized placebo-controlled, double-blind crossover study. Tumori 88:239–242

Miles CL, Fellowes D, Goodman ML, Wilkinson S (2006) Laxatives for the management of constipation in palliative care patients. Cochrane Database Syst Rev (4):CD003448

Mishra S, Bhatnagar S, Goyal GN, Rana SPS, Upadhya SP (2012) A comparative efficacy of amitriptyline, gabapentin, and pregabalin in neuropathic cancer pain: a prospective randomized double-blind placebo-controlled study. Am J Hosp Palliat Med 29:177–182

Moore RA, Wiffen PJ, Derry S, McQuay HJ (2011) Gabapentin for chronic neuropathic pain and fibromyalgia in adults. Cochrane Database Syst Rev (3):CD007938

Moore RA, Derry S, Aldington D, Cole P, Wiffen PJ (2012) Amitriptyline for neuropathic pain and fibromyalgia in adults. Cochrane Database Syst Rev (12):CD008242

Morley JS, Makin MK (1998) The use of methadone in cancer pain poorly responsive to other opioids. Pain Rev 5:51–58

Nauck F, Ostgathe C, Dickerson ED (2001) A German model for methadone conversion. Am J Hosp Palliat Care 18:200–202

Nauck F, Ostgathe C, Klaschik E, Bausewein C, Fuchs M, Lindena G, Neuwohner K, Schulenberg D, Radbruch L (2004) Drugs in palliative care: results from a representative survey in Germany. Palliat Med 18:100–107

Ostgathe C, Voltz R, Van Aaken A, Klein C, Sabatowski R, Nauck F, Gaertner J (2012) Practicability, safety, and efficacy of a "German model" for opioid conversion to oral levomethadone. Support Care Cancer 20:2105–2110

Paice JA (2003) Mechanisms and management of neuropathic pain in cancer. J Support Oncol 1:107–120

Pergolizzi J, Boger RH, Budd K, Dahan A, Erdine S, Hans G, Kress HG, Langford R, Likar R, Raffa RB, Sacerdote P (2008) Opioids and the management of chronic severe pain in the elderly: consensus statement of an International Expert Panel with focus on the six clinically most often used World Health Organization Step III opioids (buprenorphine, fentanyl, hydromorphone, methadone, morphine, oxycodone). Pain Pract 8:287–313

Portenoy RK, Hagen NA (1990) Breakthrough pain: definition, prevalence and characteristics. Pain 41:273–281

Rao RD, Flynn PJ, Sloan JA, Wong GY, Novotny P, Johnson DB, Gross HM, Renno SI, Nashawaty M, Loprinzi CL (2008) Efficacy of lamotrigine in the management of chemotherapy-induced peripheral neuropathy: a phase 3 randomized, double-blind, placebo-controlled trial, N01C3. Cancer 112:2802–2808

Raphael J, Ahmedzai S, Hester J, Urch C, Barrie J, Williams J, Farquhar-Smith P, Fallon M, Hoskin P, Robb K, Bennett MI, Haines R, Johnson M, Bhaskar A, Chong S, Duarte R, Sparkes E (2010) Cancer pain: part 1: Pathophysiology; oncological, pharmacological, and psychological treatments: a perspective from the British Pain Society endorsed by the UK Association of Palliative Medicine and the Royal College of General Practitioners. Pain Med 11:742–764

Raptis E, Vadalouca A, Stavropoulou E, Argyra E, Melemeni A, Siafaka I (2014) Pregabalin Vs. opioids for the treatment of neuropathic cancer pain: a prospective, head-to-head, randomized, open-label study. Pain Pract 14:32–42

Rayment C, Hjermstad MJ, Aass N, Kaasa S, Caraceni A, Strasser F, Heitzer E, Fainsinger R, Bennett MI, European Palliative Care Research (2013) Neuropathic cancer pain: prevalence, severity, analgesics and impact from the European Palliative Care Research Collaborative-Computerised Symptom Assessment study. Palliat Med 27:714–721

Richardson PG, Briemberg H, Jagannath S, Wen PY, Barlogie B, Berenson J, Singhal S, Siegel DS, Irwin D, Schuster M, Srkalovic G, Alexanian R, Rajkumar SV, Limentani S, Alsina M, Orlowski RZ, Najarian K, Esseltine D, Anderson KC, Amato AA (2006) Frequency, characteristics, and reversibility of peripheral neuropathy during treatment of advanced multiple myeloma with bortezomib. J Clin Oncol 24:3113–3120

Ripamonti C, Groff L, Brunelli C, Polastri D, Stavrakis A, De Conno F (1998) Switching from morphine to oral methadone in treating cancer pain: what is the equianalgesic dose ratio? J Clin Oncol 16:3216–3221

Rodriguez CG, Lyras L, Gayoso LO, Sepulveda JM, Samantas E, Pelzer U, Bowen S, van Litsenburg C, Strand M (2013) Cancer-related neuropathic pain in out-patient oncology clinics: a European survey. BMC Palliat Care 12:41

Ross FB, Smith MT (1997) The intrinsic antinociceptive effects of oxycodone appear to be kappa-opioid receptor mediated. Pain 73:151–157

Saari TI, Fechner J, Ihmsen H, Schuttler J, Jeleazcov C (2012) Analysis of total and unbound hydromorphone in human plasma by ultrafiltration and LC-MS/MS: application to clinical trial in patients undergoing open heart surgery. J Pharm Biomed Anal 71:63–70

Sawynok J (2013) Topical analgesics for neuropathic pain: preclinical exploration, clinical validation, future development. Eur J Pain 18(4):465–481

Smith EM, Pang H, Cirrincione C, Fleishman S, Paskett ED, Ahles T, Bressler LR, Fadul CE, Knox C, Le-Lindqwister N, Gilman PB, Shapiro CL, Alliance for Clinical Trials in Oncology (2013) Effect of duloxetine on pain, function, and quality of life among patients with chemotherapy-induced painful peripheral neuropathy: a randomized clinical trial. JAMA 309:1359–1367

Stute P, Soukup J, Menzel M, Sabatowski R, Grond S (2003) Analysis and treatment of different types of neuropathic cancer pain. J Pain Symptom Manage 26:1123–1131

Treede RD, Jensen TS, Campbell JN, Cruccu G, Dostrovsky JO, Griffin JW, Hansson P, Hughes R, Nurmikko T, Serra J (2008) Neuropathic pain: redefinition and a grading system for clinical and research purposes. Neurology 70:1630–1635

Urch CE, Dickenson AH (2008) Neuropathic pain in cancer. Eur J Cancer 44:1091–1096

Vadalouca A, Moka E, Argyra E, Sikioti P, Siafaka I (2008) Opioid rotation in patients with cancer: a review of the current literature. J Opioid Manag 4:213–250

van Oosterhout AG, van de Pol M, ten Velde GP, Twijnstra A (1996) Neurologic disorders in 203 consecutive patients with small cell lung cancer. Results of a longitudinal study. Cancer 77:1434–1441

Vedeler CA, Antoine JC, Giometto B, Graus F, Grisold W, Hart IK, Honnorat J, Sillevis Smitt PA, Verschuuren JJ, Voltz R, Paraneoplastic Neurological Syndrome (2006) Management of paraneoplastic neurological syndromes: report of an EFNS Task Force. Eur J Neurol 13:682–690

WHO (1998) Symptom relief in terminal illness. WHO, Geneva

Wiffen PJ, Derry S, Moore RA (2013) Lamotrigine for chronic neuropathic pain and fibromyalgia in adults. Cochrane Database Syst Rev (12):CD006044

Yan PZ, Butler PM, Kurowski D, Perloff MD (2013) Beyond neuropathic pain: gabapentin use in cancer pain and perioperative pain. Clin J Pain 30(7):613–629

Zeppetella G, O'Doherty CA, Collins S (2000) Prevalence and characteristics of breakthrough pain in cancer patients admitted to a hospice. J Pain Symptom Manage 20:87–92

Radiation Therapy in Patients with Non-curable Cancer

"Non-curable" Does Not Mean "Non-treatable": The Role of Radiation Oncology in the Palliative Treatment of Cancer

Clemens Friedrich Hess, Andrea Hille, and Hendrik A. Wolff

Contents

6.1   Introduction

During the past decades, cure rates of cancer patients have steadily increased – up to about 50 %. The other half of the patients suffer from locoregional relapse or distant metastases. In addition, with more effective systemic treatment, the lifetime with recurrent disease will be considerably longer. Most of these recurrences will cause significant symptoms, which are often accompanied by a considerable reduction in the quality of life (Lutz et al. 2014; Hartsell and Santosh 2013; Nicols et al. 2013; Rajendran et al. 2013; Konski et al. 2005).

Anticancer therapies like chemotherapy, immunotherapy, targeted substances, and radioisotopes but also endoscopic or surgical interventions may deliver a substantial symptomatic benefit to patients suffering from advanced conditions. These

C.F. Hess, MD, PhD (✉) • A. Hille, MD • H.A. Wolff, MD
Department of Radiotherapy and Radiation Oncology, University Medical Center, Göttingen, Germany
e-mail: cfhess@med.uni-goettingen.de; ahille@med.uni-goettingen.de; hendrik.wolff@med.uni-goettingen.de

© Springer-Verlag Berlin Heidelberg 2015   79
B. Alt-Epping, F. Nauck (eds.), *Palliative Care in Oncology*,
DOI 10.1007/978-3-662-46202-7_6

benefits are described elsewhere in detail. In this respect, anticancer therapies may be an important and indispensable component of palliative care concepts (as a palliative care approach may accordingly be an important component of interventional oncological concepts for patients suffering from incurable disease).

In particular, radiation therapy (RT) denotes a paradigmatic treatment modality that may reduce many tumor-related symptoms. Notably, symptoms from clearly localized tumor manifestations can be efficiently treated by a precise RT. Moreover, in the case of whole-brain RT (WBRT) for brain metastases, even a whole organ can be treated without relevant side effects (Lutz et al. 2014; Nicols et al. 2013; Sheehan et al. 2014; Graham et al. 2010; Andrews et al. 2004; Aoyama et al. 2006). Therefore, this chapter will focus on palliative radiotherapy concepts for patients suffering from incurable disease.

Radiation therapy has become more efficient and much better tolerable with increasing precision of RT planning and administration, with new insights into the radiobiological effects of tumors and normal tissues, and with the additional application of systemic – and radiosensitizing – drugs. Personalized concepts that prescribe individualized target volumes make increased single and total doses available more often. With hypofractionated and accelerated schedules, treatment durations have been considerably shortened – to a single day, for example, in radiosurgery for brain metastases. These very short treatments may be applied even in patients who live far away from radiation units. In many circumstances, they help severely ill patients to optimally utilize their remaining life span (Sheehan et al. 2014; Timmermann et al. 2014; Wu et al. 2003; Lutz et al. 2011).

In recurrent or metastatic cancer, severe pain or neurological symptoms are observed more often. Other symptoms include tumor bleeding or stenoses of visceral organs, caused by the obstruction of airways, the gastrointestinal tract, or of the ureters. In the case of an underlying localized lesion, RT is often the most effective and most tolerable treatment modality – widely independent of the underlying disease and its specific histology. With very few exceptions, such as lymphoma or testis tumors, these patients are generally not curable, and an effective relief of symptoms is the predominant goal of treatment. In selected patients with oligo-symptomatic disease, RT may also help to prolong survival time (Lutz et al. 2014; Hartsell and Santosh 2013; Nicols et al. 2013; Rajendran et al. 2013; Salama and Milano 2014; Siddiqui et al. 2014; Milano et al. 2009).

6.2 Management of Pain and Bone Destructions

In most patients with recurrent or metastatic cancer, pain is the first and often the leading symptom. In particular, unusual and persistent pain in patients with prior cancer diagnosis (especially in those with diseases of a poor prognosis) is highly suspicious of tumor recurrence. Early and adequate clinical and image-guided diagnosis is very important for diagnosing and treating the underlying cause. Often, cross-sectional imaging such as computed tomography (CT) or magnetic resonance imaging (MRI) is needed to detect the pain-causing tumors (Hartsell and Santosh 2013).

Most frequently, cancer pain is caused by skeletal metastases, located most often in the spine, pelvis, or long bones. Soft-tissue tumors may accompany bone manifestations but may also occur outside the skeleton, for instance, in the retroperitoneum. To diagnose osseous tumors, CT is often sufficient, while for soft-tissue tumors, MRI is appropriate. After delineating localized metastases, the corresponding pain symptoms can usually be effectively treated by RT. In 80 % of the patients, cancer-related pain was considerably reduced, predominantly at the end of the RT series (Fig. 6.1). This series typically includes only ten daily fractions of 3 Gy, with the target volumes concentrating on the pain-related lesions. Soft-tissue tumors may require slightly higher total doses, but the entire treatment time normally does not exceed 3 weeks. In specific cases – for example, in patients with a very limited expected life span – shorter treatment schedules (e.g., 4×5 Gy) or even single doses of 6 Gy or 8 Gy can be successfully applied. Soft-tissue tumors may also be adequately treated by high-dose rate (HDR) brachytherapy (BT), with or without concomitant hyperthermia (HT). Again, the time for these treatments should be limited to 1–3 weeks (Lutz et al. 2011, 2014; Hartsell and Santosh 2013; Rajendran et al. 2013; Wu et al. 2003).

In osteolyses with impending fracture, stabilization after RT typically needs at least 6–8 weeks. If the patients have not been treated by prior stabilizing surgery, patients should be informed about external stabilizing methods. Even without operative procedures, relevant fractures after RT for bone metastases are rare and occur in less than 10 % of all patients. Consequently, surgery should be limited to patients with oligometastases, good prognosis, or underlying diseases with relatively radioresistant histology, such as melanoma, sarcoma, or renal cell carcinoma. In addition, surgery may be necessary in patients for whom a second curative approach may be advisable or for whom repeated pathologic evaluation is needed for systemic treatment. However, RT without surgery may be adequate for many patients with bony destructions, particularly for those with multiple metastases and those with a very limited prognosis. During and after RT, adequate systemic treatment

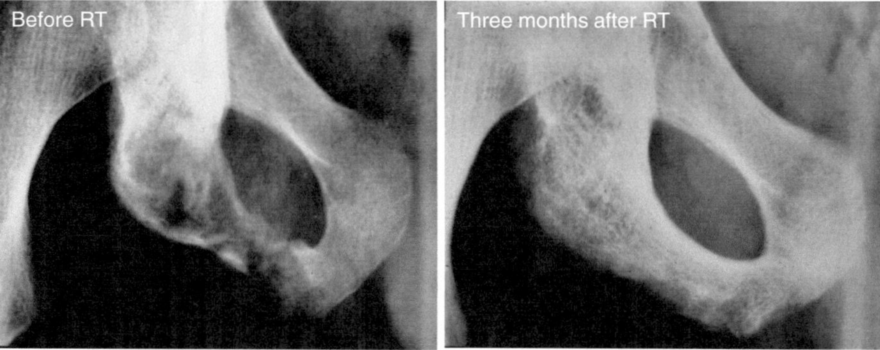

Fig. 6.1 Bone metastasis before and after RT. At the end of the 2-week RT series, severe pain was significantly reduced. Three months later, complete stabilization of the involved bone can be observed

(including bisphosphonates) is mandatory. The need for analgesics is often reduced, with a significant reduction in about 80 % of patients until 2 weeks after the end of the RT series (Lutz et al. 2014; Nicols et al. 2013; Siva et al. 2010; Schlampp et al. 2014; Van der Linden et al. 2004; Nathan et al. 2005; Chew et al. 2011).

6.3 Neurological Symptoms

6.3.1 Brain Metastases

Similar to tumor-related pain, neurological symptoms can be successfully treated by RT. In particular, an entire organ can be safely covered by palliatively effective radiation doses with WBRT. This is particularly indicated in patients with multiple brain metastases. Again, relatively short treatment schedules – such as 30 Gy in 2 weeks – are of the utmost importance as these patients often have a very limited life expectancy. This means that potential long-term RT side effects such as a decline in neurocognitive function are often hardly relevant (Lutz et al. 2014; Nicols et al. 2013; Sheehan et al. 2014; Michaelson and Smith 2005; Aoyama et al. 2007; Kocher et al. 2011; Chang et al. 2009; Mahmood et al. 2010; Son et al. 2012).

In specific cases, higher single or total doses should be given to individual metastases, which may be responsible for severe neurological symptoms. Such a localized dose escalation can be realized by modern radiation techniques of high conformity (high-precision RT, see Fig. 6.2). In particular, these strategies should be considered in histologies of presumably reduced radiation sensitivity such as melanoma, sarcoma, or renal cell carcinoma (Sheehan et al. 2014; Andrews et al. 2004; Kocher et al. 2011).

In patients with single brain metastases, prior surgery significantly improves patient outcome. In the case of increased surgical risk, the application of high single RT doses (stereotactic radiosurgery, SRS) is as efficient as operative resection (Fig. 6.3). Radiosurgery can be realized by different RT methods: There is no significant difference in efficacy, tolerability, or safety between the different types of radiosurgery ("Gamma Knife," "Linac Knife" with specific linear accelerators, or the "CyberKnife"). These treatments may also be considered for a limited number of brain metastases (<5). Most importantly, these numbers should be clearly documented by MRI. Additional WBRT reduces the relapse risk in the brain, but not the overall survival time (Nicols et al. 2013; Sheehan et al. 2014; Andrews et al. 2004; Aoyama et al. 2006, 2007; Kocher et al. 2011; Central Nervous System 2011).

Repeated RT for recurrent brain metastases may be safely applied. This is particularly valid after initial RS. Repeated WBRT is relatively safe even after initial WBRT. Additional doses >20 Gy should be given after initial WB doses of 30–35 Gy. About 70 % of patients experience neurologic improvement. Median survival may be improved, particularly in patients without progressive extracerebral disease and those with a relatively long prior period of disease control (Nicols et al. 2013; Sheehan et al. 2014; Mahmood et al. 2010).

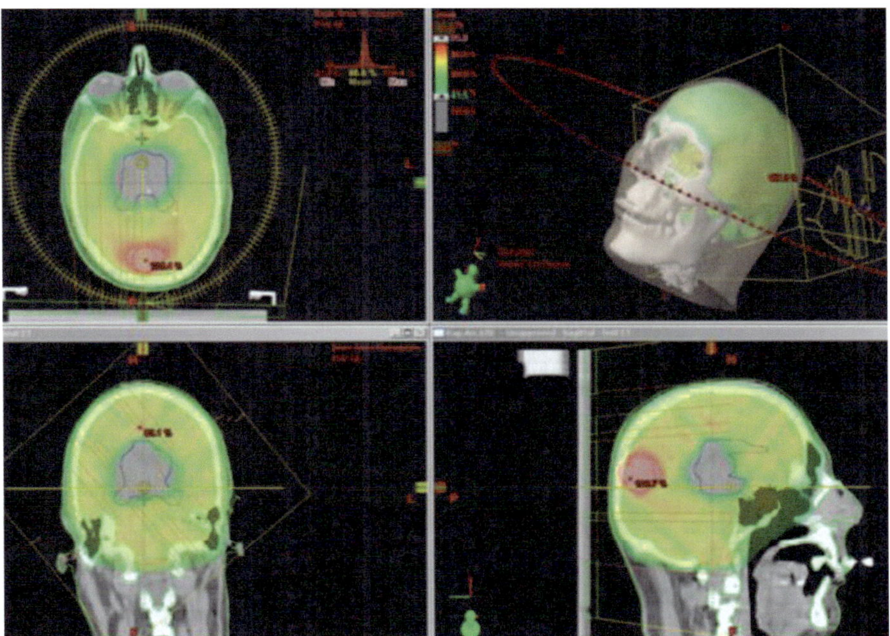

Fig. 6.2 High-precision RT of brain metastases. In a patient with multiple brain metastases, WBRT is combined with dose escalation in selected metastases (*red volumes*). In addition, a concomitant boost that spares the hippocampus is expected to limit potential neurocognitive RT effects (*blue-colored volume*)

In most patients with brain metastases, concomitant corticosteroids should be given. They should be adapted to clinical symptoms, however. They can normally be continuously reduced until the end of the RT series. There is no conclusive evidence that the use of concurrent radiosensitizers may further improve median survival times – with the possible exception of temozolamide. Other radiosensitizers may possibly further improve patients' symptoms or may be indicated for progressive extracerebral disease. In this case, attention should be paid to increased toxicity – particularly for the additional application of specific immunotherapy in malignant melanoma (Nicols et al. 2013).

Whereas focal neurological deficits are rarely related to RT for brain metastases (even in the case of repeated RT), hair loss and a neurocognitive decline are the most frequent late effects of RT. Neurocognitive effects are more often associated with WBRT than with local RT (such as RS), with higher single and total doses and with a relatively long period of disease control. A progressive neurocognitive decline, however, is much more often caused by progressive brain disease; therefore, initial or repeated RT should not be withheld in most patients with brain metastases. Anticonvulsants should be restricted to patients with prior seizures because they may often lead to neurocognitive decline (Nicols et al. 2013; Kocher et al. 2011).

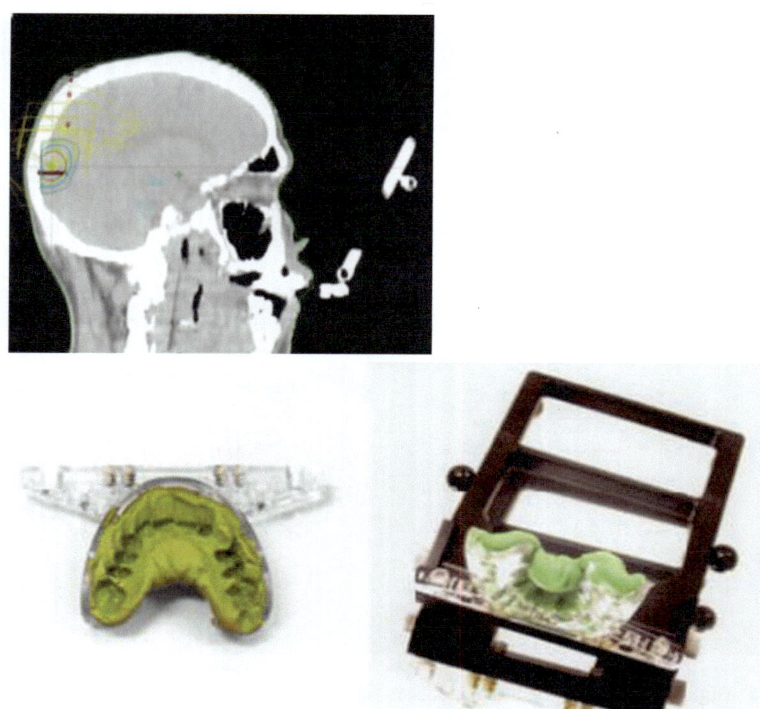

Fig. 6.3 Radiosurgery in brain metastases. Noninvasive stereotactic RT uses individually adapted bite blocks and specific navigation systems

6.3.2 Spinal Cord Compression and Related Symptoms

Tumor-related paraplegia is one of the severest symptoms in patients with metastatic disease. Therefore, early detection and treatment of all signs of myelopathy is of the utmost importance. Besides early surgery, RT is the most important treatment modality. In most patients, new onset back pain is the first symptom of incipient myelopathy. Therefore, myelopathy should be suspected in all patients with new or progressively worsening back pain, particularly in patients with prior high-risk breast or prostate cancer or patients with lung cancer. Even longtime smokers without a cancer history carry a significant risk. In these symptomatic patients, adequate cross-sectional imaging should be promptly initiated. While CT may often be appropriate to diagnose back pain, additional or initial MRI is mandatory for patients with CT-suspected spinal cord compression or for patients with weakness, sensory deficits, or autonomic dysfunction. Since spinal metastases are often multifocal, cross-sectional imaging should cover the entire spine (Nicols et al. 2013).

Optimizing ambulatory outcome is the main goal of treatment in all patients suspected of having spinal cord compression. Rapid diagnostic work-up until initiation of treatment is mandatory, since the rapidity of symptom onset is the most important predictor for the subsequent ambulatory status. Other predictive factors are pre-therapy ambulatory status and radiosensitive histology such as lymphoma, testicular tumors, or small cell carcinoma.

Immediate application of a high dose of dexamethasone, which may be even given before conclusive diagnosis, significantly improves ambulatory outcome. In addition, decompressive and stabilizing surgery within 24 h of diagnosis has been shown to positively affect treatment outcome in all operable patients. Posttreatment ambulatory status, pain, and dexamethasone and morphine doses have been significantly reduced by early surgery, even in diseases with radiosensitive histology. Additional radiotherapy is applied to further improve patient outcome and to reduce the risk of recurrence in the spine. Radiotherapy alone may be adequate only in inoperable patients or in those with multiple spinal lesions or a very poor prognosis (Nicols et al. 2013; Patchell et al. 1990).

Whether with or without prior surgery, a total dose of 30 Gy in ten fractions is the most frequently employed fractionation scheme. Other schedules such as 20 Gy in four fractions or a single dose of 8 Gy have been shown to produce similar results in terms of posttreatment ambulatory rates, motor function improvements, and pain relief. However, in-field recurrences were more frequent in patients receiving short-term (hypofractionated) schedules instead of the standard scheme of 30 Gy in ten fractions. In contrast to recurrent bone metastases, these recurrences may be detrimental because they may lead to durable paraplegia. Therefore, hypofractionation should be restricted to patients with an otherwise progressive disease and very limited life expectation. In patients with a newly diagnosed disease, an otherwise unpredictable clinical course, oligometastatic disease, or good prognostic features, even higher total doses may be appropriate to achieve long-term tumor control. In these patients, again, specific techniques of high-precision RT should be administered (Fig. 6.4) to minimize the risk of radiation-induced myelopathy. This is particularly important since an increasing percentage of patients with spinal cord compression may profit from improved effects of systemic tumor treatment.

In pediatric patients with spinal cord compression, RT is applied less frequently. Depending on the underlying disease, chemotherapy may be able to improve the related symptoms, with or without surgery. Radiotherapy is restricted to specific cases such as Ewing sarcoma or ineffective prior non-RT treatment. Adult patients with intramedullary spinal cord metastases are treated in a similar way as those with spinal cord compression, but surgery carries a high risk of morbidity, with RT being the preferred treatment in most cases. Patients with leptomeningeal carcinomatosis have a very poor prognosis, with systemic and/or intrathecal chemotherapy as the treatment of choice. In these patients, RT is restricted to WBRT for symptomatic brain metastases or to RT of localized symptomatic spinal metastases. Doses and fractionation schedules follow the same principles as in spinal cord compression (Nicols et al. 2013).

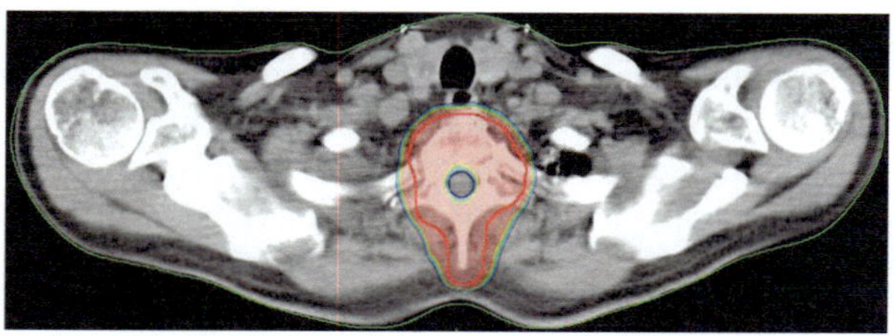

Fig. 6.4 Myelon-sparing for re-irradiation of bone metastases

6.3.3 Symptoms Related to the Involvement of Cranial and Peripheral Nerves

Cranial nerve symptoms may be caused by leptomeningeal carcinomatosis. They are most often not a result of brain, but of skeletal metastases. Using high-resolution CT or skeletal scintigraphy with single-photon emission CT (SPECT), osseous lesions to the base of the skull can be detected in most patients. Most frequently, breast or prostate cancer or multiple myeloma are the underlying diseases, with additional skeletal metastases in the spine or other signs of progressive disease, such as highly elevated serum levels of prostate-specific antigen. In more than 80 % of these cases, RT doses of 30 Gy in ten fractions lead to significant improvement of symptoms Dröge et al. (2014). Surgery, which may be critical in this region, can therefore safely be restricted to the very few patients in whom RT is expected to be ineffective (Patchell et al. 2005).

Plexopathy or infiltrations of peripheral nerves may result in considerable alterations of the corresponding nerves. Often starting with increasing pain, severe plegia can occur if the underlying cause is diagnosed too late. Again, cross-sectional imaging should be initiated with the first signs of potential metastatic involvement. Since these symptoms are often due to soft-tissue recurrences, MRI is the adequate modality to guide subsequent treatment. In these patients, surgery without considerable side effects may be difficult. Depending on the underlying disease and the general status of the patients, adaptive doses between 30 and 50 Gy in 2–5 weeks should be given, possibly accompanied by systemic (radiosensitizing) chemotherapy. Interstitial brachytherapy with or without hyperthermia may be applied as well in selected cases (Fig. 6.5).

6.4 Symptoms Related to Visceral Bleeding or Stenosis

Severe bleeding or stenosis of visceral organs may result in life-threatening situations. Often they are caused by soft-tissue tumors, either from locoregional recurrences or from metastatic disease. Multidisciplinary management is mandatory to save the patients' life and to reduce symptomatic disease. In many cases, such as in ileus due to intestinal stenosis, surgery is the preferred treatment modality. In other circumstances such as ureter stenosis, minimally invasive procedures such as the administration of a double-J catheter may be adequate. In severe bleeding, interventional radiology with the intravasal application of coils may be very helpful. These methods – if applicable – usually lead to an immediate improvement of symptoms.

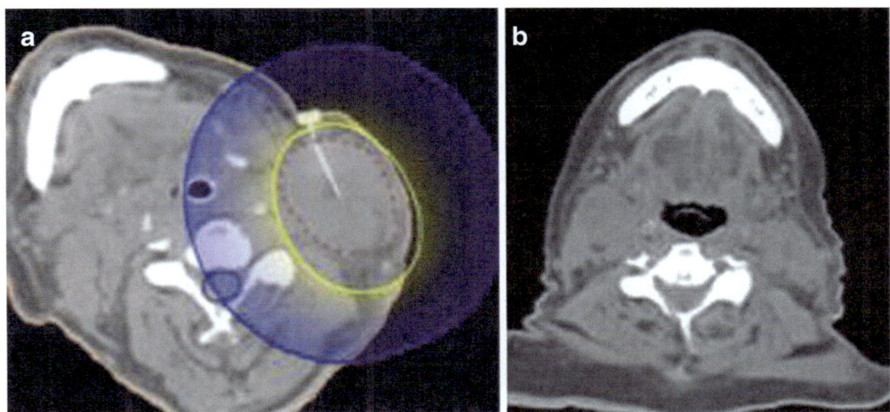

Fig. 6.5 Combined interstitial brachytherapy and hyperthermia is applied using catheters that have been inserted under CT guidance (**a**). Six weeks after this 2-week treatment, painful neck metastases, which had occurred 2 years after initial high-dose radiochemotherapy for advanced oropharyngeal cancer, are in complete remission (**b**)

If surgical or minimally invasive procedures cannot be successfully applied, RT can be an effective alternative. This is particularly true for bleeding symptoms of the upper airways or the uterus, or for stenosis symptoms of the esophagus. Radiotherapy should be initiated early in severe bleeding, with high single doses of between 3 and 10 Gy. Depending on the particular situation, percutaneous RT or BT may be given. Bleeding symptoms are often reduced after a few days of treatment, while stenosis-related symptoms may need several weeks to improve. The overall treatment strategy should be adapted early after initial symptomatic success. In particular, target volumes, planned total doses, treatment techniques, and additional oncological treatment should be reevaluated. This is most important if curative goals should be realistic. This may be the case, for example, in primary diagnosis or isolated local relapse of cervical or rectum cancer, but also in highly radio- and chemosensitive tumors (Rajendran et al. 2013).

6.5   Oligosymptomatic Disease

Occasionally, RT may be medically sensibly applied even in patients with asymptomatic metastatic disease. Data increasingly show that local treatment of a limited number of metastases – either by surgery or by RT – may substantially prolong patients' lives or improve their quality of life. Such treatments may be particularly helpful in patients with a prior long period of stable disease and in those with good performance status. Frequently, the underlying diseases are colorectal or renal cancer or sarcomas. But patients suffering from breast or prostate cancer may also profit from local treatment in selected metastatic circumstances (Rajendran et al. 2013; Timmermann et al. 2014; Salama and Milano 2014; Siddiqui et al. 2014; Milano et al. 2009; Rodrigues et al. 2011; Singh et al. 2004; Quian 2011).

Since medium or long-term success of these approaches is, however, not proven by evidence-based medicine, strict control of treatment toxicity is mandatory. With modern methods of high-precision treatment, RT is increasingly an attractive alternative to invasive open surgery or minimally invasive modalities (Fig. 6.6). Radiotherapy may be applied to a great variety of tumor locations (Table 6.1). It is generally associated with very low toxicity and treatment durations shorter than 2 weeks. In some cases, RT may need inpatient care, but most often, outpatient treatment is possible.

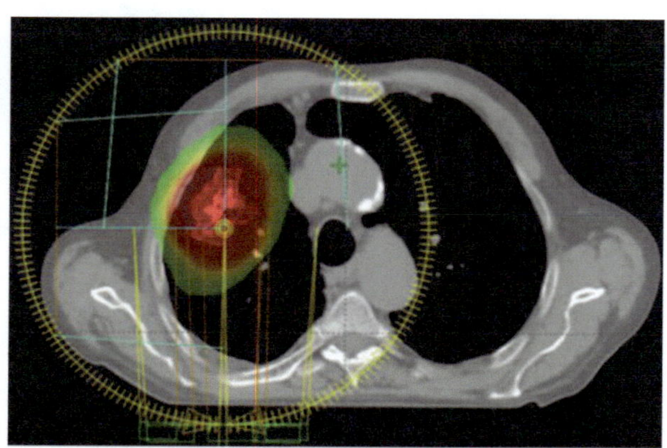

Fig. 6.6 Stereotactic body irradiation for lung metastases

Table 6.1 High-precision radiotherapy for diverse cancer entities

Tumor	IMRT/IGRT	Stereotactic RT	Brachytherapy	Medical therapy
Brain tumor	+	+	+	Temozolomide chemotherapy
Head and neck cancer	+	(+)	+	Chemotherapy/ immunotherapy
Lung cancer	+	+	+	Chemotherapy
Esophageal cancer	+	(+)	+	Chemotherapy
Breast cancer	+	−	IORT	Chemotherapy/ hormonal therapy
Pancreatic/gastric cancer	+	+	−	Chemotherapy/ immunotherapy
Rectal cancer	+	(+)	(+)	Chemotherapy
Cervical cancer	+	(+)	+	Chemotherapy
Prostate cancer	+	(+)	+	Hormonal therapy (tentative)
Sarcoma	+	(+)	+	Chemotherapy (tentative)
Metastases (all locations)	+	+	+	Related to the underlying tumor

6.6   Specific Technical Considerations in Palliative Radiotherapy

Compared with RT with a curative intent, target volumes in palliative RT are commonly restricted to tumor manifestations that are actually responsible for the patients' symptoms. Additional volumes of "adjuvant" RT should only be considered in treatments with curative intent or (rarely) in patients with oligosymptomatic disease. In these patients, additional surgical or medical approaches should be discussed as well (Lutz et al. 2014; Rajendran et al. 2013).

In addition to improving the symptoms, control of acute toxicity is of utmost importance. With the limitation of total doses, often to a maximum of 30 Gy, radiation-induced symptoms are rare and treatment duration can be limited to 2 weeks at most. In selected patients with soft-tissue tumors, oligometastases, or potentially curative diseases, the total RT doses or durations may be increased. In all patients, treatment techniques should minimize doses to normal, particularly to early-reacting organs such as the mucosa of nearby organs. In some patients, dose limitations to the lung, liver, or kidneys may be important Fairchild et al. (2008). In re-irradiation conditions, doses to the myelon or to the nerval plexus deserve special attention. Therefore, detailed three-dimensional RT planning and administration of modern techniques such as image-guided RT (IGRT) and intensity-modulated RT (IMRT) with "VMAT" or "RapidArc" technology considerably help in reaching the treatment goal. Similarly, three-dimensional BT with sophisticated CT planning – with or without additional hyperthermia – may be useful (Sheehan et al. 2014; Timmermann et al. 2014; Quian 2011; Norihisa et al. 2008; Scorsetti et al. 2011; Perez and Emami 1989; Wootton et al. 2011).

References

Andrews DW, Scott CB, Sperduto PW et al (2004) Whole brain radiation therapy with and without stereotactic radiosurgery boost for patients with one to three brain metastases: phase III results of the RTOG 9508 randomized trial. Lancet 363:1665–1672

Aoyama H, Shirato H, Tago MK et al (2006) Stereotactic radiosurgery plus whole-brain radiation therapy vs stereotactic radiosurgery alone for treatment of brain metastases. JAMA 295:2483–2491

Aoyama H, Tago M, Kato N et al (2007) Neurocognitive function in patients with brain metastases who received either who whole brain radiotherapy plus stereotactic radiosurgery of radiosurgery alone. Int J Radiat Oncol Biol Phys 68:1388–1395

Central Nervous System Cancers (2011) NCCN Clinical practice Guidelines in Oncology. V.2.2011. www.nccn.org/professionals/physician_gls/PDF/cns.pdf

Chang EL, Wefel JS, Hess KR et al (2009) Neurocognition in patients with brain metastases treated with radiosurgery or radiosurgery plus whole-brain irradiation: a randomized controlled trial. Lancet Oncol 10(11):1037–1044

Chew C, Craig I, Edwards R et al (2011) Safety and efficacy of percutaneous vertebroplasty in malignancy: a systematic review. Clin Radiol 66:63–72

Dröge LH, Hinsche T, Canis M, Alt-Epping B, Hess CF, Wolff HA (2014) Fractionated external beam radiotherapy of skull base metastases with cranial nerve involvement. Strahlenther Onkol 190(2):199–203. doi:10.1007/s00066-013-0460-9

Fairchild A, Harris K, Barnes E et al (2008) Palliative thoracic radiotherapy for lung cancer: a systematic review. J Clin Oncol 26(24):4001–4011. doi:10.1200/JCO.2007.15.3312

Graham PH, Bucci J, Broen L (2010) Randomized comparison of whole brain radiotherapy, 20 Gy in four daily fractions versus 40 Gy in 20 twice-daily fractions, for brain metastases. Int J Radiat Oncol Biol Phys 77(3):648–654

Hartsell W, Santosh Y (2013) Palliation of bone metastases. In: Perez and Brady's: principles and practice of radiation oncology, 6th edn. Wolters Kluwer/Lippincott Williams & Wilkins, Philadelphia

Kocher M, Soffietti R, Abacioglu U et al (2011) Adjuvant whole-brain radiotherapy versus observation after radiosurgery or surgical resection of one to three cerebral metastases: results of the EORTC 22952–26001 study. J Clin Oncol 29(2):134–141

Konski A, Feigenberg S, Chow E (2005) Palliative radiation therapy. Semin Oncol 32:156–164

Lutz S, Berk I, Chang E et al (2011) Palliative radiotherapy for bone metastases: an ASTRO evidence-based guideline. Int J Radiat Oncol Biol Phys 79:965–976

Lutz ST, Jones J, Chow E (2014) Role of radiation therapy in palliative care of the patient with cancer. J Clin Oncol 32:2913–2919

Mahmood U, Kwok Y, Regine WF et al (2010) Whole-brain irradiation for patients with brain metastases: still the standard of care. Lancet Oncol 11:221–222

Michaelson MD, Smith MR (2005) Bisphosphonates for treatment and prevention of bone metastases. J Clin Oncol 23:8219–8224

Milano MT, Zhang H, Metcalf SK et al (2009) Oligometastatic breast cancer treated with curative-intent stereotactic body radiation therapy. Breast Cancer Res Treat 115:601–608

Nathan SS, Healey JH, Mellano D et al (2005) Survival in patients operated on for pathologic fractures: implication for end-of-life orthopedic care. J Clin Oncol 23:6072–6082

Nicols E, Patchel RA, Regine WF, Kwok Y (2013) Palliation of brain and spinal cord metastases. In: Perez and Brady's: principles and practice of radiation oncology, 6th edn. Wolters Kluwer/Lippincott Williams & Wilkins, Philadelphia

Norihisa Y, Nagata Y, Takayama K et al (2008) Stereotactic body radiotherapy for oligometastatic lung tumors. Int J Radiat Oncol Biol Phys 72:398–403

Patchell RA, Tibbs PA, Walsh JW et al (1990) A randomized trial of surgery in the treatment of single metastases to the brain. N Engl J Med 322:494–500

Patchell RA, Tibbs PA, Regine WF et al (2005) Direct decompressive surgical resection in the treatment of spinal cord compression caused by metastatic cancer: a randomized trial. Lancet 366:643–648

Perez CA, Emami B (1989) Clinical trials with local (external and interstitial) irradiation and hyperthermia. Current and future perspectives. Radiol Clin North Am 27:525–542

Quian J (2011) Interventional therapies of unresectable liver metastases. J Cancer Res Clin Oncol 137:1763–1772

Rajendran RR, Jabbari S, Hartsell WF (2013) Palliation of visceral recurrences and metastases and treatment of oligometastatic disease. In: Perez and Brady's: principles and practice of radiation oncology, 6th edn. Wolters Kluwer/Lippincott Williams & Wilkins, Philadelphia

Rodrigues G, Videtic GMM, Sur R et al (2011) Palliative thoracic radiotherapy in lung cancer: an American Society for Radiation Oncology evidence-based clinical practice guideline. Pract Radiat Oncol 1:60–71

Salama JK, Milano MT (2014) Radical irradiation of extracranial oligometastases. J Clin Oncol 32:2902–2912

Schlampp I, Rieken S, Gabermehl D et al (2014) Stability of spinal bone metastases in breast cancer after radiotherapy. Strahlenther Onkol 190:792–797

Scorsetti M, Bignardi M, Alongi F et al (2011) Stereotactic body radiation therapy for abdominal targets using volumetric intensity modulated arc therapy with Rapid Arc: feasibility and clinical preliminary results. Acta Oncol 50:528–538

Sheehan JP, Yen CP, Loeffler JS (2014) Cranial stereotactic radiosurgery: current status of the initial paradigm shifter. J Clin Oncol 32:2836–2846

Siddiqui F, Liu AK, Watkins-Bruner D et al (2014) Patient-reported outcomes and survivorship in radiation oncology: overcoming the cons. J Clin Oncol 32:2920–2927

Singh D, Yi WS, Brasacchio RA et al (2004) Is there a favorable subset of patients with prostate cancer who develop oligometastases? Int J Radiat Oncol Biol Phys 58:3–10

Siva S, MacManus M, Ball D (2010) Stereotactic radiotherapy for pulmonary oligometastases: a systematic review. J Thorac Oncol 5:1091–1099

Son CH, Jimenez R, Niemierko A et al (2012) Outcomes after whole brain re-irradiation in patients with brain metastases. Int J Radiat Oncol Biol Phys 82(2):e167–e172

Timmermann RD, Herman J, Cho LC (2014) Emergence of stereotactic body radiation therapy and its impact on current and future clinical practice. J Clin Oncol 32:2847–2853

Van der Linden Y, Dijkstra PD, Kroon HM et al (2004) Comparative analysis of risk factors for pathological fracture with femoral metastases. J Bone Joint Surg Br 86:566–573

Wootton JH, Prakash P, Hsu IC, Diederich CJ (2011) Implant strategies for endocervical and interstitial ultrasound hyperthermia adjunct to HDR brachytherapy for the treatment of cervical cancer. Phys Med Biol 56:3967–3984

Wu JS, Wonf R, Johnston M et al (2003) Meta-analysis of dose-fractionation radiotherapy trials for the palliation of painful bone metastases. Int J Radiat Oncol Biol Phys 55:594–605

Symptom Management: The Nursing View

Philip J. Larkin

7

Contents

7.1 Introduction

The role of nursing as fundamental to the delivery of palliative and end-of-life care has an historical basis in the practice of hospice care from the Middle Ages to the early writings of the founder of the modern hospice movement, Cicely Saunders. Notwithstanding her own professional background as a nurse, she identified the impact of nursing on the care of dying people in her earliest writing, and it should not be forgotten that one of her first publications on the topic of pain and symptom management was for the British journal, Nursing Times, in 1959 (Saunders and Clark 2006). Contemporary nursing practice has developed a professional

P.J. Larkin, PhD, MSc
School of Nursing, Midwifery and Health Systems, UCD Health Sciences Centre,
University College Dublin, Dublin, Ireland

Our Lady's Hospice and Care Services, Harold's Cross, Dublin, Ireland
e-mail: philip.larkin@ucd.ie

© Springer-Verlag Berlin Heidelberg 2015
B. Alt-Epping, F. Nauck (eds.), *Palliative Care in Oncology*,
DOI 10.1007/978-3-662-46202-7_7

leadership with respect to palliative care and symptom management, notably in the United Kingdom and the United States, where advanced clinical roles of clinical nurse specialist and advanced nurse practitioner have contributed to new and innovative pathways of care for cancer patients with a defined symptom burden. In this chapter, an understanding of the eclectic role of palliative care nursing is given, and the unique nursing contribution to the management of symptoms for the oncology patient with palliative care needs is discussed. In particular, palliative nursing practice in the management of three symptoms that are known to impact significantly on the cancer patients' life quality is addressed: the assessment and treatment of opioid-induced constipation, management of fungating malignant wounds and care of the patient with 'death rattle' at the end of life. These symptoms, though not exhaustive, represent the potential of the nursing contribution to the care of cancer patients with advanced and life-limiting illness. This chapter begins with a brief exploration of the philosophy and practice of palliative care nursing.

7.2 Understanding the Components of Palliative Care Nursing

One of the challenges in defining palliative care nursing is that, ostensibly, all nurses provide care for people with life-limiting conditions and in end-of-life scenarios. The ability to care compassionately and competently (both terms that need definition) is a prerequisite for professional nursing discipline, irrespective of the area of practice.

One model that has provided both an historical and contemporary framework for palliative nursing practice is that of Davies and Oberle (1990). As a seminal piece of work, this model, derived from a grounded theory study with a US expert community nurse, served as a template for both practice and education of nurses. Identifying support as the core component of practice, it defined (and later refined) a set of interrelated attributes that define the supportive role of the nurse (Oberle and Davies 1992; Pavlish and Ceronsky 2009). Table 7.1 below presents these attributes and the philosophical and practice-based principles that they underpin.

Table 7.1 Dimensions of the supportive role of the nurse in palliative care

Attribute	Focus on palliative care nursing practice
Valuing	Reflects concepts of humanity and worth in the individual
Connecting	Considers the deepening relationship between nurse and patient as illness progresses
Empowering	Focused on independence and enabling
Doing for	Regarding the physical aspects of caregiving derived from knowledge and practice
Finding meaning	Enabling the patient to make sense of the end of life through honesty and sensitivity
Preserving one's own integrity	The balance of the professional nurse and the nurse as a person, which underpins the ideals of respect and authenticity

Adapted from Davies and Oberle (1990)

Although the model clearly influenced the way in which palliative care nursing practice and education developed internationally (Walker et al. 2000; Widger et al. 2009; Becker 2010; Baldwin 2011), it was developed at a time when palliative care was largely equated with the care of the dying, specifically in relation to cancer, and so does not reflect current definitions, which frame the breadth of application for palliative care (World Health Organisation 2002). Furthermore, the model predates the development of expert nursing practice and roles such as nurse practitioner and advanced practitioner, which have become much more evident in palliative care. A more recent reading of Davies and Oberle's original work and a revision of the model to incorporate this from a British perspective have been offered by Newton and McVicar (2013). The revised model reflects the expansion of palliative care services beyond hospice care, such as hospital-based teams, the range of higher education and practice opportunities available to nurses (e.g. advanced practice and nurse consultancy) and the complexity of managing complex and challenging symptomology alongside the holistic application of principles of care and comfort (Clarke et al. 2002; Seymour et al. 2002; Skilbeck and Payne 2003; NICE 2004; Becker 2009).

The revised model, based on data derived from a predominantly qualitative mixed-method design (Newton and McVicar 2013), confirmed that the attributes of the original model were still current, but it identified two additional domains of *displaying expertise* and *influencing other professionals* as components of contemporary practice. Within *displaying expertise*, the ability to manage complexity in clinical decision-making and communication is explored. *Influencing other professionals* reflects the roles of negotiation, education, expert guidance and an inherent sense that palliative care contributes to the development of care across the health spectrum. Practical application of expert practice, such as assessment, care planning and evaluation, was evident within the original attributes and so included in the attribute descriptors listed in Table 7.1.

It is noted that the expansion of specialist palliative care nursing practice is, to some extent, an Anglo-Saxon model. In many European countries, the professional status of nursing is variable, and there has been limited opportunity for expansion of practice and higher education. One approach adopted by the European Association for Palliative Care (EAPC) led to a set of guidelines for practice and education based on a stepwise approach from generalist to specialist (De Vlieger et al. 2004). No less than Newton and McVicar's (2013) work, this framework is now 10 years old and a revision is timely. What has become evident in recent times is the focus towards competency, and again, European initiatives of the EAPC have addressed this (Gamondi et al. 2012a, b).

7.3 New Challenges for Palliative Care Nursing: Expert Practice and Clinical Competency

The complexity of palliative care symptom management has created opportunity for nurses working in this field to enhance clinical knowledge and skills in order to advance and expand their practice. Although roles may differ, the clinical nurse specialist, advanced nurse practitioner and, in some countries, nurse consultant may undertake a range of activities including history taking, physical examination, ordering and interpreting diagnostic tests and prescription of medication. There is increasing evidence of these roles in palliative care and oncology nursing and the impact on the outcome for the patient (Dyer et al. 2012; O'Connor and Peters 2009; Skalla 2006). Advanced practice usually requires the candidate to have at least master's level education and a professionally accredited certification relative to health assessment. The emphasis on an interdisciplinary team as the medium for palliative care planning is essential to the delivery of advanced nursing practice, particularly where palliative care provides a consultancy model to the patient's responsible clinical team and is not the sole provider of care. Historically, many nurses in palliative care came from an oncology background, providing a common ground for understanding the journey of the cancer patient through curative, supportive and eventually palliative treatment. Increasingly, the expansion of palliative care beyond cancer has resulted in nurses coming with diverse expert backgrounds (such as Intensive Care Nursing, Public Health Nursing), which, though valuable, may require further skills update in relation to current oncology nursing practice.

Competency is complex to define, reflecting both the ability to perform a task and the skills and attributes necessary to do that. Gamondi et al. (2012a, b) defined four key questions to address this (see Box 7.1):

> **Box 7.1. Key Questions on Competency for Palliative Care**
> What is the current position of palliative care within the national health system?
> What is the capacity of the individual to achieve competency?
> What resources are available to enable the individual to learn and practice skills?
> Are baseline standards available against which competency can be determined?

Clearly, additional to this is the status of nursing. Stoof et al. (2002) identified the need for critical thinking, problem-solving and outcome assessment skills, in addition to judgement and wisdom in devising the intervention and evaluation of care. All of these are now global prerequisites of nurses' professional training. In some countries where expert roles are now integral to practice, higher level academic education has enabled nurses to expand their role to include nurse-based clinics and nurse prescribing (Andrews and Morgan 2012; Owens and Cleaves 2012). Based on this and international variation in the service delivery of palliative care, the definition offered by Parry (1996) may fit the diversity of nursing provision within palliative care (see Box 7.2).

> **Box 7.2. Definition of a Competency**
> A competency is: a cluster of related knowledge, skills and attitudes that affects a major part of one's job (a role or responsibility), that correlates with performance on the job, that can be measured against well-accepted standards, and that can be improved via training and development. (Parry 1996)

The challenge in determining appropriate competencies for palliative care nursing lies in the fact that core skills and attributes for practice are often difficult to measure, standardise and teach. As an example, there would be an expectation that nurses are compassionate in the way they deliver palliative care, but this is hard to quantify in terms of improved patient outcomes. Similarly, there are many examples of the importance of relationship in palliative and end-of-life care literature, particularly from the perspective of the nurse (Abma 2005; Brännstörm et al. 2005). However, the quality of relationship can be equally difficult to determine, although it has been explored (Walshe and Luke 2010). Defining the contribution of nursing to symptom management arises from the holistic and integrative concepts of physical, psychological, social and spiritual care demonstrated in Cicely Saunders' 'Total Pain' approach. Nursing practice involves attention to multiple perspectives at the same time and, as will be demonstrated through a description of common clinical symptoms, often requires the combined efforts of a team of practitioners with a common goal: the alleviation of symptom burden. The three symptoms chosen (constipation, malignant fungating wounds and the 'death rattle') reflect not only those that are commonly managed in general nursing practice, but those for which palliative care nursing has a particular role, especially in the oncology setting. Key to the success of quality symptom management for nurses is their close proximity to the patient in the clinical area over time and therefore the ability to monitor progress, assess effectiveness of an intervention and effect change swiftly where necessary. Hence, an important role for the palliative care nurse working from an advanced consultancy role is their ability to impart the skills of assessment to their oncology nurse colleagues and to act as both guide and mentor in that respect.

7.4 Nursing Contribution to the Palliative Care Management of Constipation

Constipation is a consistent health problem. Bowel management is often a core skill of the professional nurse, and the responsibility of nurses in this regard is well reported (Landers et al. 2012; Woolery et al. 2008). Constipation is a common problem for palliative care patients with advanced cancer, and much of the evidence for its assessment and management derives from the oncology setting (Connolly and Larkin 2012). The subjective nature of the symptom makes it difficult to define, although criteria for definition are available (Sykes 2010; Drossman and moderator 2006). Although causes can be varied and associated with environmental and social factors such as privacy, diet and exercise, in the cancer patient with advanced disease, these may be a direct result of their tumour, surgical intervention as a necessary part of treatment, secondary effects of disease (such as hypercalcaemia) or medication. In the latter category, the physiological impact of opioids on the gut is often the most significant factor for constipation in the palliative care patient (Lentz and McMillan 2010). Attention to the factors noted above is rarely sufficient for managing constipation in a palliative context, and its management will require careful attention to medication management and clinical intervention to alleviate the symptom.

Assessment is key to management, and the nurse should consider the pre-illness bowel pattern as well as the current presentation. A number of validated tools have been developed to assist in the assessment process and should be used where possible (Clark et al. 2010). One example of such is the Victoria Bowel Performance Scale (Hawley and Baldwin 2012; Hawley et al. 2011). The assessment, which may involve physical examination and possibly digital rectal examination (termed DRE), should consider issues of posture, gait, tenderness, distension, pain, faecal loading and impaction. Concurrent other symptoms such as nausea and vomiting, which may indicate high colonic impaction or possibly malignant intestinal obstruction (MIO), should be noted. A detailed description of faeces is also indicated in order to determine consistency, size, smell, the presence of fresh or occult blood, ease of passage and evidence of 'overflow' (watery stool, which may indicate a higher colonic impaction) and is important in determining the most appropriate clinical intervention (Larkin et al. 2008). Radiological examination may be a helpful discriminator in determining the choice and targeting of treatment options (Moylan et al. 2010).

The principal application of treatment involves a prophylactic and systematic three-line approach commencing with oral laxatives and a stool softener and stimulant in combination. The effective use of senna as a particular choice in the care of children with cancer has been recently reported (Feudtner et al. 2013). A second-line approach may include the addition of enemata or suppositories, and a more recent intervention that has obtained increasing interest in palliative care is the use of a peripherally specific opioid antagonist such as methylnaltrexone (Larkin et al. 2008; Clemens and Klaschik 2010; Jones et al. 2011). As this acts on the μ-opioid receptor in the gut but not in the CNS, it can offer a third-level intervention where conventional treatments are unsuccessful.

For the patient with palliative care needs, certain caveats apply in the management of constipation. Bulking agents such as bran added to diet are unpalatable and may have an opposite effect to that desired, leading to obstruction and hence, are best avoided in palliative care patients (Connolly and Larkin 2012). The balance of laxative therapy against progressive disease means that the ability to take increasing doses of liquids can be challenging. The use of rectal interventions needs to be managed with caution, particularly where there is a risk of disease infiltration to the bowel wall or rectum. Enema may cause abdominal and rectal cramping and should be used cautiously. However, as death approaches and goals of management shift, restlessness may indicate the necessity for a rectal intervention to address faecal loading (Connolly and Larkin 2012). However, the management of the symptom in a palliative context is approached, and the focus should be on a shared management strategy between the patient, carer and professional to ensure an optimal outcome (Andrews and Morgan 2013).

7.5 The Nursing Contribution to the Management of Malignant Wounds

The significance of effective wound management as a critical aspect of palliative care is acknowledged and notably its ability to act as a prognostic factor in advanced disease (Maida 2013). The ability to address the consequences of a malignant wound provides insight into the holistic 'total pain' approach of palliative nursing care. In addition to the physical aspects of management, such as pain or the risk of bleeding, the challenge of malodour and exudate also reflects the need to plan for the psychological consequences that this distressing symptom can produce (Grocott et al. 2013; Probst et al. 2013; Alexander 2009a, 2009b, 2009c). As an area with a growing body of research evidence, the range of symptoms that can be exacerbated by a malignant or fungating wound is notable. Depression, shame, loss of confidence, poor sleep pattern, anorexia and nausea are all indicated in the literature (Gibson and Green 2013; Probst et al. 2012, 2013; Lo et al. 2012). Therefore, a multidisciplinary approach including the family in all aspects of individualised planning is important. Such planning includes an understanding that the wound may not be able to heal and that clinical decisions in terms of treatment choices that may apply to wounds in other contexts may well not apply here.

There is an increasing body of evidence in the palliative assessment and management of wounds. One, the Toronto Symptom Assessment System for Wounds, modelled on the Edmonton Symptom Assessment Scale (ESAS), has proven effective in understanding the global impact of pain and distress associated with wounds and as a tool to assist palliation (Maida 2013; Maida et al. 2009).

Studies reported in nursing and allied literature draw particular reference to the burden to both patient and carer of living with a malignant fungating wound. Probst et al. (2012) undertook a phenomenological study with seven carers to understand the experience of living with a cancer patient who has a malignant wound. The presence of a wound became a visible reminder of the cancer diagnosis, and carers were often left to manage the consequences of the wound (discharge, odour) themselves. The offensive nature of the wound often led to isolation of both patient and carer, particularly where healing was challenging. This impact on quality of life was further explored by Lo et al. (2012) in a descriptive cross-sectional multi-centre study of cancer and palliative care patients in Taiwan. Using the Taiwanese version of the McGill Quality of Life questionnaire, statistically significant correlations were found between life quality and pain, dressing comfort, dressing change, bleeding and malodour. Gibson and Green (2013) noted how the devastation of a malignant wound can be alleviated by effective nursing interventions that incorporate sensitive communication as well as therapeutic skills. Furthermore, the palliative management of malignant wounds is an excellent example of the interface between causative therapy and palliative care and how an appropriate palliative approach can underpin the healing process (Maida 2013; Alvarez et al. 2007). Attention to the principles of wound healing, such as correcting underlying pathology and supportive nutrition, can be supplemented by using the lens of a palliative care approach, which would advocate a balanced approach to the management of the wound. In this, the degree of clinical intervention needs to be considered in the context of declining health status, the ability to manage a treatment regimen and the need to ensure comfort where the complete healing of the wound may not be possible.

For palliative care nurses, attention to issues of pain, risk of bleeding and managing malodour and exudate would be a generic part of practice. Wound pain may be experienced as both nociceptive and neuropathic (Ngugi 2007), enhanced through infection, swelling or indeed poor technique in dressing management (Alexander 2009a). The use of topical analgesia has something of a limited evidence base, particularly in the context of malignant wounds (Alexander 2009c). However, it remains a part of practice. The use of topical opioids at 0.1 %w/w (i.e. 1 mg opioid to 1 g of the carrier gel weight for weight) has been recommended (Naylor 2005), and the limited bioavailability in topical form does not appear to impact significantly on the total opioid requirement (Ribiero et al. 2004). Recognising the total pain experience, one case study demonstrated a decrease in pain scores when malodour was successfully treated (Bale et al. 2005), and so multiple factors may contribute to the experience and resolution of pain. Since the evidence for topical analgesic approaches is weak, the need to manage systemic analgesia to address wound pain as part of the overall symptomatology is essential. The use of complementary therapies may be of benefit, particularly the use of aromatherapy (Alvarez et al. 2007). The impact of pruritus, though not strictly pain but a high indicator of discomfort, is also noted in the literature as a significant feature that needs to be managed in the treatment of malignant wounds. Such options include oral medication, systemic corticosteroids, histamine receptor blockers and ultraviolet therapy (Adderley and Smith 2007; Holme et al. 2001).

The friability of tissue associated with tumour infiltration, coagulopathy and the development of abnormal vasculature can lead to bleeding and resistant haemostasis (Alexander 2009a). Bleeding may be minor and localised, moderate or heavy, indicative of a larger and perhaps catastrophic bleed, which needs palliative care emergency management.

Localised bleeding may occur when a dressing has adhered to a wound and needs to be changed. The need for careful and gentle intervention to loosen the dressing using warmed saline to avoid further tissue trauma is advocated (McMurray 2003). It is argued that sufficient pressure is needed to cleanse the wound and reduce trauma (McDonald and Lesage 2006), although this needs to be set against the palliative nature of the wound and the need for a gentle intervention.

Where bleeding is minimal, the judicious use of ice, local pressure or haemostatic alginate may be helpful. In moderate cases of bleeding, again alginates may be used but should be managed cautiously where there is any risk that alginate fibres may irritate friable tissues. Although the evidence is clearly dated and points to the need for further research, the use of surgical sponge, a natural fluid absorber that can be secured with a secondary dressing, has been identified as an option for practice (Grocott 1998). In the event of heavy bleeding, it may be possible to pre-empt this and prevent excessive blood loss. The use of adrenaline-soaked swabs has been reported but needs to be used with caution since it can cause ischaemia and necrosis (Alexander 2009c).

The risk of catastrophic bleeding is an excellent example of the palliative nursing role in the care and support of both patient and family when there is an eminent risk of death. Anticipation is the key to successful management. All patients and families need a clear strategy for dealing with both the event and consequences of this event. Dark towels are commonly used to manage blood loss and minimise its presence. Decisions need to be made about actions should a bleed occur (e.g. whether a transfer to the hospital is preferred). Depending on local practice, an 'emergency pack' usually containing a prescribed dose of analgesic and sedative may be available in the home. The palliative care nurse may have a range of roles here, from advocacy in relation to clinical decisions to managing the traumatic event and its aftermath.

The problem of exudate and odour highlights the psychological and social impact of a fungating wound for the person living with it. The destruction of flesh and consequent smell in terms of the patient's isolation, stigma and reaction from others, especially when the wound is visible and cannot be covered can be devastating at a critical time in the patient's life. Malodour is often the most distressing of symptoms for both patient and family, and nurses have a specific responsibility to address this problem. The cause of malodour may be related to aerobic and/or anaerobic bacteria accumulation and the smell of necrotic flesh, blood or soiled dressings, or it may arise where a fistula is formed, notably in the perineal or genital area (Nazarko 2006).

Whereas the evidence for topical analgesia is poor, the use of topical applications and metronidazole (nitroimidazole) in particular would seem to be the treatment of choice (Alexander 2009b). Although the early evidence for its use has been demonstrated through randomised studies (Bower et al. 1992; Hampson 1996), the small sample sizes and inadequate power of these studies mean that significant conclusions cannot be reached. This said, the use of metronidazole is common practice and usually effective. There are some challenges in terms of possible systemic side effects, particularly affecting the gastrointestinal tract, when used in high doses over a prolonged period. However, it seems that this would not be a problem in the normally affective dose range used in malodour treatment. There is a need for further research in the area to support what is largely practice-based and anecdotal evidence.

Exudate is often an important cause of malodour, as well as being potentially detrimental to the wound structure itself. A significant challenge is that dressings are usually designed to work in a moist healing environment with cure as the ultimate outcome. A fungating wound may be excessively moist and cure unlikely, with comfort management as the better option. The protection of skin is an important consideration. The size of commercial dressings may not conform appropriately to the wound, provide adequate layers for removal of exudate or be removed easily (Alexander 2009b).

In terms of dressing choice, there is a substantive body of literature in the field and an equal amount of debate as to the most appropriate choice. Generally, choice is dependent on wound size, risk of bleeding and degree of malodour and exudate. However, it should be noted that little of the research evidence has focused on malignant wounds. For malodour, there is increased interest in dressings impregnated with silver, which inhibit bacterial growth (Ovington 2004). The use of iodine has received a very mixed review, as has the use of charcoal, although combined charcoal-silver dressings have benefits in managing both odour and exudate (Lee et al. 2006). Debridement is rarely used in a malignant wound due to its friability and the evident distress to the patient. Similarly, decisions about the use of topical antiseptics should be made based on the overall health status of the patient and thorough wound assessment. In practice, cleansing with normal saline is often effective and outweighs the risk of using specific cleansing products with limited evidence base. There are also a number of alternative approaches using essential oils or products such as honey, sugar paste and yoghurt (Alexander 2009b; Mercier and Knevitt 2005). From a palliative nursing perspective, the appropriate decision is always one that causes least impact on the quality of life of the patient. A complex dressing regimen that restricts patients' activities may be unfavourable. Dressings can be expensive and so may not be cost-effective or add to the patient burden. The management of the wound requires innovation and adaptability. For example, products used in the management of ostomy may be helpful in successful dressing adherence. However, the nurse manages wound care, and the principle for best practice should include an approach that promotes comfort, provides a dressing that is aesthetically pleasing, does not require excessive intervention to achieve treatment goals and is cognisant of minimising pain and discomfort during dressing procedures.

7.6 The Nursing Contribution to the Management of the 'Death Rattle'

Noisy breathing, termed 'death rattle', is used to describe the oscillation of secretions in the upper airways of patients in the terminal stages of life. Although its exact cause remains unproven, it is usually associated with dying patients who are unable to expectorate. 'Death rattle' is often seen as a predominant clinical sign to indicate to both clinicians and families that the patient's life is ending (Wildiers et al. 2009). It is reported in between 25 and 90 % of patients and ranks highly alongside pain and agitation as prominent symptoms to manage in the terminal stages of life. Its treatment is a balance between nursing measures to assert comfort, including repositioning, and the use of medication to inhibit secretions (Wee and Hillier 2012). It is considered to be a traumatic event and one frequently remembered by clinical staff and families long after the patient's death (Wee et al. 2006a, 2008). However, it has also been shown that the perception of distress for relatives may be less than assumed, and for some, 'death rattle' is a helpful indicator of progression and timeframe (Wee et al. 2006a, b).

The management of the symptom usually requires a combination of anticholinergic medication, administered by either subcutaneous injection or infusion, repositioning of the patient to allow drainage of secretions and concomitant oral care management and the judicious use of oral catheter nasopharyngeal suctioning. The latter is increasingly unfavourable in practice on the grounds that it does not necessarily alleviate the symptom, may cause distress to the patient and needs particular skills in terms of application and assessment of need.

The key medications of choice in current practice are either hyoscine hydrobromide or hyoscine butylbromide with the use of glycopyrronium as a relatively recent addition. Atropine has also been reported but would seem to be less evident in practice. Decisions on the choice of medication may be dictated by cost and availability as the evidence would not indicate the clinical benefit of one over the other. However, there is also an increasing debate about the benefit and use of anticholinergic medication and presence in end-of-life care pathways and strategies given its limited efficacy (Hirsch et al. 2012).

An updated Cochrane review by Wee and Hillier (2012) has reviewed current evidence about treatment choices and management. Randomised controlled trials (RCTs), controlled before and after studies, and interrupted time-series studies were included. However, only four studies were identified that met the criteria with insufficient data for analysis. Studies compared various medication choices in a variety of combinations (atropine, hyoscine hydrobromide, hyoscine butylbromide and glycopyrronium), and with the exception of one non-placebo-controlled trial using glycopyrronium, which seemed to reduce the sound of noisy breathing, there was no evidence to support the use of any specific medication over placebo. The authors considered these conclusions to be consistent with those of the original 2008 review.

One more recent small-scale study in a palliative care population has suggested that 'death rattle' is not associated with respiratory distress. In a prospective, two-group observation study ('death rattle' vs. no 'death rattle'), no evidence was found that indicated that anticholinergic medication provided any significant benefit, and so this study questioned the validity of the use of such medication at the end of life (Campbell and Yarandhi 2013). The Wildiers et al. (2009) study reported earlier and cited in the 2012 Wee and Hilliers' Cochrane review would have reached similar conclusions. It is worth noting that this study, a prospective randomised multi-centred trial, was undertaken within a cancer population. As may be suspected, those with lung cancer had the least favourable response to medication. Furthermore, this paper highlighted the challenge in parameters for outcome measures of effectiveness across studies. Since different indicators of a positive outcome varied considerably, cross-comparison of findings is difficult.

From a palliative nursing perspective, a number of factors determine the care response. Firstly, the unconscious status of the patient at the time of the 'death rattle' needs an increased vigilance in terms of changing goals of care in the last days of life, advising and guiding the family as respiratory and circulatory changes occur and, in remembering the 'personhood' of the patient, working respectfully to include the patient in conversations and decisions made. This is based on the often-cited idea that the patient's hearing remains patent even if unconscious. Whether this is actually the case is not relevant to the palliative care nursing intervention, which should be based on meticulous attention to detail in all things, including the sensitivity of communication. A recent Japanese nursing study (Shimizu et al. 2013) reported on a nationwide cross-sectional survey of bereaved caregivers regarding the experience of being present to 'death rattle' and views on the care strategy used. The findings indicated that care needed to be planned to facilitate greater repositioning of the patient in a timely fashion, constant communication with the family about decisions (particularly where suctioning was ordered and anticholinergic medication regimens altered) and prospective guidance on the meaning and expectation of 'death rattle' for the finality of death.

With these studies in mind, it is clear that nurses present to patients and families in the dying phase of life have specific responsibilities in the care and management of potentially distressing symptoms such as 'death rattle'. The key is communication between clinical team and family, with the nurse acting as a conduit between parties to facilitate clarity around decision-making and rationale for treatment choices, interventions or non-intervention as appropriate. Reflecting the earlier discussion on competency, the palliative care nurse should be able to demonstrate core skills in communication, and the ability to successfully manage the last days of life in an holistic family-orientated way would be an indicator of expert practice.

Conclusion

This chapter has considered only three symptoms demonstrating the unique nursing contribution to palliative care and has been set within the oncology context in relation to the supportive evidence. The choice was made to demonstrate the range of skills and application to practice needed by a palliative care nurse, including direct care, clinical assessment, judgement and decision-making and consultancy. Palliative care nursing is developing its own body of research and evidence to support its practice but remains in its infancy in terms of professional recognition and development in many countries. Perhaps the most significant contribution that palliative care nursing brings to the team is their proximity to patients and families through a significant transition and to support other colleagues for whom palliative care nursing is not the totality of their work to adapt their care to this unique situation. Clinical expertise in palliative care nursing is underpinned by not just knowledge, skills and attitudes but also by clinical wisdom to know what is the right thing to do in a particular situation. This can be summarised as the ability to intervene wisely, manage appropriately and withdraw sensitively when death occurs and bereavement support becomes the focus of care.

References

Abma TA (2005) Struggling with the fragility of life: a relational-narrative approach to ethics in palliative nursing. Nurs Ethics 12(4):337–348

Adderley U, Smith R (2007) Topical agents and dressings for fungating wounds. Cochrane Database Syst Rev (2):CD003948

Alexander S (2009a) Malignant fungating wounds: key symptoms and psychosocial issues. J Wound Care 18(8):325–329

Alexander S (2009b) Malignant fungating wounds: managing malodour and exudate. J Wound Care 18(9):374–382

Alexander S (2009c) Malignant fungating wounds: managing pain, bleeding and psychosocial issues. J Wound Care 18(10):418–425

Alvarez O, Kalinski C, Nusbaum J et al (2007) Incorporating wound healing strategies to improve palliation in patients with chronic wounds. J Palliat Med 10(5):1161–1189

Andrews A, Morgan G (2012) Constipation management in palliative care: treatments and the potential of Independent Nurse Prescribing. Int J Palliat Nurs 18(1):17–22

Andrews A, Morgan G (2013) Constipation in palliative care: treatment options and consideration for individual patient management. Int J Palliat Nurs 19(6):268–273

Baldwin MA (2011) Attributes of palliative caring. In: Baldwin MA, Woodhouse J (eds) Key concepts in palliative care. Sage Publications Ltd, London, pp 7–11

Bale S, Tebble N, Price P (2005) A topical metronidazole gel used to treat malodorous wounds. Br J Nurs 13(11):S4–S11

Becker R (2009) Palliative care 2: exploring the skills that nurses need to deliver high quality care. Nurs Times 105:18–20

Becker R (2010) Palliative nursing skills: what are they? In Fundamental aspects of palliative care nursing: an evidence based handbook for student nurses, 2nd edn. Quay Books, London, pp 17–28

Brännstörm M, Brulin C, Norberg A, Barnoy K, Stronaberg G (2005) Being a palliative care nurse for persons with severe congestive heart failure in advanced homecare. Eur J Cardiovasc Nurs 4(4):314–323

Bower M, Stein R, Evans TR et al (1992) A double-blind study of the efficacy of metronidazole gel in the treatment of malodourous fungating tumours. Eur J Cancer, 28A, 4(5):888–889

Campbell ML, Yarandhi HN (2013) Death rattle is not associated with patient respiratory distress: is pharmacologic treatment indicated? J Palliat Med 16(10):1255–1259

Clark K, Urban K, Currow DC (2010) Current approaches to diagnosing and managing constipation in advanced cancer and palliative care. Palliat Med 13(4):473–476

Clarke D, Seymour J, Douglas H, Bath P, Beech N, Corner J, Halliday D, Hughes P, Haviland J, Normand C, Marples R, Skilbeck J, Webb T (2002) Clinical nurse specialists in palliative care (2): explaining diversity in the organization and costs of Macmillan nursing service. Palliat Med 16:375–385

Clemens KE, Klaschik E (2010) Managing opioid-induced constipation in advanced illness. Focus on methylnaltrexone bromide. Ther Clin Risk Manage 3(6):77–82

Connolly M, Larkin P (2012) Managing constipation: a focus on care and treatment in the palliative setting. Br J Community Nurs 17(2):60–67

Davies B, Oberle K (1990) Dimensions of the supportive role of the nurse in palliative care. Oncol Nurs Forum 17:87–93

De Vlieger M, Gorchs N, Larkin P, Porchet F (2004) Palliative nurse education; towards a common language. Palliat Med 18(5):401–403

Drossman DA, moderator (2006) AGA Clinical Symposium – Rome III: new criteria for the functional GI disorders. Program and abstracts of Digestive Disease Week, Los Angeles, 20–25 May 2006

Dyer S, Lesperance M, Sharon R, Sloan J, Colon-Etero G (2012) A nurse practitioner directed intervention improves quality of life of patients with metastatic cancer. Results of a randomized pilot study. J Palliat Med 15(8):890–895

Feudtner C, Freedman J, Kang T, Womer JW, Dingwei D, Faerber J (2013) Comparative effectiveness of senna to prevent problematic constipation in pediatric oncology patients receiving opioids: a multicenter study of clinically detailed administrative data. J Pain Symptom Manage. http://dx.doi.org/10.1016/j.jpainsymman.2013.09.009

Gamondi C, Larkin P, Payne S (2012a) Core competencies in palliative care: an EAPC White Paper on palliative care education: part 1. Eur J Palliat Care 20(2):86–91

Gamondi C, Larkin P, Payne S (2012b) Core competencies in palliative care: an EAPC White Paper on palliative care education: part 2. Eur J Palliat Care 20(3):140–145

Gibson S, Green J (2013) Review of patient's experiences of fungating wound and associated quality of life. J Wound Care 22(5):265–266

Grocott P (1998) Controlling bleeding in fragile fungating tumours. J Wound Care 7(7):342

Grocott P, Gethin G, Probst S (2013) Malignant wound management in advanced illness: new insights. Curr Opin Support Palliat Care 7(1):101–105

Hampson JP (1996) The use of metronidazole in the treatment of malodorous wounds. Wound Care 5(9):421–426

Hawley PH, Baldwin C (2012) Long-term 'real-life' usefulness of the Victoria Bowel Performance Scale. J Pain Symptom Manage 44(3):e2–e3

Hawley P, Bowich D, Kirk C (2011) Implementation of the Victoria Bowel Performance Scale. J Pain Symptom Manage 42(6):946–953

Hirsch CA, Mariott JF, Faul CM (2012) Influences on the decision to prescribe or administer anticholinergic drugs to treat death rattle: a focus group study. Palliat Med 23(8):732–738

Holme SA, Pease NJ, Mills CM (2001) Crotamiton and narrow-band UVB phototherapy: novel approaches to alleviate pruritus of breast carcinoma skin infiltration. J Pain Symptom Manage 23(4):803–805

Jones CB, Goodman ML, Drake R, Tookman A (2011) Laxatives or methylnaltrexone for management of constipation in palliative care patients (review). Cochrane Database Syst Rev (1):CD003448

Landers M, McCarthy G, Savage E (2012) Bowel symptom experiences and management following sphincter saving surgery for rectal cancer: a qualitative perspective. Eur J Oncol Nurs 16:293–300

Larkin PJ, Sykes NP, Centeno C et al (2008) The management of constipation in palliative care: clinical practice recommendations. Palliat Med 22(7):796–807

Lee G, Anand SC, Rajendran S, Walker I (2006) Overview of current practice and future trends in the evaluation of dressings for malodorous wounds. J Wound Care 15(8):344–346

Lentz J, McMillan SC (2010) The impact of opioid-induced constipation on patients near the end of life. J Hosp Palliat Nurs 12(1):29–38

Lo SF, Hayter M, Hu WY, Tai CY, Hsu MY, Li YF (2012) Symptom burden and quality of life in patients with malignant fungating wounds. J Adv Nurs 68(6):1312–1321

Maida V (2013) Wound management in patients with advanced illness. Curr Opin Support Palliat Care 7(1):73–79

Maida V, Ennis M, Kuziernsky C (2009) The Toronto Symptom Assessment System for Wounds: a new clinical and research tool. Adv Skin Wound Care 22(10):468–474

McDonald A, Lesage P (2006) Palliative management of pressure ulcers and malignant wounds in patients with advanced illness. J Palliat Med 9(2):285–295

McMurray V (2003) Managing patients with fungating malignant wounds. Nurs Times 99(13):55

Mercier D, Knevitt A (2005) Using topical aromatherapy for the management of fungating wounds in a palliative care unit. J Wound Care 14(10):497–501

Moylan S, Armstrong J, Diaz-Saldano D, Saker M, Yerkes EB, Ludgren BW (2010) Are abdominal X-rays a reliable way to assess for constipation? J Urol 184(Suppl):1692–1698

Naylor WA (2005) A guide to wound management in palliative care. Int J Palliat Nurs 11(11): 572–579

Nazarko L (2006) Malignant fungating wounds. Nurs Residential Care 8(9):402–406

Newton J, McVicar A (2013) Evaluation of the currency of the Davies and Oberle (1990) model of supportive care in specialist and specialised palliative care settings in England. J Clin Nurs. doi:10.1111/jocn.12301

Ngugi V (2007) Managing neuropathic pain in end-stage carcinoma. End Life Care 1(1):38–46

NICE (2004) Guidance on cancer services: improving supportive clinical and palliative care for adults with cancer. National Institute for Clinical Excellence, London

O'Connor M, Peters L (2009) Palliative care nurse consultants in acute hospitals in Australia. J End Life Care 3(1):48–53

Oberle K, Davies B (1992) Support and caring: exploring the concepts. Oncol Nurs Forum 19:763–767

Ovington L (2004) Silver: fact-or fiction. Ostomy Wound Manage 50(9A):1S–105S

Owens AL, Cleaves J (2012) Then and now: updating clinical nurse advancement programs. Nursing 42(10):17–27

Parry SB (1996) The quest for competences: competency studies can help you make HR decision, but the results are only as good as the study. Training 33:48–56

Pavlish C, Ceronsky L (2009) Oncology nurses' perceptions of nursing roles and professional attributes in palliative care. Clin J Oncol Nurs 13:404–412

Probst S, Arber A, Trojan A, Faithfull S (2012) Caring for a loved one with a malignant fungating wound. Support Care Cancer 20(12):3065–3070

Probst S, Arber A, Faithfull S (2013) Malignant fungating wounds: the meaning of living in an unbounded body. Eur J Oncol Nurs 17(1):38–45

Ribiero MDC, Joel SP, Zeppetella G (2004) The bioavailability of morphine applied topically to cutaneous ulcers. J Pain Symptom Manage 27(5):434–439

Saunders C, Clark D (2006) Cicely Saunders – selected writings 1958–2004. Oxford University Press, Oxford

Seymour J, Clark D, Hughes P, Bath P, Beech N, Corner J, Douglas H, Halliday D, Haviland J, Marples R, Normand C, Skilbeck J, Webb T (2002) Clinical nurse specialists in palliative care (3): issues for the Macmillan nurse role. Palliat Med 16:386–394

Shimizu Y, Miyashita M, Morita T, Sato K, Tsuneto S, Shima Y (2013) Care strategy for death rattle in terminally ill cancer patients and their family members: recommendations from a cross-sectional nationwide survey of Bereaved Family Members' Perceptions. J Pain Symptom Manage. http://dx.doi.org/10.1016/j.jpainsymman.2013.07.010

Skalla KA (2006) Blended role: advanced practice nursing in palliative care of the oncology patient. J Hosp Palliat Nurs 8(3):155–163

Skilbeck J, Payne S (2003) Emotional support and the role of clinical nurse specialists in palliative care. J Adv Nurs 43:521–530

Stoof A, Martens RL, Jeroen JG et al (2002) The boundary approach of competence: a constructivist aid for understanding and using the concept of competence. Hum Resour Dev Rev 1(3):345–365

Sykes NP (2010) Constipation and diarrhea. In: Walsh D (ed) Palliative medicine. Saunders, Philadelphia, pp 846–854

Walker A, Wilkes L, White K (2000) How do patients perceive support from nurses? Prof Nurse 16:902–904

Walshe C, Luker KA (2010) District nurses' role in palliative care provision: a realist review. Int J Nurs Stud 47:1167–1183

Wee B, Hillier R (2012) Interventions for noisy breathing in patients near to death. Cochrane Database Syst Rev (1):CD005177. doi:10.1002/14651858.CD005177.pub2

Wee BL, Coleman PG, Hillier R, Holgate SH (2006a) The sound of death rattle: are relatives distressed by hearing this sound? Palliat Med 20:171–175

Wee BL, Coleman PG, Hillier R, Holgate SH (2006b) The sound of death rattle II: how do relatives interpret the sound? Palliat Med 20:177–181

Wee B, Coleman PG, Hillier R, Holgate SH (2008) Death rattle: its impact on staff and volunteers in palliative care. Palliat Med 22:173–176

Widger K, Steele R, Oberle K, Davies B (2009) Exploring the supportive care model as a framework for paediatric palliative care. J Hosp Palliat Nurs 11:209–216

Wildiers H, Dhaenekint C, Demulenaere P, Clement PMJ, Desmet M, van Nuffelen R, Gielen J, van Droogenbroeck E, Geurs F, Lobelle J-P, Menten J (2009) Atropine, hyoscine butylbromide, or scopolamine are equally effective for the treatment of death rattle in terminal care. J Pain Symptom Manage 38(1):124–133

Woolery M, Bisanz A, Lyons HF, Gaido L, Yenulevich M, Fulton S, McMillan SC (2008) Putting evidence into practice®: evidence-based interventions for the prevention and management of constipation in patients with cancer. Clin J Oncol Nurs 12(2):317–337

World Health Organisation (2002) WHO definition of palliative care. Available at: http://www.who.int/cancer/palliative/definition/en/. Accessed 20th Dec 2013

Part III

The Final Phase

The Liverpool Care Pathway for the Dying Patient

8

Andrew F. Khodabukus and John E. Ellershaw

Contents

8.1 Introduction

Despite continuing advances in the treatment of people with cancer, death due to cancer remains a frequent occurrence for many cancer types. Therefore, caring for people with cancer during the dying phase of their illness is a fundamental aspect of oncology and palliative care. Good-quality care of the dying embodies what good-quality palliative care should be: an impeccable assessment, a rigorous approach to symptom control and a recognition that the duty of care extends beyond the individual. Care of the dying needs to be prompt, individually tailored, comprehensive

A.F. Khodabukus, BSc, MBChB (⊠)
Royal Liverpool and Broadgreen University Hospitals NHS Trust, Liverpool, UK
e-mail: andrew.khodabukus@rlbuht.nhs.uk

J.E. Ellershaw, MA, FRCP
Marie Curie Palliative Care Institute Liverpool, Liverpool, UK
e-mail: J.E.Ellershaw@liverpool.ac.uk

© Springer-Verlag Berlin Heidelberg 2015
B. Alt-Epping, F. Nauck (eds.), *Palliative Care in Oncology*,
DOI 10.1007/978-3-662-46202-7_8

and compassionate. Failure to meet these standards leaves little time for correction and can have a long-lasting impact for grieving relatives.

In this chapter we will examine what constitutes the best care for the dying person with cancer, encompassing clinical assessment, communication, spirituality and care planning in life and death. Within that approach we will discuss the Liverpool Care Pathway for the Dying Patient (LCP), which aims to promote the best possible care for an individual and their relatives in the last hours and days of life.

8.1.1 Recognising Dying

Anticipating that death can occur and is approaching can help optimise the care and experience when someone with cancer enters the dying phase. People with advanced cancer often show a constellation of features suggestive of advancing disease (Glare and Christakis 2013). These include a worsening Eastern Cooperative Oncology Group (ECOG) performance status as shown by increasing levels of fatigue and reduced mobility. There is a lack of response to chemotherapy, targeted treatments and radiotherapy.

The classic illness trajectory for people with cancer is of a precipitous decline in function at 8–12 weeks prior to death (Costantini et al. 2008; Glare and Christakis 2013). This is in contrast to other classifications or illness trajectory which includes sudden death, organ failure and frailty (Lunney et al. 2003). As ever, the art of the clinician is to interpret these models when faced with an individual who does not necessarily correlate with the median or average person in these models.

What is the purpose of attempting prognostication when there are no further oncological therapeutic agents? In essence, the events or symptoms described can all act as prompts to explore cancer patients' preferences for what happens when they are dying. It offers the individual the opportunity to prepare and talk about their worsening health, dying and death with their relatives and carers. This preparation lays the groundwork for the best care for the dying person.

Recognising that someone is in the last few hours or days of life is always complex (MCPCIL 2012). A review of the published literature concluded that there is a lack of specific scientific literature to support a "diagnosis of dying" despite a number of studies describing the phenomena of dying (Eychmüller et al. 2013). These phenomena of dying include reduced levels of consciousness, respiratory and circulatory changes and biochemical markers.

Whilst there are a number of tools to support prognostication in advanced cancer (Lau et al. 2007), the recognition that someone is dying remains a clinical judgement. Boyd and Murray (2010) suggest the following questions that can prompt a multidisciplinary dialogue about recognising dying: Could this patient be in the last days of life? Was this patient's condition expected to deteriorate in this way? Have potentially reversible causes of deterioration been excluded? Is further life-prolonging treatment inappropriate?

A multidisciplinary team approach to this judgement – led by the most senior doctor ultimately responsible for the patient's care – maximally enhances the quality of the judgement made. This should include the patient where possible and appropriate and always those that personally know the patient best, usually relatives or carers. No judgement can be absolute and the team looking after the patient has to be able to deal with a number of uncertainties.

Table 8.1 Ten key elements of care for the dying person (Ellershaw and Lakhani 2013)

1. Recognition that the person is dying
2. Communication with the person (where possible) and always with family and loved ones
3. Spiritual care
4. Anticipatory prescribing for symptoms of pain, respiratory tract secretions, agitation, nausea and vomiting, dyspnoea
5. Review of clinical interventions should be in the person's best interests
6. Hydration review, including the need for commencement or cessation
7. Nutritional review, including commencement or cessation
8. Full discussion of the care plan with the person and relative or carer
9. Regular reassessment of the person
10. Dignified and respectful care after death

Uncertainty is an integral part of dying in common with other areas of medicine (Montgomery 2005). Uncertainties include those occasions when a patient who is thought to be dying lives longer than expected and vice versa. They also include the length of the dying phase and the manner of symptoms and death. Even in patients with advanced and advancing cancer, there will be elements of uncertainty regarding these features. Uncertainty is best managed by good communication and support for the patient and their relatives and carers and an iterative dialogue across all members of the healthcare team. This enables all care and treatment options to be properly considered and either started or stopped, as is best for the patient.

8.1.2   What Is the Best Care for the Dying Person?

Recognising that someone is dying is the first step in providing the best care for the dying person. Table 8.1 outlines the key elements of care for the dying person.

These ten elements have been derived from consensus work across nations and cultures, appraising the evidence and experience of caring for dying patients (Mason et al. 2012; Costantini and Lunder 2012; Ellershaw et al. 2013). The best care for the dying needs not only high-quality direct clinical care but also the attention to healthcare systems, education and training and research to consistently drive up standards, knowledge and practice.

One complex intervention designed to address these factors holistically that has been available to the health community over recent years has been the Liverpool Care Pathway for the Dying Patient (LCP).

8.2   The Liverpool Care Pathway for the Dying Patient

8.2.1   The Origins of the LCP

From its beginnings in Liverpool in the United Kingdom, the LCP has been adopted both nationally and internationally in a range of healthcare settings (Marie Curie Palliative Care Institute Liverpool 2012). The LCP was developed to improve care for patients dying in the hospital by identifying the best practices in caring for dying patients seen in hospices and transferring these into the hospital environment. The aim of the LCP is to provide guidance and support for symptom control, communication and monitoring and evaluation of the care process, delivery and outcome in care of the dying patient. In the next section of this chapter, we will examine the development of the LCP and the concept of "pathways" before discussing in more detail the components of the LCP to support patients dying from cancer.

8.2.2　Development of the Liverpool Care Pathway for the Dying Patient

The LCP was the result of this work to bring hospice-inspired care into the hospital environment. The work was developed in Liverpool using integrated care pathway, thus giving the name Liverpool Care Pathway. It is important to understand the concept of integrated care pathways in order to place the LCP in its fullest context.

Integrated care pathways are "a complex intervention for the mutual decision making and organisation of care processes for a well-defined group of patients during a well-defined period" (Vanhaecht et al. 2007). The late 1990s saw the widespread adoption of integrated care pathways in a number of healthcare disciplines (Vanhaecht et al. 2006), for example, the management of myocardial infarction or fractured neck of the femur. Integrated care pathways are not simply forms or checklists but include the workings of a multidisciplinary team in unique organisations within an evolving evidence base of practice. This is demonstrated in Fig. 8.1 which summarises the aims, themes and practices addressed within the LCP.

1 Aim
To improve care of the dying in the last hours or days of life

2 Key themes
To improve the knowledge related to the process of dying

3 Key sections
Initial assessment
Ongoing assessment
Care after death

4 Key domains of care
Physical
Psychological
Social
Spiritual

5 Key requirements for organisational governance
Clinical decision making
Management and leadership
Learning and teaching
Research and development
Governance and risk

Fig. 8.1 The LCP model pathway

Table 8.2 Ten-step Continuous Quality Improvement Programme

The Institute has developed a ten-step Continuous Quality Improvement Programme (CQIP) to aid the implementation, dissemination and sustainability of the LCP Model Pathway, UK, into an organisation.

Phase 1: Induction	Step 1	Establishing the project – preparing the environment
Phase 2: Implementation	Step 2	Develop the documentation
	Step 3	Base review/retrospective audit of current documentation
	Step 4	Induction/education programme – pilot site
	Step 5	Clinical implementation of the LCP in pilot sites
Phase 3: Dissemination	Step 6	Maintaining and improving competencies using reflective practice and post-pathway analysis
	Step 7	Evaluation and further training
	Step 8	Continuous development of competencies in order to embed the LCP Model within the clinical environment
Phase 4: Sustainability	Step 9	Organisational recognition that all staff who work with people who are dying are properly trained to look after dying patients and their carers within an agreed organisational/educational strategy
	Step 10	To establish the LCP within the governance/performance agenda within the organisation/institution

Essential to the methodology of the integrated care pathway is a continuous quality improvement process. The LCP is no different. It is currently in its 12th iteration and has a ten-step approach to induction, implementation, dissemination and sustainability of the integrated care pathway (Table 8.2).

The best care for the dying in patients whose care is supported by the LCP is therefore dependent on high-quality achievement of the ten steps above. The LCP is a guide to supporting care for the dying by prompting clinicians to review the care given. The LCP is not a substitute for clinical decision-making and does not recommend specific elements of healthcare. In short, the LCP can only ever be as good as the people using it. The benefits of successful use of the LCP is a cultural change in acknowledging the universality of death and that providing the best care for the dying can be one of the most rewarding experiences for any health professional.

8.3   Supporting Care with the LCP

As discussed earlier in the chapter, recognising dying – that someone is likely to be in the last hours to days of life – is essential. The LCP includes an algorithm (Fig. 8.2) to prompt the multidisciplinary team (MDT) to determine if the patient is likely to be dying. The MDT will vary between healthcare settings and institutions but should, as a minimum, include a doctor and a nurse.

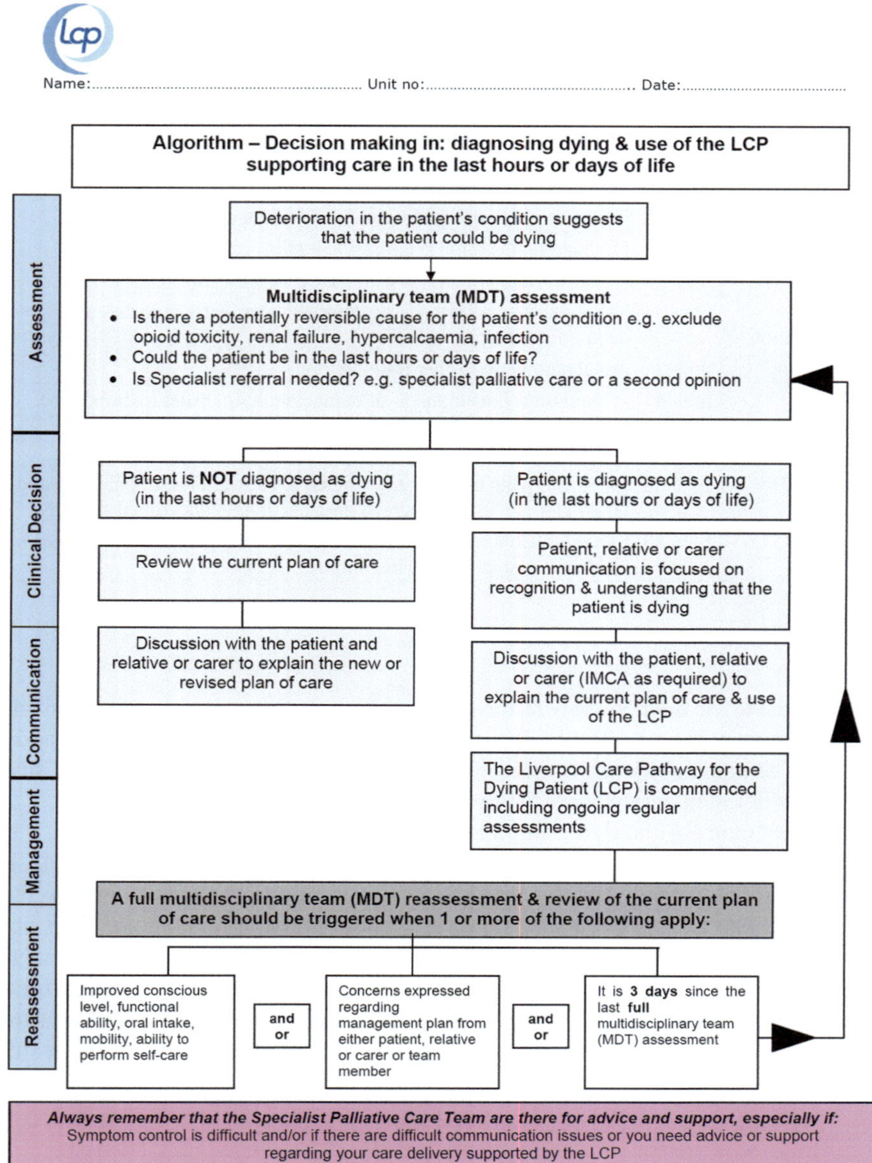

Fig. 8.2 Decision-making in recognising dying

The MDT assessment of recognition of dying should consider:

- Is there a potentially reversible cause for the patient's condition, e.g. excluding opioid toxicity, renal failure, hypercalcaemia, and infection?
- Could the patient be in the last hours or days of life?
- Is a specialist referral needed (e.g. specialist palliative care or a second opinion)?

If the considered opinion of the MDT is that yes, this person is dying, then this should be communicated if possible with the patient and always with their relative or carer. The views of all concerned and involved should be sought, listened to and documented accordingly. Where there is contention about the recognition of dying, a second opinion should be sought. The final step of the decision to support care with the LCP is a written endorsement of the time, date and signature of the most senior clinician in charge of the person's care.

Care at this point of time is framed by complexity and uncertainty. A formal, multidisciplinary review of the patient's care should take place every 3 days or sooner if concerns are expressed by professionals, the patient or relatives. The outcome of this review should be recorded within the LCP. This is in addition to the minimum four-hourly review of the patient required when supporting a patient's care with the LCP.

8.3.1   Section 1: Initial Assessment

This first phase of initial assessment covers the key goals to be considered when the patient has entered the last hours/days of life. It begins by a baseline assessment of symptom control, establishing what the current problems are so care can be planned accordingly. This is followed by a series of goals covering the commonly occurring issues to be considered. This assessment should be done by at least a doctor and a nurse.

8.3.1.1 Communication and Information: Goals 1.1–1.5 and 2

Clear and comprehensive communication is the cornerstone of providing the best care for the dying person. The aim is for the dying person and their relatives to take a full and active role in planning their future care. Their current level of understanding of what is happening should be explored.

Barriers to this communication, such as language and disability, should be identified and optimised. Accurate telephone numbers and addresses should be obtained to allow prompt update of any change in condition and for future bereavement support. At this emotionally heightened time, families sometimes change who the primary contact is from the next of kin. People's wishes for how they are told can differ with some preferring not to be informed of a death during the night.

Goal 2 addresses the facilities, such as getting food and drink or quiet areas, the relatives can use. Ideally there should be accompanied written information to act as an aide-memoire for the family.

8.3.1.2 Spirituality: Goals 3.1 and 3.2

Health professionals should understand the spiritual needs of the dying person and their relatives now, at the moment of death and after death. This can help identify important cultural and religious rites that need to be done. These should be recorded within the LCP to facilitate the right care at the right time.

8.3.1.3 Medication: Goals 4.1 and 4.2

Anticipatory medication should be available and prescribed for the five commonest symptoms experienced by dying people: pain, nausea and vomiting, breathlessness, agitation and respiratory tract secretions. These need only be given when required at a dose no greater than that needed to achieve symptom control. Doses should be titrated individually to patient need. For some people, a continuous subcutaneous infusion may be needed or already in place to manage symptoms. If this is now needed due to the change in clinical condition, it should be started diligently and promptly.

8.3.1.4 Current Interventions: Goals 5.1–5.3

When someone is recognised to be dying, a review of which interventions, treatments and investigations are performed should be done. The aim is twofold: to initiate some interventions and therapies to confer benefit for someone in the dying phase. Similarly, it can be appropriate to eliminate those that are not conferring benefit. Goal 5.1 specifically prompts clinicians to review the need for blood tests, intravenous antibiotics, blood glucose monitoring, routine recording of vital signs and oxygen therapy. Any one of these can be continued, discontinued or commenced and this list is not exhaustive.

Attempting cardiopulmonary resuscitation in someone who is recognised as imminently dying from an irreversible cause is deemed futile by national and continental resuscitation councils. A decision about this intervention should be recorded in Goal 5.2, with Goal 5.3 addressing the decision around deactivation of implantable cardioverter defibrillators.

8.3.1.5 Clinically Assisted Hydration and Nutrition: Goals 6 and 7

All patients who are dying should be supported to manage what they can by mouth. These goals address the provision of clinically assisted hydration and nutrition, that is, administration of prescribed fluid and nutrition by assisted enteral and parenteral means. The decision is individual to each dying person; the LCP neither precludes nor mandates medical interventions and exists to support clinical decisions. The decision should be clearly documented to support care until the next review.

8.3.1.6 Skin Care: Goal 8

Dying people are at greater risk of compromising skin integrity due to physiological changes associated with disease processes and immobility. Optimising skin integrity therefore will minimise symptoms of pain; however, some interventions designed to do this may not be suitable in someone in the last hours or days of life. This goal prompts health professionals to plan care and reassessment of pressure areas, optimal turning and the use of supportive measures such as pressure-relieving mattresses.

8.3.1.7 Explanation of Plan of Care: Goals 9.1–9.4

The purpose of these goals is to reiterate the plan of care for professionals, the patient and relatives. As described before, this needs to be done in a clear and sensitive manner. A leaflet such as the LCP front sheet and the "Coping with Dying" leaflet can help reinforce some of the conversations that will have happened with the assessment. Local versions of this can also be used. It is also important to update all health professionals involved in care, and the medical team that supports the patient in their usual place of residence, such as a general practitioner, should also be informed of the situation.

8.3.2   Section 2: Ongoing Assessment

Section two continues the focus on maximising patient comfort through ongoing review of the symptom control and psychological and spiritual goals described in the initial assessment. The frequency of monitoring is individually determined. For the duration that the patient remains supported by the LCP, assessment of these goals is performed as a minimum on a four-hourly basis where there is 24-h nursing care or at each visit in the other environments.

The recording of care is organised around goals of symptom control and support for the patient and family (Fig. 8.3). Assessments are "moment in time" reports, not a summary of the 4-h period. Often the patient and relative will be visited multiple times in that 4-h period – when problems are encountered, this is entered on the summary variance sheet to determine what action has been taken and the effect of this action. Variance is not a negative occurrence but simply provides a record of what happened, what was done about it and the outcome.

8.3.3   Section 3: Care After Death

This section concerns the factual, procedural and moreover the care needed to look after someone who has died with dignity and respect. Details of the death are recorded, including time/date and any people present at time of death. These details aid completion of the required official death certification procedures. This section also focuses on ensuring appropriate procedures for the care of the body and any belongings after death. It includes any specific religious requirements that may be

lcp

Name:………………………………………………………… Unit no:………………………………………….. Date:……………………………………

Section 2 Ongoing assessment of the plan of care – LCP DAY……..						
Undertake an MDT assessment & review of the current management plan if:						

Improved conscious level, functional ability, oral intake, mobility, ability to perform self-care

and or

Concern expressed regarding management plan from either the patient, relative or team member

and or

It is 3 days since the last **full** MDT assessment

Consider the support of the specialist palliative care team and/or a second opinion as required. Document all reassessment dates and times on page 3

Codes to be recorded at each timed assessment (a moment in time)   A= Achieved   V = Variance (exception reporting)

Record an A or a V not a signature	**0400**	**0800**	**1200**	**1600**	**2000**	**2400**
Goal a: The patient does not have pain Verbalised by patient if conscious, pain free on movement. Observe for non-verbal cues. Consider need for positional change. Use a pain assessment tool if appropriate. Consider prn analgesia for incident pain						
Goal b: The patient is not agitated Patient does not display signs of restlessness or distress, exclude reversible causes e.g. retention of urine, opioid toxicity						
Goal c: The patient does not have respiratory tract secretions Consider positional change. Discuss symptoms & plan of care with patient, relative or carer Medication to be given as soon as symptom occurs						
Goal d: The patient does not have nausea Verbalised by patient if conscious						
Goal e: The patient is not vomiting						
Goal f: The patient is not breathless Verbalised by patient if conscious, consider positional change. Use of a fan may be helpful						
Goal g: The patient does not have urinary problems Use of pads, urinary catheter as required						
Goal h: The patient does not have bowel problems Monitor – constipation / diarrhoea. Monitor skin integrity Bowels last opened:…………………………						
Goal i: The patient does not have other symptoms Record symptom here…………………………………………………. *If no other symptoms present please record N/A*						
Goal j: The patient's comfort & safety regarding the administration of medication is maintained If CSCI in place – monitoring sheet in progress S/C butterfly in place if needed for prn medication location:………………………….. The patient is only receiving medication that is beneficial at this time. *If no medication required please record N/A*						

Fig. 8.3 Ongoing assessment: goals

necessary. As in the previous sections, support of family/carers, who are now recently bereaved, is an important aspect of the LCP. It ensures that the family receives both practical information about registering the death and funeral arrangements but also continuing psychological support and bereavement advice. It concludes with ensuring that all health professionals inside and outside the organisation, who were involved in this person's care, are informed of their death.

8.4   Summary

Providing the best possible care for the dying for an individual and their relatives consists of a series of skills honed through education, training and experience and supported by a healthcare environment where care for the dying is embedded as a priority. It requires the concerted application of the elements we have discussed in this chapter; it will not happen by default. Dying is a universal experience, and when it happens, sometimes after several years of oncological therapy, it should not be regarded as a failure. To do so could deny this person the opportunity to complete their lives in the manner best suited to them and their relatives and carers.

The LCP and its Continuous Quality Improvement Programme recognise that just as dying is complex, so is healthcare. The LCP will only make that difference as part of an embedded mature culture of learning, improvement and person-centred care. Providing that care for dying people encapsulates the best actions, intentions and vocation of health professionals.

References

Boyd K, Murray S (2010) Recognising and managing key transitions in end of life care. Br Med J 341:c4683

Costantini M, Lunder U (2012) OPCARE9 – a European perspective in the last days of life. Eur J Palliat Care 19(4):175–177

Costantini M, Beccaro M, Higginson IJ (2008) Cancer trajectories at the end of life: is there an effect of age and gender? BMC Cancer 8:127. doi:10.1186/1471-2407-8-127

Ellershaw J, Lakhani M (2013) Best care for the dying patient. BMJ 347:f4428 doi:10.1136/bmj.f4428

Ellershaw J, Fürst CJ, Lunder U, Boughey M, Eychmüller S, Hannam Hodgson S, Faksvåg Haugen D, Marshall B, Walker H, Wilkinson S, Voltz R, van Zuylen L (2013) Care of the dying and the LCP in England: an international perspective. Eur J Palliat Care 20(3):120–123

Eychmüller S, Domeisen Benedetti F, Latten R, Tal K, Walker J, Costantini M (2013) 'Diagnosing dying' in cancer patients – a systematic literature review. Eur J Palliat Care 20(6):292–296

Glare P, Christakis NA (2013) Prognosis in advanced cancer. Oxford University Press, Oxford, United Kingdom

Lau F, Cloutier-Fisher D, Kuziemsky C, Black F, Downing M, Borycki E, Ho F (2007) A systematic review of prognostic tools for estimating survival time in palliative care. J Palliat Care 23(2):93–112

Lunney JR, Lynn J, Foley DJ, Lipson S, Guralnik JM (2003) Patterns of functional decline at the end of life. JAMA 289:2387–2392

Marie Curie Palliative Care Institute Liverpool (2012) LCP – International Model Pathway. http://www.mcpcil.org.uk/media/10807/lcp%20model%20pathway.pdf. Liverpool, UK

Mason S, Dowson J, Gambles M, Ellershaw J (2012) OPCARE9—optimising research for cancer patient care in the last days of life. Eur J Palliat Care 19(1):17–19

Montgomery K (2005) How doctors think: clinical judgment and the practice of medicine. Oxford University Press, Cary

Vanhaecht K, Bollmann M, Bower K, Gallagher C, Gardini A, Guezo J, Jansen U, Massoud R, Moody K, Sermeus W, Van Zelm R, Whittle C, Yazbeck A, Zander K, Panella M (2006) Prevalence and use of clinical pathways in 23 countries – an international survey by the European Pathway Association. J Integr Pathw 10(1):28–34

Vanhaecht K, De Witte K, Sermeus W (2007) The impact of clinical pathways on the organisation of care processes. ACCO, Leuven

Further Reading

Ellershaw J, Wilkinson S (2011) Care of the dying: a pathway to excellence, 2nd rev edn. Oxford University Press, Oxford

Marie Curie Palliative Care Institute Liverpool. LCP International Programme. www.mcpcil.org.uk

The Final Phase

9

Friedemann Nauck

> *You matter because you are you. You matter to the last moment of your life, and we will do all we can to help you not only to die peacefully, but also to live until you die.*
>
> (Cicely Saunders 1976)

Contents

9.1 Introduction

Palliative care aims to improve the quality of life of patients and their families facing life-threatening illness. An overall treatment strategy not only includes prevention, assessment, and treatment of pain and other symptoms but also integrates psychological, social, emotional, and spiritual problems of the patient and his/her relatives. The large majority of patients being managed in palliative medicine are suffering from incurable, far-advanced, and progressive cancer. Pain is the

F. Nauck, MD
Department of Palliative Medicine, University Medical Center, Göttingen, Germany
e-mail: Friedemann.Nauck@med.uni-goettingen.de

© Springer-Verlag Berlin Heidelberg 2015
B. Alt-Epping, F. Nauck (eds.), *Palliative Care in Oncology*,
DOI 10.1007/978-3-662-46202-7_9

major source of anxiety and distress at the end of life, particularly in cases of end-stage cancer. As in any stage of the disease, cancer pain treatment requires standardized guidelines adapted to the WHO's three-step ladder of cancer pain relief (WHO 1996). Burdens and suffering of patients and relatives should be minimized, and physical, psychosocial, and spiritual symptoms must be treated even in the terminal phase.

It is a fact that the terminal phase is a very dynamic process. During the last days of life, it is important to redefine treatment goals, as symptoms that were previously present may increase and new symptoms may appear (Lichter and Hunt 1990; Nauck 1994, 2001; Saunders 1988; Conill et al. 1997). The dying phase has often been claimed to be underdiagnosed. In consequence, team conflicts, futile treatment, and insufficient symptom control were reported. After years of undertreated symptoms, there is now a danger of unreasonable application of high doses of strong opioids without a medical indication or the application of sedatives to cope with difficult symptoms at the end of life. Therapeutic decisions must consider probably conflicting issues of medical indication, ethics, and law. This is of particular relevance when treatment preferences of patients are not known or in contrast to those of the carers.

9.2 The Final Phase

There are different terms used worldwide to describe the different phases in end-of-life care of patients with advanced cancer and other life-limiting diseases, including terminal phase, end-stage of the disease, final phase, final stage, and last period of life. Up-to-date clear definitions of the term terminal disease are lacking, and there are no objective criteria to predict death (Lynn et al. 1997). According to the World Health Organization (WHO), palliative care is defined as: "…an approach that improves the quality of life of patients and their families facing the problem associated with life-threatening illness, through the prevention and relief of suffering by means of early identification and impeccable assessment and therapy of pain and other problems, physical, psychosocial and spiritual…" (Sepúlveda et al. 2002). Early identification and impeccable assessment and symptom control mean not least after the study of Jennifer Temel et al., where median survival in patients with metastatic non-small-cell lung cancer was longer among patients receiving early palliative care (Temel et al. 2010), that we get to know patients earlier during their course of disease when they still benefit from rehabilitation interventions (Javier and Montagnini 2011). During this phase of rehabilitation, patients benefit from the cooperation and treatment and care from oncologists and palliative care specialists. Definitions for rehabilitation in palliative medicine, for the terminal phase and the final phase, however, can be found in the literature (Javier and Montagnini 2011; Kaye 1992; Nauck et al. 2000; Jonen-Thielemann 2007). Palliative care and rehabilitation share common goals and therapeutic approaches with a multidisciplinary model of care, which aims to improve patients' levels of function and comfort months before death. Rehabilitative interventions can impact function and symptom management in terminally ill patients and improve their care. Physical function and independence should be maintained as long as possible to improve patients' quality of life and reduce the burden of care for the caregivers. Pain therapy and symptom control, psychosocial intervention, and spiritual care are the basic treatment for patients at this stage of their disease. The terminal phase can be defined as the period when day-to-day deterioration is occurring. There is weakness (sometimes profound), drowsiness, bedriddenness, poor appetite, organ failure, and finally peripheral cyanosis. It is difficult to predict when the terminal phase will be reached.

Comfort is the priority in the final phase, and opioids and sedatives are used to achieve comfort, if required (Kaye 1992). The final phase is described as the last 3 days of life (Nauck et al. 2000). It is difficult to predict that a patient is about to die, even for doctors and nurses working in the field of palliative medicine. Also, not only treatment decisions depend on the question of patients "how much time do I have left?"

In a recent study it could be shown that prognostic scores are not able to produce a precise, reliable prognosis of survival time in patients receiving inpatient palliative care (Stiel et al. 2010). Overestimating of survival times by the factor of five has been reported for 80 % of cases (Christakis and Lamont 2000). There are different prognostic instruments used in palliative medicine: the Palliative Prognostic Index (PPI) and the Palliative Prognostic Score (PaP-S). However, until now it is not clear if the value of these instruments is to facilitate the evaluation of patient groups rather than of individual patients.

For detection of a patient's transgression from the terminal into the final phase, the use of the "surprise question" can be helpful. The physician should ask himself "Would I be surprised if this patient dies in the next year/next week/next hours?" If this is answered with "No, I would not be surprised" for the last two options, the probability is high that the patient will die within this time range. The surprise question enables the health-care professionals to assimilate communication and care planning with the prognosis of the patient (Stiel et al. 2010; Pattison and Romer 2001; Stiel and Radbruch 2014).

9.3 Symptoms in the Final Phase

The final phase is a dynamic process that may require "active" medical treatment of exacerbating, previously well-controlled symptoms like pain, dyspnea, vomiting, fear, etc. Discontinuation and change of treatment regimens, respectively, may also become necessary (Nauck et al. 2000).

Most patients in palliative care die under good symptom control, even in the outpatient setting (Maier et al. 2008). This, however, requires availability of the respective drugs and excellent expertise of the therapeutic team.

A list of signs that may indicate the final phase is provided in the Oxford Textbook of Palliative Medicine (Twycross and Lichter 1998).

> **Signs of the Last Days of Life (Twycross and Lichter** 1998)
> - Arising of "new symptoms"
> - Increasing weakness
> - Essentially bedbound
> - Drowsy for extended periods
> - Disoriented for time
> - Limited attention span
> - Increasingly disinterested in food and fluid
> - Difficulty in swallowing medication

In patients with an incurable and progressive illness, this phase sometimes can be anticipated, but it is also known that a deterioration can be sudden and distressing (Twycross and Lichter 1998). The most common symptoms in the last 3 days of life of patients in a palliative care unit (PCU) in Germany, for example, were drowsiness and confusion (55 %), death rattle (45 %), restlessness and agitation (43 %), pain (26 %), dyspnea (25 %), and nausea and vomiting (14 %) (Conill et al. 1997). Other studies on the most common symptoms in the final days show similar results (Back et al. 2001; Morita et al. 1999; Hall et al. 2002; Potter et al. 2003).

If team members detect the "point of no return" and are prepared to care for the dying patient and offer sufficient symptom control in the last days of life, they have to redefine the goals of treatment. New strategies and aims have to be communicated with relatives, and it must be kept in mind that the relatives themselves may be in need of support when their loved one is close to death.

Principles of managing the last 3 days of life [mod. by (Adam 1997)]:

> - Detect the "point of no return" by reviewing the patient.
> - Review all drugs and symptoms regularly.
> - Symptom control is of utmost priority.
> - Avoid unnecessary interventions.
> - Maintain communication with patient and relatives.
> - Ensure support for family and carers.

Note: Medication that no longer has any direct benefit in the final phase may include diuretics, cardiac medication, antibiotics, antidepressants, and cytotoxic agents.

9.4 Symptom Management in the Last Days of Life

The main focus in this article will be the treatment of cancer-related pain. Dyspnea, delirium, death rattle, and other symptoms will be addressed in less detail.

9.5   Treatment of Cancer-Related Pain

Assessment and diagnosis of the cause of pain are essential before starting any pain treatment but difficult in the final phase when patients are likely unable to communicate in an adequate way. Clinical examination and information from relatives and team members are most helpful to explore pain types and pain intensity. Reasons for poor relief of pain include fear of using strong opioids, choice of the wrong opioid, underdosing, side effects, and opioid tolerance.

9.5.1   Treatment with Strong Opioids

Opioids are not the "panacea" for the relief of cancer pain, but are necessary in most cancer pain patients in the last days of their life. Oral morphine (Hanks 1996) still remains the opioid of choice worldwide, but in some countries there are a large number of alternative opioids available in a range of different formulations, e.g., fentanyl, hydromorphone, methadone, oxycodone, or buprenorphine. There are no differential indications for choosing the "right opioid" at the "right time." Nevertheless, clinical experience shows an advantage of hydromorphone or methadone in some patients.

At the very end of life, many patients are no longer able to swallow tablets or solutions, and the route of administration of strong opioids must be changed, for example, to subcutaneous or intravenous application. Even in the last days of life, opioid rotation can lead to improved pain control with less toxicity in some patients.

9.5.2   Choice of Route

In the treatment of pain in the final stage, it is helpful that opioids can be administered in many different routes (oral, subcutaneous, intravenous and transdermal, buccal/transmucosal, rectal, topical, and epidural or spinal). Not all strong opioids can be given by all routes because of their particular pharmacological characteristics (for instance, oral bioavailability or first-pass effect of the liver), and not all are available in all preparations.

The choice of an alternative route will depend on the need for rapid titration in cases of severe pain and on patient preferences. Some believe that a change in route rather than changing an opioid is the most logical means of instigating an opioid rotation in an attempt to improve pain control or lessen toxicity (Enting et al. 2002). If patients are unable to take drugs orally, the subcutaneous administration is easy to initiate, including in the home care setting. Only few drugs are licensed for the subcutaneous route of delivery, but off-label use (with regard to the route of administration) of other opioids has become a daily routine in palliative care and is known to deliver good results with no detrimental effects on patient safety.

Opioid administration by the parenteral route facilitates rapid titration and offers a shorter time to peak analgesic effect. This is an advantage for patients with severe pain or unstable pain in the last days of life. In Germany, for example, an increasing number of patients have intravenous port-a-caths, allowing easy administration of pain medication.

There is an ongoing discussion about the indication of transdermal application of fentanyl or buprenorphine in the last days of life. Profuse sweating may lead to failure of the patch to adhere to the skin, and the transdermal absorption of these drugs can be seriously impaired by circulatory disorder. If there is need for rapid titration of analgesics for moderate-to-severe pain, transdermal opioids should not be used. It also should not be initiated in the final phase, because of the time taken to reach an effective plasma concentration (Hardy and Nauck 2009). In unproblematic cases with stable pain intensity, however, the transdermal application can be continued until death and will offer a convenient alternative to parenteral drug delivery.

Transmucosal, buccal, and intranasal lipid-soluble opioids are commercially available in some countries. Their rapid onset of analgesia has been shown to be effective for breakthrough pain (Zeppetella and Ribeiro 2006; Mercadante et al. 2009).

The concept of titration for oral, subcutaneous, and intravenous formulations (1/6 of the daily dose for breakthrough pain) is not used for the calculation of the required dose of transmucosal, buccal, and intranasal lipid-soluble formulations of fentanyl. Therefore, the dose has to be titrated for each individual patient and independently from the daily opioid dose. The use of these formulations in dying patients, however, still remains a subject of controversial discussions.

9.5.3 Dose Titration

There is no explicit inclusion of recommendations for dying patients in the guidelines on the use of morphine (Hanks 1996). But it is general practice in the treatment of patients in all stages of their disease that opioids should be given regularly by the clock in opioid-naïve patients starting on a low dose of an immediate-release strong opioid (Tables 9.1 and 9.2). These titration schemes apply not only to morphine but also to other opioids with predictable kinetics, such as hydromorphone or oxycodone, but do not apply to drugs with unique pharmacology, for example, methadone. A number of different dosing strategies have been recommended for this drug (Mercadante et al. 2009; Nauck et al. 2001).

Patients in the final phase of their illness and with severe pain may require titration with parenteral opioids. An appropriate starting dose for opioid-naïve patients is subcutaneous morphine 5 mg, given every 4 h (or subcutaneous hydromorphone 1 mg given every 4 h) or 10–20 mg subcutaneous or intravenous morphine per 24 h (or equivalent dose of fentanyl or hydromorphone). The dose can then be increased according to pain scores. If the patient is still in pain, increase the dose by 25–50 %. If the patient is experiencing side effects, reduce by 25 %.

For potential episodes of breakthrough pain, rescue medication needs to be provided. There is no standard as to the dose of breakthrough medication. Current practice is to give one-sixth of the total daily dose of the regular strong opioid.

Table 9.1 Titration of morphine – recommendations for the final phase

Opioid-naïve patients
Use of immediate-release preparations to titrate, e.g., morphine ampoules given every 4 h SC
Start at a low dose, usually 5 mg every 4 h (2.5 mg in the elderly)
Prescribe breakthrough (PRN) immediate-release morphine at the same dose as the 4 hourly dose, given as often as required (up to hourly)
There is no limit to the number of extra doses that can be administered. Take the number of breakthrough doses into account when adjusting the total daily dose
Increase the 4 hourly doses by approximately 30–50 % every 24–48 h until pain is controlled
Patient still on opioids
Patient is already on a slow-release morphine preparation and is in severe pain, titrate by converting back to an immediate-release preparation given every 4 h, and increase the 4-hourly dose by approximately 30–50 %, until pain is controlled
Note
IV infusion of opioids may be preferable in patients who already have an indwelling line, have generalized edema, develop severe site reactions, and have coagulation disorders or poor peripheral circulation
The 24-h dose of parenteral morphine is one-half to one-third of the total daily oral dose of morphine
Breakthrough doses (equivalent to the 4-hourly parenteral dose) can be offered every 30 min
Assess the number of breakthrough doses required each day and change the 24-h dose accordingly
A small proportion of patients develop intolerable side effects to morphine. In such patients, a change to an alternative opioid should be considered

IR immediate release, *SC* subcutaneous, *IV* intravenous, *PRN* pro re nata/as required

Table 9.2 Pain management in the last 3 days of life

Drug	Dose	Route of administration
Morphine	Start with 2.5–5–10 mg/4 h	Oral/rectal
	0.5–1.0 mg/h	Continuously subcutaneous or intravenous
	Individual dose titration!	
Hydromorphone	Start with 0.5–1–2 mg/4 h	Oral
	0.1–0.25 mg/h	Continuously subcutaneous or intravenous
	Individual dose titration!	
Oxycodone	Start with 1.25–2.5–5 mg/4 h	Oral
	0.25–0.5 mg/h	Continuously subcutaneous or intravenous
	Individual dose titration!	
Fentanyl	Only if the patient is already using patches!	Transdermal

9.5.4 Opioid Rotation

Opioid rotation or switching of opioids is a common practice in cancer pain therapy, to improve pain control or reduce toxicity, or both. In many countries a large number of different opioids and opioid formulations are now available. A systematic review of the published literature found no controlled evidence to support the practice of opioid rotation, but clinical experience and uncontrolled evidence showed improvements in side effects and/or pain control when rotating from one opioid to another (Quigley 2004).

9.6 Careful Monitoring of Pain Treatment

In the final phase pain control may need adjustments. It has been shown that nearly 50 % of patients under strong opioids received an unchanged dose of analgesics during the final phase (Lichter and Hunt 43 %, WHO 1996). In other patients the dose of morphine had to be increased, because of insufficient pain control. In one-fourth of our patients, we have to decrease the dose of strong opioids during the last hours of life, to achieve good symptom control (Conill et al. 1997). Main reasons for opioid reduction are side effects, e.g., sedation or myoclonus. These side effects are more often observed in patients with renal failure or when the opioid is given in combination with drugs/substances that have extrapyramidal side effects, e.g., metoclopramide.

9.7 Treatment of Dyspnea

Dyspnea is a common symptom during the final days or weeks of life and described as shortness of breath or air hunger. It is often associated with an increased respiratory rate, compared with anxiety and agitation, and may predict short survival. Dyspnea may be caused by pleural effusion, pulmonary edema, infection, ascites, cardiac cause, anemia, and many other reasons. The underlying cause of dyspnea is in the final phase mostly no longer treatable.

Treatment with opioids decreases the perception of air hunger, regardless of the underlying pathophysiology and without causing respiratory depression (Thomas and von Gunten 2002).

The main therapeutic strategy in the final phase is to reduce the breathing rate by low doses of opioids, such as morphine 2.5–5 mg orally all 4 h, which may provide good relief in opioid-naïve patients. Higher doses may be indicated in patients with more severe dyspnea or in patients treated with opioids for pain. Supplemental oxygen is only useful in hypoxemic patients (Booth et al. 2004). There are some alternative strategies, such as positioning, a cool fan toward the patient's face, repositioning the patient into an upright position, or physiotherapy. Cognitive behavioral therapies such as breathing control exercises and relaxation or psychosocial support may be only effective in some patients in the final phase because of limited capacity to participate in these techniques. Antibiotics may provide relief from infectious sources of dyspnea and reduce symptoms of pulmonary secretion. But these drugs should not be given in the last hours of life. In some patients glucocorticoids or bronchodilators can provide relief, but potential side effects include increase of anxiety or psychotropic effects. In some patients anxiety may be treated by lorazepam 12.5 mg every 8 h. If dyspnea is refractory to opioids and other treatments, palliative sedation with benzodiazepines or neuroleptics may be indicated.

9.8   Treatment of Delirium

Delirium with agitation, hallucinations, and restlessness is common during the final days of life (Lawlor and Bruera 2002). Delirium may be caused by metabolic changes (e.g., hypercalcemia, opioid metabolites); dehydration; drugs such as corticosteroids, opioids, and anticholinergic agents; or drug interactions. A full bladder, pain, dyspnea, and withdrawal from alcohol or benzodiazepines are also known to cause dyspnea.

Treatment includes stopping unnecessary medications, reversing metabolic abnormalities (if consistent with the goals of care), and treating the symptoms of delirium.

Delirium can be treated with haloperidol, 1–4 mg (orally, intravenously, or subcutaneously). Other drugs that may be effective are benzodiazepines (such as lorazepam) or atypical antipsychotics. In intractable cases of delirium, palliative sedation may be justifiable. Family members and professional carers observing delirium may experience considerable distress, and particularly relatives will need thorough information and support.

9.9   Death Rattle

Death rattle occurs when saliva accumulates in the oropharynx and upper airways in a patient who is too weak to clear the throat. Rattle is an indicator of impending death, with an incidence of approximately 50 % in people who are actively dying. There are two different types of rattle which can be identified: type 1, where rattle is caused by salivary secretions, and type 2, where rattle is caused by deeper bronchial secretions (Wildiers and Menten 2002).

The pharmacological treatment of rattle includes antimuscarinic agents such as scopolamine or glycopyrrolate to reduce secretion. Scopolamine is available in transdermal formulations. Glycopyrrolate (Robinul) is available for parenteral administration. Doses typically range from 0.1 mg to 0.2 mg IV or SC every 4 h.

If the cause of rattle is deep fluid accumulation, there is no effective treatment in the last hours of life, which is more stressful for relatives than for the patient. Sometimes opioids in small doses or change of position on the side (30°) is helpful to reduce rattle.

9.10   Treatment of Other Symptoms

Other symptoms, such as nausea, vomiting, and constipation, occur less frequently in the final phase, but complementary and nursing care are essential components of symptom control. This includes mouth care for management of a sore or dry mouth, quark poultices for lymphedema, and bed baths and rubs for profuse sweating and itching; also compresses, acupressure, or acupuncture can be useful. The combination of various treatment approaches not only broadens the range of effects but also may have a positive influence on the occurrence of side effects of medical treatment.

9.11   Palliative Sedation

Palliative sedation is an important and necessary therapy in the care of selected palliative care patients with otherwise refractory distress. The use of palliative sedation requires due caution and good clinical practice and is particularly controversial for psychosocial and existential symptoms. Harmful and unethical practice may undermine the credibility and reputation of the responsible clinicians and institutions as well as the discipline of palliative medicine more generally (Cherny et al. 2009). The framework for the use of sedation in palliative care recommended by the European Association for Palliative Care may be a useful resource to get a guideline (Cherny et al. 2009).

Relatives need continuous information and professional guidance when palliative sedation is used.

References

Adam J (1997) The last 48 hours. BMJ 315:1600–1603

Back IN, Jenkins K, Blower A et al (2001) A study comparing hyoscine hydrobromide and glycopyrrolate in the treatment of death rattle. Palliat Med 15(4):329–336

Booth S, Wade R, Johnson M et al (2004) The use of oxygen in the palliation of breathlessness. A report of the expert working group of the Scientific Committee of the Association of Palliative Medicine. Respir Med 98(1):66–77

Cherny NI, Radbruch L, Board of the European Association for Palliative Care (2009) European Association for Palliative Care (EAPC) recommended framework for the use of sedation in palliative care. Palliat Med 23(7):581–593

Christakis NA, Lamont EB (2000) Extent and determinants of error in doctors' prognoses in terminally ill patients: prospective cohort study. BMJ 320:469–473

Conill C et al (1997) Symptom prevalence in the last week of life. J Pain Symptom Manage 14(6):328–331

Enting RH, Oldenmenger WH, van der Rijt CC, Wilms EB, Elfrink EJ, Elswijk I et al (2002) A prospective study evaluating the response of patients with unrelieved cancer pain to parenteral opioids. Cancer 94(11):3049–3056

Hall P, Schroder C, Weaver L (2002) The last 48 hours of life in long-term care: a focused chart audit. J Am Geriatr Soc 50(3):501–506

Hanks GW (1996) Morphine in cancer pain: modes of administration. Expert Working Group of the European Association for Palliative Care. BMJ 312(7034):823–826

Hardy J, Nauck F (2009) Opioids for cancer pain. In: Walsh TD, Caraceni AT, Fainsinger R, Foley KM, Glare P, Goh C, Lloyd-Williams M, Nunez Olarte J, Radbruch L (eds) Palliative medicine. Saunders Elsevier, Philadelphia, pp 1404–1411. ISBN 978-0-323-056748

Javier NS, Montagnini ML (2011) Rehabilitation of the hospice and palliative care patient. J Palliat Med 14(5):638–648

Jonen-Thielemann I (2007) Sterbephase in der Palliativmedizin. In: Aulbert E, Nauck F, Radbruch L (eds) Lehrbuch der Palliativmedizin. 2. vollst. überarb. u. erw. Aufl., Schattauer, Stuttgart, pp 176–209

Kaye P (1992) Terminal phase. In: Kaye P (ed) Notes on symptom control in hospice and palliative care. Hospice Education Institute, Essex, pp 296–300

Lawlor PG, Bruera ED (2002) Delirium in patients with advanced cancer. Hematol Oncol Clin North Am 16(3):701–714

Lichter I, Hunt E (1990) The last 48 hours of life. J Palliat Care 6(4):7–15

Lynn J et al (1997) Prognoses of seriously ill hospitalized patients on the days before death: implications for patient care and public policy. New Horiz 5:56–61

Maier R, Maier A, Müller-Busch C (2008) Outpatient opiate therapy in cancer patients during their last days of life. Schmerz 22(2):148, 150–155

Mercadante S, Radbruch L, Davies A, Poulain P, Sitte T, Perkins P, Colberg T, Camba MA (2009) A comparison of intranasal fentanyl spray with oral transmucosal fentanyl citrate for the treatment of breakthrough cancer pain: an open-label, randomised, crossover trial [In Process Citation]. Curr Med Res Opin (England) 25(11):2805–2815

Morita T, Tsunoda J, Inoue S et al (1999) Contributing factors to physical symptoms in terminally-ill cancer patients. J Pain Symptom Manage 18(5):338–346

Nauck F (1994) Der Patient in der Finalphase. In: Klaschik E, Nauck F (eds) Palliativmedizin Heute. Springer, Berlin/Heidelberg/New York/London/Paris/Tokyo/Hong Kong/Barcelona/Budapest, pp 42–50

Nauck F (2001) Symptom control in the terminal phase. Schmerz 15(5):362–369

Nauck F, Klaschik E, Ostgathe C (2000) Symptoms and symptom control during the last three days of life. Eur J Palliat Care 7(3):81–84

Nauck F, Ostgathe C, Dickerson ED (2001) A German model for methadone conversion. Am J Hosp Palliat Care 18(3):200–202

Pattison M, Romer AL (2001) Improving care through the end of life: launching a primary care clinic-based program. J Palliat Med 4(2):249–254

Potter J, Hami F, Bryan T et al (2003) Symptoms in 400 patients referred to palliative care services: prevalence and patterns. Palliat Med 17(4):310–314

Quigley C (2004) Opioid switching to improve pain relief and drug tolerability. Cochrane Database Syst Rev (3):CD004847

Saunders C (1976) Care of the dying – 1 The problem of euthanasia. Nursing Times July 1, pp 1003–1005

Saunders C (1988) Pain and impending death. In: Wall P, Melzack R (eds) Textbook of pain. Churchill Livingstone, Edinburgh/New York, pp 624–631

Sepúlveda C, Marlin A, Yoshida T, Ulrich A (2002) Palliative care: the World Health Organization's global perspective. J Pain Symptom Manage 24:91–96

Stiel S, Radbruch L (2014) Prognosestellung bei schwer kranken Menschen. Palliativmedizin 15(03):109–121

Stiel S, Bertram L, Neuhaus S, Nauck F, Ostgathe C, Elsner F, Radbruch L (2010) Evaluation and comparison of two prognostic scores and the physicians' estimate of survival in terminally ill patients. Support Care Cancer 18(1):43–49

Temel J, Greer J, Muzikansky A, Gallagher E, Admane S, Jackson V, Dahlin C, Blindermann C, Jacobsen J, Pirl W, Billings A, Lynch T (2010) Early palliative care for patients with metastatic non-small-cell lung cancer. N Engl J Med 363:733–742

Thomas JR, von Gunten CF (2002) Clinical management of dyspnoea. Lancet Oncol 3(4):223–228

Twycross G, Lichter I (1998) The terminal phase. In: Doyle D, Hanks GWC, MacDonald N (eds) Oxford textbook of palliative medicine, 2nd edn. Oxford University Press, Oxford/New York/Tokyo, pp 977–990

WHO (1996) Cancer pain relief, with a guide to opioid availability, 2nd edn. World Health Organisation (WHO), Geneva

Wildiers H, Menten J (2002) Death rattle: prevalence, prevention and treatment. J Pain Symptom Manage 23(4):310–317

Zeppetella G, Ribeiro MD (2006) Opioids for the management of breakthrough (episodic) pain in cancer patients. Cochrane Database Syst Rev (1):CD004311

Part IV

Pharmacological Aspects

Constanze Rémi and Claudia Bausewein

Contents

10.1   A Short Introduction on Pharmacokinetics

Pharmacokinetics describes the pathway of a drug through the body. The pharmacokinetic properties of a drug are described by the time-dependent processes liberation, absorption, distribution, metabolism, and elimination ("LADME"; Table 10.1).

Knowledge about the pharmacokinetic properties of a drug is crucial for an effective drug therapy because adequate drug doses must be delivered to the target site before a drug can unfold its pharmacodynamic properties (therapeutic effect) at the anticipated site of action. The pharmacokinetic characteristics of a drug determine the optimal therapeutic regimen, especially the route and frequency of drug administration. Pharmacokinetic properties of one drug can vary with different formulations. This allows one to be more flexible within a therapeutic regimen, but also requires an increased level of attention in prescribing and administering a drug

C. Rémi, MSc (✉) • C. Bausewein, MD, PhD, MSc
Department of Palliative Medicine, University of Munich, Munich, Germany
e-mail: Constanze.Remi@med.uni-muenchen.de; claudia.bausewein@med.uni-muenchen.de

© Springer-Verlag Berlin Heidelberg 2015
B. Alt-Epping, F. Nauck (eds.), *Palliative Care in Oncology*,
DOI 10.1007/978-3-662-46202-7_10

Table 10.1 Pharmacokinetic processes

Description	Might be influenced by
*L*iberation of the drug from the dosage form	Changes in gastric pH (drug–drug or drug–food interactions), drug formulation
*A*bsorption of the drug into the systemic circulation	Changes in gastric emptying, intestinal transit, drug complexation (drug–drug or drug–food interactions)
*D*istribution of the drug within the body	Nutritional status, comorbidities, age
*M*etabolism (biotransformation) of the drug by the liver, kidney, or other tissues	Drug interactions, hepatic impairment, renal impairment
*E*limination of the drug from the body	Hepatic impairment, renal impairment

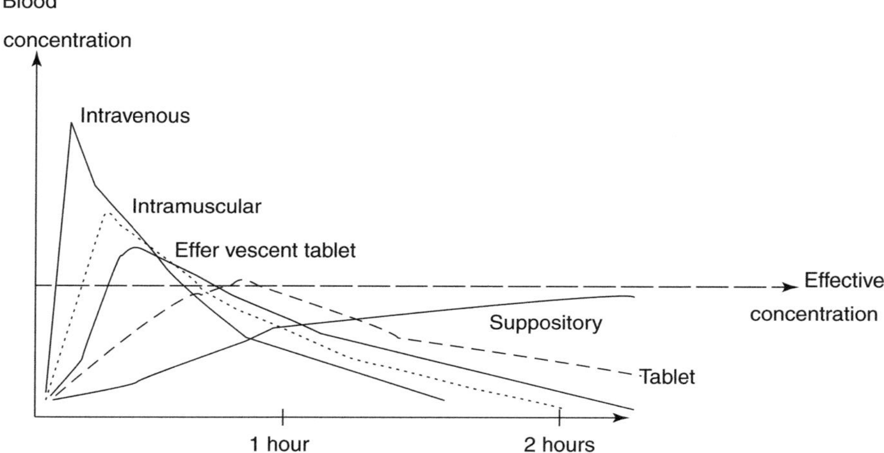

Fig. 10.1 Blood concentrations depending on mode of application (based on first order kinetics in a one-compartement model; adapted from (Garrett E.R. 1994)

that is available in different formulations. Pharmacokinetics can change significantly in certain patient populations, especially in the elderly and in patients with organ failure (see below). Depending on the mode of administration, different plasma concentration time curves can be achieved, and, accordingly, onset and duration of action may vary as well as the side-effect profile. An i.v. bolus of morphine, for example, will result in a steep increase in morphine blood levels, a high peak concentration, and a fast onset of action (Fig. 10.1). At the same time, the risk of central side effects such as respiratory depression or sedation might increase. The drug will also be eliminated faster from systemic circulation, with a shorter duration of action than for other methods of administration. In contrast to the concentration time curve after an i.v. bolus of morphine, the drug first needs to be liberated from its formulation after oral administration. After this process, differences in membrane permeability contribute to the varying degrees of drug absorption throughout the gastrointestinal tract (Fleisher et al. 1999). After absorption, the drug passes the liver before morphine and its active and inactive metabolites are distributed in the body and reach their site of action.

To achieve the best therapeutic results, it is essential to combine the best pharmacokinetic and pharmacodynamic properties of a drug and different drug formulations, for instance, use slow-release formulations for baseline therapy and short-acting formulations for breakthrough situations.

10.2 Routes of Drug Administration

Many drugs are available in a variety of different formulations that offer the option to individualize a therapeutic regimen to current circumstances and patients' needs. The modes of administration vary from oral to sublingual, intranasal, and parenteral routes such as intravenous, subcutaneous, or intramuscular. Some drugs are absorbed transdermally or find their way into the body through inhalation into the lungs.

The potential routes of drug administration are determined by drug properties and therapeutic considerations such as intended onset of action, duration of action, chronic use, and local or systemic effects. Various factors influence the choice of the route of drug administration in clinical practice, for instance:

- Availability of different drug formulations and their license status.
- Desired onset of action and duration of therapy.
- Drug properties; certain cytotoxic drugs are highly irritant and/or have a high osmolality and must therefore be administered via a central line.
- Setting and resources.

Every route of drug administration has its advantages and disadvantages (see Table 10.2). The intravenous route ensures a rapid onset of action and a high bioavailability. At the same time, it is always associated with the need for trained staff, higher staff utilization, and the need for additional equipment. Furthermore, it bears a higher risk of infectious complications, can be more cost intense, and might be a potential barrier for care at home. In oncology, many patients receive their cytotoxic drugs via a portacath, which then can be easily used in palliative care. Patient choice has also to be taken into account. It has to be acknowledged that the preferred route of drug administration might change in certain circumstances and as the disease progresses and patients become unable or are unwilling to take their medication orally. Therefore, drugs will almost always be administered via the parenteral route in the terminal phase, with intravenous and subcutaneous administration as the most preferred routes.

The most suitable route of administration certainly depends on the actual needs, problems, and phase of the illness of a patient: whereas a more noninvasive route of administration (e.g., oral) with high autonomy might be most appropriate for a fully ambulant patient, this might change when a patient becomes weaker or swallowing drugs becomes an unsurmountable burden. A comparison of different routes of drug administration in cancer pain management found that efficacy and safety of rectal, transdermal, subcutaneous, and intravenous routes of drug administration are

Table 10.2 Routes of drug administration

Route	Advantage	Disadvantage
Oral	Most frequently used Noninvasive Convenient Well known Economic Various drug formulations (e.g., immediate release, extended release) available High stability of solid dosage forms Relatively easy to use Safe and acceptable	Dependent on capability to swallow Dependent on gastrointestinal drug absorption Drug–drug and drug–food interactions might impact on onset of action and bioavailability Depending on drug formulation: relatively slow onset of action Highly dependent on patient compliance
Sublingual	Rapid absorption Convenience of drug administration Decreased need for swallowing Avoidance of first-pass metabolism	Limited to special formulations (Inadvertent) swallowing might result in loss of effect → Increased need for patient education
Intranasal	Rapid absorption Convenience of drug administration No need for swallowing Avoidance of first-pass metabolism	Limited to drugs with eligible properties Only applicable for small volumes Local tolerability
Inhalational	Rapid delivery (similar to parenteral route)[a] First-pass metabolism avoided	Limited to drugs with adequate properties Availability of suitable dosage form Need for special equipment
Rectal	Drug administration in patients who are unable to swallow Local and/or systemic effects	Availability of suitable dosage form Unpredictable drug absorption Patient acceptability Carer acceptability
Topical/Transdermal	Local drug administration without or little systemic effects (topical) Continuous (systemic) drug delivery possible (transdermal) Noninvasive Lower frequency of drug administration For patients unable to swallow	Increased need of explanation Transdermal: low flexibility in available dosage regimen Mostly slow onset of action

Table 10.2 (continued)

Route	Advantage	Disadvantage
Parenteral	**Parenteral**	**Parenteral**
	Rapid onset of action Avoidance of gastrointestinal tract Administration of drugs that are poorly absorbed or unstable in the gastrointestinal tract High bioavailability Independent of level of consciousness	Higher staff utilization Training of staff Supporting equipment required High requirements for parenteral drug preparation (e.g., aseptic working) High risk of infection compared with other routes Potentially painful Lack of flexibility with continuous infusion regimen Combination of different drugs is challenging Lack of compatibility data for some mixtures
Intravenous	**Intravenous**	**Intravenous**
	High control over circulating drug levels Intermittent and continuous administration of (large volumes of) drugs and fluids possible	Availability of parenteral drug formulation
Subcutaneous	**Subcutaneous**	**Subcutaneous**
	Intermittent and continuous administration of drugs and fluids possible	Unlicensed for most drugs Only small volumes Lack of pharmacokinetic data (e.g., bioavailability → conversion from p.o. to s.c.)
Intramuscular	**Intramuscular**	**Intramuscular**
	Long-acting formulations available	More likely to be painful Restricted to intermittent injections and small volumes

[a]If drug properties allow direct absorption at the site of administration

comparable and are all good alternatives for cancer patients if the oral route is not possible (Radbruch et al. 2011). Clinical characteristics for the various routes are considered in Table 10.3.

Drug therapy, including routes of drug administration, always needs to be planned in anticipation of complications that might occur in the near future. Patients'

Table 10.3 Clinical characteristics of various routes of administration (Davies et al. 2011)

	Onset of action	Sustained action	i.v. access and maintenance required	Injection frequency	Sites	Effect on mobility	Complications
Oral	Gradual	Yes	No	None	n/a	None	Rare
Rectal	Gradual	Yes	No	None	n/a	None	Uncommon, local irritations
Buccal or sublingual	Moderately rapid	No	No	None	n/a	None	Rare
Intravenous	Rapid	No	Yes	Frequent, every 3–4 h	Limited due to intravenous access change every 2–3 days	Moderate, need injection every 3–4 h	Uncommon, but could be serious, infection, sepsis
Continuous intravenous	Rapid	Yes	Yes	Frequent, every 2–3 days	Limited due to intravenous access change every 2–3 days	Mild if portable pump is used	Uncommon, but could be serious, infection, sepsis
Subcutaneous	Moderately rapid	No	No	Frequent, every 3–4 h	Limited due to number of injections	Moderate, need injection every 3–4 h	Uncommon, but could be serious, abscess formation, bleeding
Continuous subcutaneous	Moderately rapid	Yes	No	Infrequent every 7 days	Unlimited, many sites with site change every 7 days	Mild if portable pump is used	Uncommon, local irritation

N/A not applicable

acceptability and preferences of different routes of drug administration can vary depending on the type of symptom as well as because of cultural differences (Simon et al. 2012; Davies et al. 2011). The care setting, including preferences of place of care and potential carers, needs to be taken into consideration as well as local infrastructure, policies, or legal aspects. In some settings, for example, it might be difficult to have intermittent regular injections administered on time, and a continuous i.v. or s.c. infusion might be more likely to provide better round-the-clock comfort. Furthermore, the care and change of the peripheral vein or port needles might not be supported because specially trained nurses or doctors might be obligatory, cartridges might only be prepared by specialized pharmacies, etc.

10.2.1 Enteral Drug Administration

Some conditions may require the placement of enteral feeding tubes such as in oropharyngeal cancer. These tubes can also be used for drug administration, although most drugs are not licensed for use via feeding tubes. Drug administration via enteral feeding tube is dependent on the type and location of the feeding tube and on drug properties (e.g., absorption site within the gastrointestinal tract) and formulation. A variety of enteral feeding tubes are available. They are typically classified by site of insertion and location of the distal tip of the feeding tube (Williams 2008). Not all drugs can be crushed, as breaking might result in reduced effectiveness, increased risk of toxicity, reduced stability, or significant changes in the pharmacokinetic profile. In cmr substances (carcinogenic, mutagenic, or toxic for reproduction), crushing can impose risk to healthcare professionals or carers that prepare the medication. Therefore, care has to be taken when converting a regimen to ensure safety and efficacy of drug administration via enteral feeding tubes. The following aspects should be considered when drug administration via a feeding tube becomes necessary (Williams 2008; Gilbar 1999):
If cmr substance, check:

- Availability of liquid formulation: check tonicity, pH, and sorbitol content.
- Solid dosage forms: check whether manipulation is possible (e.g., crushing or opening), diluent choice (preferably water), or if an extemporaneously prepared oral suspension is available.
- Absorption site.
- Alternative routes of administration and dosage forms: rectal, transdermal, and parenteral.
- Drug–formula interaction, drug–drug interactions, and drug–tube interaction.

In general, liquid medications should be preferred for enteral administration. These might be hypertonic or contain sorbitol in large amounts, which causes irritations or a laxative effect. Therefore, not all liquid drugs are suitable for every patient. Crushing of solid dosage forms is not always possible either for various reasons, such as modified-release formulation, stability issues, or toxic potential. Some drugs may interact with the tube material, for instance, phenytoin, which results in decreased bioavailability (Zhu and Zhou 2013).

All drugs have to be administered separately and the tube needs to be flushed with water before and after administration of each drug. Incorrect administration methods may result in clogged feeding tubes, decreased drug efficacy, increased adverse effects, or drug–formula incompatibilities (Williams 2008).

Whether a drug can be administered via an enteral feeding tube has to be assessed independently for every single licensed product because available formulations may vary.

Guidance on enteral drug administration is available from several organizations, for example, from the Society of Hospital Pharmacists of Australia (SHPA) (S.o.H.P.o. Australia 2011).

10.2.2 Parenteral Drug Administration

Intravenous (peripheral or central), intramuscular, and subcutaneous drug administration are common routes in oncology and palliative care. Parenteral drug administration can become necessary during the course of illness, for instance, with persistent nausea and vomiting or dysphagia. It can be a helpful temporary or permanent alternative route of drug administration. For opioid administration, the subcutaneous route is considered as an alternative route of choice for patients who are unable to receive opioids by oral or transdermal routes (Caraceni et al. 2012). In cases where the subcutaneous administration is contraindicated (e.g., because of peripheral edema, coagulation disorders, poor peripheral circulation, and need for large volumes and doses), the intravenous route can be an alternative (Caraceni et al. 2012). The intravenous route is preferable when a rapid opioid dose titration for pain control is necessary (Caraceni et al. 2012). These recommendations can probably be extrapolated for the control of other distressing symptoms, although one should bear in mind that patients referred to palliative care services will potentially already have some sort of central venous catheters (CVC).

If parenteral access by CVC already exists, the potential benefits of additional subcutaneous access should be weighed against the risks. Indications for CVCs include patients with limited venous access, patients with prolonged or continuous i.v. infusions, and patients receiving vesicants, for example, doxorubicin (Schiffer et al. 2013). There is a variety of CVC used in clinical practice. Some of the most common types are subcutaneous implanted port-chamber catheters (e.g., Port-A-Cath) and peripherally inserted central venous catheters (PICC) (Schiffer et al. 2013). CVCs might provide a higher level of comfort to the patient because of a decreased need for painful venipunctures and less mobility constraints than for peripheral vein access (Yamada et al. 2010). At the same time, CVCs bear the potential for serious complications. Late complications that are not directly associated with catheter placement include infection, thrombosis, and catheter malfunction. Infections can lead from localized entrance/exit site infections and tunnel infections to catheter-related blood-stream infections (BSI). The risk varies between catheter type and local and national standards (Schiffer et al. 2013; Chopra et al. 2012; Hansen et al. 2009). The use of anti-infective catheters, for example, is clinically effective in reducing the risk of infection. However, their use has to be integrated in the appropriate use of other practical care initiatives (Hockenhull et al. 2008). To minimize the risk for such complications, the usual requirements in catheter care also apply for palliative care patients. The presence of central venous access reduces or even eliminates the need for routine replacement of peripheral intravenous catheters. Recommendations on catheter care and the prevention of catheter-related infections have been issued by different institutions, such as the CDC guidelines for the prevention of intravascular catheter-related infections, the IDSA 2009 update of the clinical practice guidelines for the diagnosis and management of intravascular catheter-related infection, or the recommendations by the German Robert Koch Institute on the prevention on intravascular catheter-related infections (O'Grady et al. 2011; Mermel et al. 2009; Prävention Gefäßkatheterassoziierter 2002).

The subcutaneous application of drugs and fluids is common in palliative care when patients are unable to swallow and other routes of administration are not applicable, unacceptable, or not feasible in the specific setting (e.g., care at home) (Fonzo-Christe et al. 2005; Menahem and Shvartzman 2010). The subcutaneous route allows one to use infusion sites independent of veins and vein status (Mitten 2001). The most common areas suitable for subcutaneous application are the abdomen and both thighs (see Fig. 10.2). The upper arms and the anterior thoracic wall are also frequently used. Sometimes the upper areas of the back can be used for agitated patients because patients cannot pull out the s.c. needle. The infusion site should be rotated regularly. A change every 72 h is sometimes recommended. However, in some patients, and dependent on the cannulae used, changes may only be necessary every 5–7 days (Dickman et al. 2011; Morgan and Evans 2004).

Areas that should be avoided for subcutaneous access, if possible, are (Mitten 2001):

- Areas of broken skin
- Skin folds and breast tissue
- Lymphedematous areas (absorption may be reduced)
- Sites of tumor or infection
- Bony prominences
- Recently irradiated skin
- Sites near a joint

Drugs can be administered by intermittent injection or continuous infusion, for example, using infusion pumps (see below) (Menahem and Shvartzman 2010;

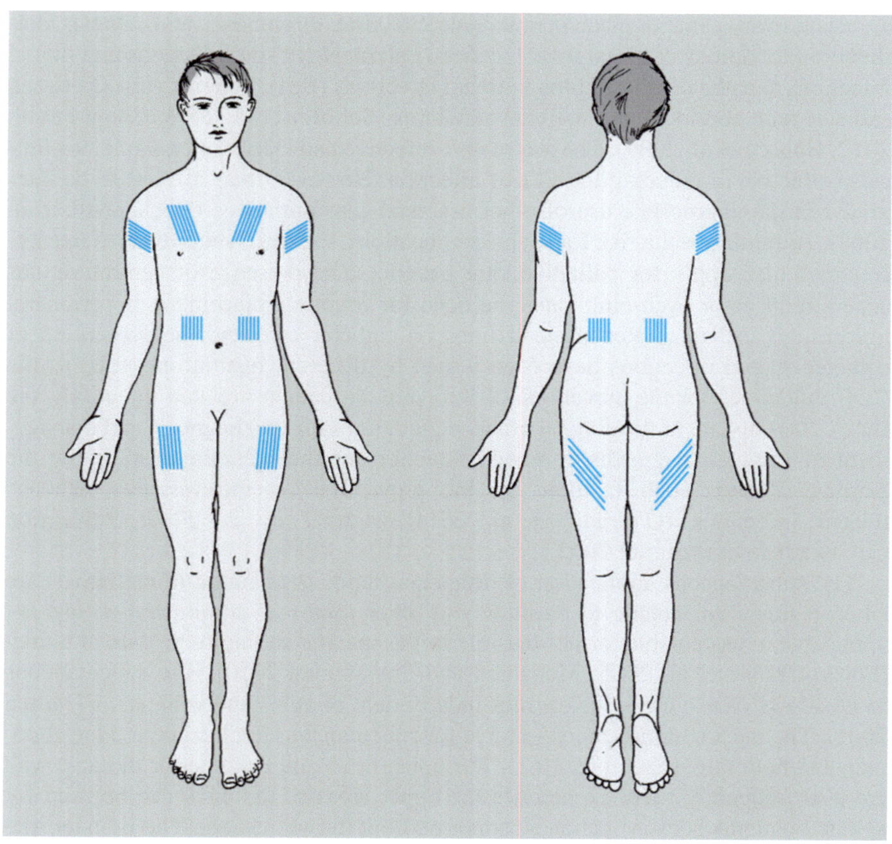

Fig. 10.2 Body map indicating areas suitable for subcutaneous access (Mitten 2001)

Herndon and Fike 2001). Only few drugs used in symptom control in palliative care are licensed for this route of administration, and therefore, a significant proportion is used off label (Fonzo-Christe et al. 2005; Hafner 2013). The applicability of parenteral drug solutions by the intravenous and intramuscular route is limited by the osmolarity and the tonicity (2011; Parenteralia 5.2/0520 2012; Jauch et al. 2007). There are no official recommendations regarding osmolarity and pH for the subcutaneous route of drug administration, and the evidence is scarce (Table 10.4) (Schneider et al. 1997).

Parenteral drug therapy is not only limited by the availability of a suitable drug formulation but also by the number of drugs that can be administered concomitantly. Compatibility data for mixtures with two and more drugs are often scarce.

Table 10.4 Infusion pumps

Mechanism	Examples	Description of operation mode	Disadvantages	Advantages
	CADD® Legacy PCA, Rhythmic®, Plus, Curlin® 6000 CMS	Drug solution delivered from a reservoir (cartridge or bag) by a pump with a set of rollers that pinches down on a length of flexible tubing (drug solution is pushed forward)	High cost of purchase Special supporting equipment needed Regular training of staff necessary Relatively heavy compared with other systems	Small and easy transportable devices available Flexible dosing regimens (e.g., rate of infusion, bolus volume) High-volume cartridges (e.g., 250 ml) available Various pump-operating programs available Automatic documentation of given doses, number of boluses, etc. Various alarm options High accuracy of infusion rate Operated by battery or other power source
Syringe driver	Sims Deltec MS26®	Normal syringe is clamped onto the device and the plunger is pressed at a precisely controlled rate	Limited to small volumes (10–30 ml) Limited boost function No lockout period High level of staff training required Power source necessary	Low cost for device and supporting medical equipment Lightweight Battery operated
	Perfusor®		High acquisition cost Stationary system Power source necessary In general no patient-controlled boost function	Low cost for supporting medical equipment Widespread use in hospitals
Elastomeric pump	Surefuser®, Easypump®	Stretchable balloon is filled and delivers drug fluid depending on wall pressure and fluid restrictor (for flow-rate control)	Relatively expensive single-use disposable system No bolus function, no changes in infusion rate possible	Helpful for short-term bridging Available for a variety of different volumes Lightweight No need for a power source Maintenance-free

10.3 Infusion Devices and Drug Compatibility

For the round-the-clock provision of a drug, a continuous infusion can be more comfortable than intermittent injections. Continuous intravenous or subcutaneous drug administration can be carried out by infusion of a drug by gravity drip or by using an (electronic) infusion pump. The use of infusion pumps is often recommended for safety and reliability reasons. However, infusion by a gravity drip may be easier and more readily available, depending on the drug to be infused and the healthcare setting. With gravity infusion, the drop factor (drops that equal 1 ml) of the tubing used needs to be identified. When using electronic pumps, the volume per time unit can be set (Menahem and Shvartzman 2010). The rate of infusion depends on the individual rate of absorption. A common rate is 2–3 ml/h or 50 ml/24 h.

The most classical infusion devices in palliative care that are used for continuous subcutaneous drug administration are syringe drivers (O'Doherty et al. 2001; Wilcock et al. 2006). Due to safety concerns, the most commonly used devices, Smiths Medical (formerly Graseby) MS26 and MS16A, are currently phased out in the United Kingdom. International standards and safety features should be acknowledged when choosing a suitable infusion device (I.E. Commission 2012).

The following factors need to be considered when choosing a device:

- Rate setting in *milliliters* (ml) per hour
- A mechanism to stop the infusion if the syringe is not properly and securely fitted
- An alarm that activates if the syringe is removed before the infusion is stopped
- Lockbox cover and/or lockout controlled by a password
- Provision of internal log memory to record all infusion device events (Patient Safety Agency) 2010)

Other systems are available, such as infusion pumps, which are used for patient-controlled analgesia (PCA), or elastomeric pumps (such as used for chemotherapy). With the use of many infusion devices, independence and mobility of the patient can be maintained because many devices are lightweight and can be worn under or over clothes. Every infusion device has its own characteristics, differs in extra equipment needed, etc. Therefore, professionals need to familiarize themselves with a few devices instead of using every new technology available.

Regardless of the infusion method, infusion settings need to be double-checked. Regular checks of the infusion device, the visual appearance of the infusion, and of the administration site have to be performed during the infusion. The infusion device and the infusion solution have to be checked in use. When mixing drugs, it is essential to consider drug compatibility. Not all drugs can be mixed in one syringe because of the risk of incompatibility. The consequences of incompatibility may be loss of therapeutic activity, production of a toxic product, and local irritations (Rose and Currow 2009). To avoid deleterious effects on the patient, the following aspects need to be acknowledged:

- Check for stability and compatibility data.
- Mixing of as few drugs as possible.

- Mixing for a period as short as possible.
- Prefer mixtures with known compatibility and stability data.
- Prefer mixing drugs with similar pH.
- Do not mix drugs with low solubility.

To reduce the number of drugs in a pump, drugs with a long duration of action should be administered once or twice daily as bolus injection, for example, dexamethasone.

For patients needing parenteral drug or infusion therapy, the route of administration and catheter type should be influenced by the drugs or solutions used, expected duration of therapy, prognosis, and the patients' or carers' ability to provide care when a catheter is used. Future needs should be considered (Schiffer et al. 2013).

10.4 Drug Therapy in Metabolic Derangements

10.4.1 Hepatic Impairment

The liver is the main site for the biotransformation of drugs and other compounds. In consequence, hepatic impairment can have great impact on the pharmacokinetics and subsequently the pharmacodynamics of certain drugs. Considering the pharmacokinetic processes described above, the changes might be the following (Schlatter et al. 2009):

- Absorption: increased bioavailability in drugs with high first-pass metabolism.
- Distribution: might be increased in patients with ascites, edema, and hypoalbuminemia. Might also decrease due to muscle loss and dehydration.
- Metabolism: decreased CYP P450 metabolism in severe impairment.
- Elimination: renal and biliary excretion might decrease due to changes in metabolism or hepatorenal syndrome.

There are many reasons for hepatic impairment (Schlatter et al. 2009; Schlatter 2008). Liver dysfunction in an oncology patient might be affected by the primary liver tumor, metastases, cirrhosis, or as a result of hepatotoxic effects of the drug treatment. Assessing the impact of liver function on drug therapy is not as straightforward as in renal impairment. The use of biochemical markers is of limited benefit. Measures used to assess the degree of liver dysfunction are the Child–Pugh classification or the Model for End-Stage Liver Disease (MELD) score (Pugh et al. 1973; Kamath et al. 2001). However, these measures have only limited usefulness in predicting the capacity of the liver to metabolize drugs (Schlatter et al. 2009). The impact of chronic liver disease on drug metabolism is easier to predict than in acute liver impairment (Sloss 2009). Portosystemic shunts can lead to a direct transport of a drug from the gut to the systemic circulation, bypassing the liver and therefore first-pass metabolism (Sloss 2009). An impact of liver disease on phase I metabolism (oxidation, reduction, e.g., CYP P450) has to be expected in extensive destructive or metastatic disease or in advanced cirrhosis (Rhee and Broadbent 2007). Phase II metabolism (conjugation) is less often affected (Rhee and Broadbent 2007).

Hepatic clearance of a compound mainly depends on three factors: blood flow to hepatocytes (→ metabolic cells), functional hepatocytes, and extent of binding to albumin and other blood compounds affected by liver disease (Sloss 2009). Hepatic clearance is defined as the volume of blood from which this substance is removed completely by the liver per time unit (Schlatter et al. 2009). According to the extent of hepatic clearance, drugs can be classified as high-, intermediate-, and low-extraction drugs. The clearance of high-extraction drugs mainly depends on and is limited by hepatic blood flow and that of low-extraction drugs on hepatocyte function. High-extraction drugs are mainly affected by portosystemic shunts and other alterations in hepatic blood flow. It is therefore recommended to reduce the initial oral drug dose. The maintenance dose has to be adapted. For parenteral therapy, only the maintenance dose has to be reduced (Schlatter et al. 2009). In patients with portosystemic shunts, the bioavailability of high-extraction drugs is assumed to be 100 %. An equation that can be used to calculate the adapted dose for high-extraction drugs is:

reduced dose=(normal dose × normal bioavailability)/100 (Delco et al. 2005).

The hepatic clearance of low-extraction drugs is primarily limited by the capacity of hepatic enzymes to metabolize the drug, primarily CYP P450. Portosystemic shunts do not have a significant impact on the systemic bioavailability of low-extraction drugs. Therefore, the initial oral dose can remain the same as in normal hepatic function. The maintenance dose may have to be reduced by about 50 %. The same applies to parenteral drug dosing (Schlatter 2008). Intermediate-extraction drugs are influenced by both hepatic blood flow and enzymatic capacity, although not to the same extent. Therefore, a lower starting dose is advisable in oral dosing; the maintenance dose should be reduced by about 50 % (Schlatter et al. 2009; Schlatter 2008). In cholestasis, biliary excretion of drugs can be reduced.

The net effect of pharmacokinetic changes will most likely be an increase in drug exposure due to a higher extent of absorption and a decrease in elimination. Subsequently, higher systemic drug exposure can increase the risk of adverse drug reactions. Furthermore, patients might be more susceptible to central nervous effects including side effects of a drug due to changes in pharmacokinetics and body composition (e.g., loss of integrity of the blood–brain barrier) (Rhee and Broadbent 2007).

Guidance on analgesic drug dosing in liver failure can be found in Table 10.5. More information on drug use in hepatic impairment is available at http://livertox.nih.gov/index.html.

10.4.2 Renal Impairment

Renal impairment mainly occurs in the elderly with the consequence that it affects both the pharmacokinetic and pharmacodynamic properties of many drugs. Some drugs are converted into active metabolites, which are dependent on the kidney for elimination, and these accumulate in patients with diminished kidney function (Drayer 1976). This may lead to increased side effects and toxicity that can potentially harm the patients. Prolonged half-life and a longer time to reach steady state are other potential problems.

Table 10.5 Drug dosing of analgesics and coanalgesics in hepatic or renal impairment (Schlatter et al. 2009; Schlatter 2008; Tegeder et al. 1999; Ashley and Currie 2009; Aronoff et al. 2007)

Drug	Renal impairment	Hepatic impairment	Comments
Paracetamol (acetaminophen)	Dose ↓ or dosing interval ↑	Dose ↓ or dosing interval ↑	Hepatic metabolism; renal elimination
	GFR 10–50 ml/min: every 6 h	Try to avoid if possible	Low hepatic extraction. Careful when used concomitantly with other hepatotoxic drugs or substances
	GFR < 10 ml/min: interval at least 8 h		
Ibuprofen	No adjustments; avoid if possible	Mild to moderate impairment: no adjustments	Hepatic metabolism; low hepatic extraction. Metabolites inactive; predominantly renal elimination; may decrease renal function
	Severe impairment: contraindicated	Severe impairment: contraindicated	
Diclofenac	No adjustments; avoid if possible	Mild to moderate impairment: no adjustments	Hepatic metabolism; low hepatic extraction. Metabolites inactive; predominantly renal elimination; may decrease renal function
	Severe impairment: contraindicated	Severe impairment: contraindicated	
Tramadol	GFR 20–50 ml/min: no adjustments	Dose ↓ or dosing interval ↑	Hepatic metabolism; metabolites partially pharmacologically active (O-desmethyltramadol); low hepatic extraction; predominantly renal elimination
	GFR 10–20 ml/min: 50–100 mg every 8 h initially; titrate according to response and tolerability	Severe impairment: contraindicated	Avoid if possible in renal failure
	GFR <10 ml/min: 50 mg every 8 h; avoid if possible		
Morphine	GFR 20–50 ml/min: 75 % of normal dose	Careful dosing	Hepatic metabolism; metabolites partially pharmacologically active (e.g., morphine-3-glucuronide M3G and morphine-6-glucuronide M6G); high hepatic extraction; renal elimination
	GFR 10–20 ml/min: use low doses and extended intervals; titrate according to response and tolerability		Avoid if possible in renal failure
	GFR < 10 ml/min: use low doses and extended intervals; titrate according to response and tolerability		

(continued)

Table 10.5 (continued)

Drug	Renal impairment	Hepatic impairment	Comments
Oxycodone	GFR 20–50 ml/min: no adjustments	Careful dosing	Hepatic metabolism; metabolites partially pharmacologically active (oxymorphone, noroxycodone); low hepatic extraction; renal and fecal elimination
	GFR 10–20 ml/min: no adjustments		
	GFR <10 ml/min: start with low doses and titrate according to response and tolerability		
Hydromorphone	GFR 20–50 ml/min: no adjustments	Careful dosing	Hepatic metabolism; metabolite might be pharmacologically active (hydromorphone-3-glucuronide); predominantly renal elimination
	GFR 10–20 ml/min: start with low doses and titrate according to response and tolerability		
	GFR <10 ml/min: start with low doses and titrate according to response and tolerability		
Fentanyl	GFR 20–50 ml/min: no adjustment	Careful dosing	Hepatic metabolism; metabolites inactive; high hepatic extraction; predominantly renal elimination
	GFR 10–20 ml/min: 75 % of normal dose		
	GFR <10 ml/min: 50 % of normal dose		
Amitriptyline	No adjustments	Dose ↓	Hepatic metabolism; metabolites pharmacologically active; intermediate hepatic extraction; elimination predominantly fecal
Duloxetine	GFR 20–50 ml/min: no adjustment	Contraindicated	Hepatic metabolism; metabolites inactive; high hepatic extraction predominantly renal elimination
	GFR 10–20 ml/min: start with low doses and titrate according to response and tolerability		
	GFR <10 ml/min: start with low doses and titrate according to response and tolerability		

Mirtazapine	GFR 20–50 ml/min: no adjustment	Careful dosing	Hepatic metabolism; metabolites partially active; intermediate hepatic extraction; renal and biliary elimination
	GFR 10–20 ml/min: no adjustment		
	GFR <10 ml/min: start with low doses and titrate according to response and tolerability		
Buprenorphine	GFR 20–50 ml/min: no adjustments	Dose ↓	Hepatic metabolism; metabolites partially pharmacologically active (e.g., norbuprenorphine); predominantly fecal elimination (about 27 % renal)
	GFR 20–50 ml/min: no adjustments, avoid very high doses		
	GFR <10 ml/min: start with low doses and titrate according to response and tolerability, avoid very high doses		
Pregabalin	GFR 30–60 ml/min: initial dose 75 mg daily, titrate according to tolerability and response	No adjustments	Hardly metabolized; renal elimination
	GFR 15–30 mg/min: Initial dose 25–50 mg daily, titrate according to tolerability and response		
	GFR <15 ml/min: Initial dose 25 mg daily, titrate according to tolerability and response		
Gabapentin	GFR 30–60 ml/min: start with low doses and titrate according to response and tolerability	No adjustments	Not metabolized; renal elimination
	GFR 15–30 mg/min: start with low doses and titrate according to response and tolerability		
	GFR <15 mg/min: 300 mg on alternate days or 100 mg		
	At night initially, increase according to tolerability		

The estimated glomerular filtration rate (eGFR) is widely used to estimate the extent of renal impairment. The only measurement of creatinine and urea is not sufficient to estimate the kidney function because creatinine levels in particular depend on the muscle mass of the individual, and this is often decreased in the elderly. Individual dose adjustments of drugs and reductions are necessary to avoid drug-related problems in advanced kidney failure. The range of necessary dose adjustment depends on the range of the therapeutic index, for instance, whether it is a wide range of margins, as with many antibiotics, or a narrow range, as with digoxin and aminoglycoside antibiotics (Brater 2009).

The need for dose reduction in renal impairment depends on the extent to which the drug and any active metabolite are renally excreted and how serious undesirable effects of the drug may be (Twycross and Wilcock 2012). The following principles of dose adjustment should be followed in patients with renal impairment (Twycross and Wilcock 2012):

- For drugs with minimal undesirable effects, a simple scheme for dose reduction is sufficient, that is, start low and monitor for efficacy and toxicity.
- For drugs with a narrow safety margin, dose adjustments should be based on a measure of renal function, for instance, creatinine clearance, which is often estimated using the Cockcroft–Gault formula.
- For drugs where both efficacy and/or toxicity are closely related to serum concentration, ongoing treatment must be adjusted according to clinical response and serum concentration, for example, gentamicin.

To safely prescribe drugs in renal impairment, both the dose and the application interval can be adjusted (Brater 2009). If the dose is adjusted, the interval between doses is kept the same as in a patient with normal renal function, and the individual dose is reduced in proportion to the decrease in clearance. If the interval is adjusted, each individual dose is kept the same as in a patient with normal renal function, and the interval between doses is increased so that the total daily dose is reduced in proportion to the decrease in clearance (Brater 2009). Both methods can also be combined with each individual dose and the interval between doses being adjusted so that the total daily dose is reduced in proportion to the decrease in clearance (Brater 2009).

In palliative care, renal failure is relevant to a number of drugs such as analgesics, opioids, anticonvulsants, or antidepressants. Table 10.5 gives an overview of relevant drugs and necessary adjustments.

References

Aronoff GR, Bennett WM, Burns JS (2007) Anagesics and Sedatives, hypnotics, and other drugs used in psychiatry. In: A.C.o. Physicians (ed) Drug prescribing in renal failure, 5th edn. American College of Physicians, Philadelphia
Ashley C, Currie A (2009) The renal drug handbook, 3rd edn. Radcliffe Publishing Ltd., Oxford
Brater DC (2009) Drug dosing in patients with impaired renal function. Clin Pharmacol Ther 86(5):483–489

Caraceni A et al (2012) Use of opioid analgesics in the treatment of cancer pain: evidence-based recommendations from the EAPC. Lancet Oncol 13(2):e58–e68

Chopra V et al (2012) Bloodstream infection, venous thrombosis, and peripherally inserted central catheters: reappraising the evidence. Am J Med 125(8):733–741

Davies A et al (2011) Multi-centre European study of breakthrough cancer pain: pain characteristics and patient perceptions of current and potential management strategies. Eur J Pain 15(7): 756–763

Delco F et al (2005) Dose adjustment in patients with liver disease. Drug Saf 28(6):529–545

Dickman A, Littlewood C, Varga J (2011) The syringe driver: continuous subcutaneous infusions. In: Palliative care, 3rd edn. Oxford University Press, Oxford

Drayer DE (1976) Pharmacologically active drug metabolites: therapeutic and toxic activities, plasma and urine data in man, accumulation in renal failure. Clin Pharmacokinet 1(6): 426–443

Fleisher D et al (1999) Drug, meal and formulation interactions influencing drug absorption after oral administration: clinical implications. Clin Pharmacokinet 36(3):233–254

Fonzo-Christe C et al (2005) Subcutaneous administration of drugs in the elderly: survey of practice and systematic literature review. Palliat Med 19:208–219

Garrett E.R. (1994) The Bateman function revisited: a critical reevaluation of the quantitative expressions to characterize concentrations in the one compartment body model as a function of time with first-order invasion and first-order elimination. J Pharmacokinet Biopharm 22(2): 103–128

Gilbar PJ (1999) A guide to enteral drug administration in palliative care. J Pain Symptom Manage 17(3):197–207

Hafner K (2013) Off-Label-Use von Arzneimitteln in der Palliativmedizin. In: Mathematisch-Naturwissenschaftlichen Fakultät. Rheinische Friedrich-Wilhelms-Universität Bonn, Bonn, p 270

Hansen S et al (2009) National influences on catheter-associated bloodstream infection rates: practices among national surveillance networks participating in the European HELICS project. J Hosp Infect 71(1):66–73

Herndon CM, Fike DS (2001) Continuous subcutaneous infusion practices of United States hospices. J Pain Symptom Manage 22(6):1027–1034

Hockenhull JC et al (2008) The clinical effectiveness and cost-effectiveness of central venous catheters treated with anti-infective agents in preventing bloodstream infections: a systematic review and economic evaluation. Health Technol Assess 12(12):154

I.E. Commission (ed) (2012) IEC 60601-2-24 EN-medical electrical equipment – part 2–24: particular requirements for the safety of infusion pumps and controllers, 1st edn. IEC, Geneva

Infusionzubereitungen in Europäisches Arzneibuch 7.0 Ausgabe Grundwerk, Band 1 (2011) p 1100

Jauch KW et al (2007) 9 Technik und Probleme der Zugänge in der parenteralen Ernährung. Aktuel Ernahrungsmed 32(S 1):S41–S53

Kamath PS et al (2001) A model to predict survival in patients with end-stage liver disease. Hepatology 33(2):464–470

Menahem S, Shvartzman P (2010) Continuous subcutaneous delivery of medications for home care palliative patients-using an infusion set or a pump? Support Care Cancer 18(9):1165–1170

Mermel LA et al (2009) Clinical practice guidelines for the diagnosis and management of intravascular catheter-related infection: 2009 update by the Infectious Diseases Society of America. Clin Infect Dis 49(1):1–45

Mitten T (2001) Subcutaneous drug infusions: a review of problems and solutions. Int J Palliat Nurs 7(2):75–85

Morgan S, Evans N (2004) A small observational study of the longevity of syringe driver sites in palliative care. Int J Palliat Nurs 10(8):405–412

NPSA (National Patient Safety Agency) (2010) Safer ambulatory syringe drivers. In: Rapid response report RRR019. Available from: www.npsa.uk

O'Doherty CA et al (2001) Drugs and syringe drivers: a survey of adult specialist palliative care practice in the United Kingdom and Eire. Palliat Med 15(2):149–154

O'Grady NP et al (2011) Guidelines for the prevention of intravascular catheter-related infections. Clin Infect Dis 52(9):e162–e193

Parenteralia 5.2/0520 (2012) Arzneibuchkommentar Gesamtwerk einschliesslich 43. Aktualisierungslieferung, Wissenschaftliche Verlagsgesellschaft Stuttgart, Govi-Verlag GmbH, Stuttgart, Eschborn

Pugh RN et al (1973) Transection of the oesophagus for bleeding oesophageal varices. Br J Surg 60(8):646–649

Radbruch L et al (2011) Systematic review of the role of alternative application routes for opioid treatment for moderate to severe cancer pain: an EPCRC opioid guidelines project. Palliat Med 25(5):578–596

Rhee C, Broadbent AM (2007) Palliation and liver failure: palliative medications dosage guidelines. J Palliat Med 10:677–685

RKI (2002), Prävention Gefäßkatheterassoziierter Infektionen - Empfehlung der Kommission für Krankenhaushygiene und Infektionsprävention beim Robert Koch-Institut (RKI). Bundesgesundheitsblatt 45:907–924

Rose M, Currow DC (2009) The need for chemical compatibility studies of subcutaneous medication combinations used in palliative care. J Pain Palliat Care Pharmacother 23(3):223–230

S.o.H.P.o. Australia (2011) Australian don't rush to crush handbook, 1st edn. SHPA, Collingwood

Schiffer CA et al (2013) Central venous catheter care for the patient with cancer: American Society of Clinical Oncology clinical practice guideline. J Clin Oncol 31(10):1357–1370

Schlatter C (2008) Dosisanpassung bei Leberinsuffizienz. PZ Prisma 15(4):213–224

Schlatter C et al (2009) Pharmacokinetic changes of psychotropic drugs in patients with liver disease: implications for dose adaptation. Drug Saf 32(7):561–578

Schneider JJ, Wilson KM, Ravenscroft PJ (1997) A study of the osmolality and pH of subcutaneous drug infusion solutions. Aust J Hosp Pharm 27:29–31

Simon ST et al (2012) Acceptability and preferences of six different routes of drug application for acute breathlessness: a comparison study between the United Kingdom and Germany. J Palliat Med 15(12):1374–1381

Sloss A (2009) Prescribing in liver disease. Aust Prescriber 32:32–35

Tegeder I, Geisslinger G, Lotsch J (1999) Therapy with opioids in liver or renal failure. Schmerz 13(3):183–95

Twycross R, Wilcock A (eds) (2012) Palliative care formulary (PCF 4), 4th edn. Nottingham: palliativedrugs.com

Wilcock A et al (2006) Drugs given by a syringe driver: a prospective multicentre survey of palliative care services in the UK. Palliat Med 20(7):661–664

Williams NT (2008) Medication administration through enteral feeding tubes. Am J Health Syst Pharm 65(24):2347–2357

Yamada R et al (2010) Patient-reported usefulness of peripherally inserted central venous catheters in terminally Ill cancer patients. J Pain Symptom Manage 40(1):60–66

Zhu LL, Zhou Q (2013) Therapeutic concerns when oral medications are administered nasogastrically. J Clin Pharm Ther 38(4):272–276

Drug Interactions in Palliative Cancer Care and Oncology

11

Theresa Stehmer and Stephen A. Bernard

Contents

T. Stehmer, PharmD
Department of Pharmacy, Duke University Hospital, Durham, NC 27710, USA
e-mail: theresa.stehmer@duke.edu

S.A. Bernard, MD (✉)
University of North Carolina, Chapel Hill, NC 27514, USA
e-mail: bernmed@med.unc.edu

© Springer-Verlag Berlin Heidelberg 2015
B. Alt-Epping, F. Nauck (eds.), *Palliative Care in Oncology*,
DOI 10.1007/978-3-662-46202-7_11

11.1   Introduction

Drug interactions (DIs) in palliative care have become more complex as the discipline has expanded into the outpatient arena as either a freestanding palliative care clinic or embedded within the existing oncology clinic structure. A survey in 2010 of outpatient palliative care in the United States showed that half of NCI Cancer Centers and a third of the non-NCI Cancer Centers had an outpatient palliative care clinic with most being freestanding and 10–25 % being in an oncology clinic (Hui et al. 2010). Patients in the outpatient oncology setting may be on active therapy with antineoplastics. Medications for symptom management must now be evaluated for interactions against both old and new drugs used in oncology.

Frequently palliative care practitioners are not familiar with agents used in oncology and oncologists have only a modest knowledge of agents used in palliative care (Langler et al. 2013). The consequences of unappreciated DI can be significant—a case report of docetaxel and a protease inhibitor given concomitantly caused the patient to require hospitalization for 26 days for severe and prolonged neutropenia (Hewish et al. 2009). Both use the CYP3A4 pathway.

11.2   Drug Interactions: General

Drug interactions are classified as drug-nutrient interactions, drug-drug interactions which are the most common, and drug-herbal interactions which are also increasingly occurring as patients take complementary and alternative medications in the treatment of cancer or its symptoms. These interactions can produce pharmacokinetic effects (decreased therapeutic effect of a key drug due to failure to metabolize to an active compound) or pharmacodynamic effects (additive side effects). In a general medical population, but especially in patients with cancer, age, number of drugs, and complexity of care have been shown to increase the likelihood of drug interactions in both the inpatient and outpatient settings (Hines and Murphy 2011; Blower et al. 2005).

11.3   Drug Interactions: Frequency

The frequency of drug interactions in general varies by the groups studied with fatal interactions in patients with cancer occurring in 4 % of the patients in one series and 18 % of a general medical population. Warfarin accounted for most of the interactions in the general medical population (Juurlink et al. 2003; Buajordet et al. 2001).

In populations of patients with cancer, survey articles using differing methods to screen for interactions show that there is a potential interaction in 20–40 % for different groups of patients and in different countries, both developed and developing (Admassie et al. 2013; Beijnen and Schellens 2004; Tavakoli-Ardakani et al. 2013).

In a recent survey of reports in the literature, the frequency of potential interactions in oncology populations was 12–63 % (Riechelmann and Del Giglio 2009). Several issues arise in an oncology population that make drug interactions more likely—60 % in a recent review were over the age of 65; renal and hepatic clearance are diminished; older patients are often taking medication for other conditions, 5–10 medications on average; and the likelihood of drug-drug interactions increases with an increase in the number of medications (Blower et al. 2005; Admassie et al. 2013; Buajordet et al. 2001; Fainsinger et al. 1995).

Many drugs in oncology have a small therapeutic window or narrow therapeutic index—the concentration to achieve antitumor effects is not far from that which produces adverse events making the consequences of a drug interaction more significant.

11.3.1 Drug Interactions: Palliative Care and Oncology

Similar concerns are seen in populations of patients in a palliative care setting—many are at or older than 65; polypharmacy is the norm; and renal and hepatic clearance are often increasingly impaired as the patient approaches death (Lill et al. 2000; Hines and Murphy 2011).

Gaertner reviewed 200 patients in a palliative care setting and found 631 interactions in 151 charts; these were mainly pharmacodynamic—two drugs acting on the same receptor (Caraco 1996; Caruso 1998; Gaertner et al. 2012; Goey et al. 2013; Peng et al. 2005; Rahimi and Abdollahi 2012; Sinclair 1973).

Charts on 364 patients that were close to death in 2 inpatient hospices were reviewed utilizing the system developed by Hansten-ORCA. Sixty-one percent of patients had a potential drug-drug interaction; 43 % were classified as needing monitoring or adjustment (Hansten et al. 2001; Frechen et al. 2012). In 4 % the use of the drug was contraindicated as a precaution. No class 1 (contraindicated due to the likelihood of serious events) observations were seen. The major predictor for these interactions was polypharmacy with an odds ratio of 1.5 (95 % CI=.4–.6). The patients ranged in age from 36 to 99 with a median age of 74 but age alone was not predictive (Frechen et al. 2012).

The drugs most commonly involved in therapeutically relevant potential DDIs were antipsychotics, antiemetics (e.g., metoclopramide, antihistamines), antidepressants, insulin, glucocorticoids, cardiovascular drugs, and, in particular, nonsteroidal anti-inflammatory drugs (NSAIDs). The most prevalent potential adverse effects were additive pharmacodynamic effects: anticholinergic, antidopaminergic, cardiac (QT interval prolongation), and gastrointestinal and renal toxicity from NSAID-associated toxicity. Pharmacodynamic interactions accounted for 88 % of the potential drug-drug interactions (Frechen et al. 2012).

In the outpatient setting, the population is more likely to be ambulatory but also older and on active treatment. Medications used to manage symptoms from treatment are added to medication to manage symptoms of the underlying malignancy. Estimates of potential interactions were surveyed in the oncology setting in 405 ambulatory adult patients with solid tumors (Riechelmann et al. 2007). There were

Table 11.1 Drugs used in palliative care and oncology

Palliative care	Oncology	Oncology support
Opioids	Alkylators	Immunosuppressants
Antipyretics	Hormones	Antifungals
Anti-inflammatories	Topoisomerase inhibitors	Antibiotics
Antidepressants	Tyrosine kinase inhibitors	Antivirals
Antiemetics	Anti-VEGF	Anticoagulants
	Sonic Hedgehog inhibitors	
	MEK, MTOR inhibitors	Antiretrovirals
Antianxiety	Vaccines	
Hypnotics	Combined antibody-chemotherapy	Stem cells
Antidiarrheals	Microtubule inhibitors	
Laxatives	Anti-fols	
Appetite stimulants	Pyrimidine antagonists	
Psychostimulants	Purine antagonists	
	Radiation	
Nutrients		
Herbs		

276 combinations with the potential to interact in 27 % of the patients. Nine percent of the potential interactions were classified as serious and 77 % were moderate (Riechelmann et al. 2007). Oncology drugs included cyclophosphamide and cisplatin and accounted for 13 % of the interactions. Drugs most commonly associated with interactions included antihypertensive agents (angiotensin-converting enzyme inhibitors, beta-blockers, and hydrochlorothiazide), aspirin, warfarin, corticosteroids, phenytoin, and prochlorperazine (Riechelmann et al. 2007). Riechelmann has also surveyed ambulatory palliative care patients at Princess Margaret Hospital who were not on anticancer therapy (Riechelmann et al. 2008). In a convenience sample of 372 patients, the median age was 66; and the median number of medications was 6. Over 33 % of the patients had cardiovascular disease, 14 % had diabetes, and 5–10 % of the patients had respiratory, hepatic, or thromboembolic disease or hypothyroidism. Classes of drugs that were being taken included opioids (67 %), laxatives (54 %), acetaminophen (40 %), and corticosteroids (38 %). Riechelmann found that 31 % of the patients had a potential drug interaction with 59 % being moderately severe and 10 % major (Table 11.1) (Riechelmann et al. 2008).

11.4   Mechanisms of Drug-Drug Interactions

Drug-drug interactions can be broken down into (a) pharmacokinetic effects which arise when the absorption, distribution, metabolism, and elimination of a drug are influenced by another drug; (b) pharmacodynamic effects that can either be additive, synergistic, or antagonistic; and (c) pharmaceutical effects that arise when drugs are incompatible either physically or chemically (Beijnen and Schellens

2004). A newer concept in drug-drug interactions is inverse agonism—ligands bind to receptors where there is spontaneous activity and inhibit or upregulate the activity (Blower et al. 2005). Upregulation in the case of kappa opioid receptors by naloxone may occur and lead to tolerance and the potential for a rebound effect (Blower et al. 2005).

Absorption of drugs is in part determined by both food in the stomach or bowel which represents the potential for a food-nutrient interaction and in part determined by enzymes in the bowel lining, especially those of the cytochrome P450 system (CYP3A4) and the P-glycoprotein family.

Metabolism of drugs occurs primarily by the CYP450 system that is in the liver and small intestinal epithelium. This system consists of 57 enzymes that are responsible for the phase I metabolism of most drugs—hydroxylation, oxidation, or reduction that lead to activation or creation of toxic metabolites. Phase II reactions, such as glucuronidation or sulfation, generally lead to inactive compounds which are water soluble and allow renal excretion (Beijnen and Schellens 2004; Blower et al. 2005; Glotzbecker et al. 2012; Wilkinson 2005). Six of the CYP enzymes (named by number for family, letter for subfamily, and number for specific isoform) account for most of the activity—CYP1A2, CYP2C9, CYP2C19, CYP2D6, CYP2E1, and CYP3A4. All of these are found in the liver with CYP3A4 having the greatest proportion (Ott et al. 2010). CYP3A4 is also found in intestinal epithelium. CYP3A4 accounts for 70 % of all drug metabolism in the intestine and 60 % in the liver (Glotzbecker et al. 2012). Oral drugs are acted on by CYP3A4 in the intestinal epithelium and in the liver leading to changes in first-pass metabolism. Those given intravenously are affected by hepatic CYP3A4. A single glass of grapefruit juice for 1–2 days can inhibit CYP3A4 sufficiently to cause a decrease in blood pressure and an increase in pulse in patients on felodipine, a calcium channel blocker (Wilkinson 2005). However, because of the large amount of CYP3A4 in the liver, considerable inhibition or induction must occur to affect metabolism (Blower et al. 2005).

Several of the CYP isoforms show genetic polymorphism—CYP1A2, CYP2C9, CYP2C19, CYP2D6, CYP2E1, and CYP3A5 enzymes (Glotzbecker et al. 2012). Variations in inheritance worldwide have led to populations of individuals that are either poor metabolizers, intermediate metabolizers, rapid metabolizers (usual), or ultrarapid metabolizers (Bernard et al. 2006; Blower et al. 2005; Wilkinson 2005).

11.5 Drug-Nutrient Interactions

The impact of food and pH is increasingly important in oncology. Older drugs such as warfarin are associated with several interactions once the food—e.g., cruciferous vegetables with high concentrations of vitamin K—is absorbed (Pronsky and Crowe 2014). Absorption of newer oral drugs may be affected by fat in the diet or by the acidity of the stomach (Product Information: STIVARGA® oral tablets, regorafenib oral tablets. Bayer HealthCare Pharmaceuticals Inc. (per FDA), Wayne, NJ, 2012) (Caraci et al. 2011; Tawbi et al. 2013; Sonpavde and Hutson 2007; Egorin et al. 2009) (Product Information: VOTRIENT oral tablets, pazopanib oral tablets.

GlaxoSmithKline (Per FDA), Research Triangle Park, NC, 2012). These interactions are discussed in detail in Sect. 11.14—New Drugs.

11.6 Drug Interactions: Herbal

Herbal preparations are in widespread use. A survey from the United States in 2007 showed that 44 % of adults had used complementary and alternative medicine (CAM) therapies (http://nccam.nih.gov/news/camstats/2007/camsurvey_fs1.htm).

Surveys from other countries have shown use in 48 % of patients in a German oncology clinic, 78 % of patients on palliative chemotherapy in Norway, 67 % of patients on curative therapy from the same Norwegian clinic, and 3–25 % of patients in a review of survey literature from the United Kingdom (Zeller et al. 2013; Engdal et al. 2008; Gratus et al. 2009).

One of the most commonly used herbs, St. John's wort, contains hyperforin, a strong inducer of CYP3A4 with chronic administration and an inhibitor with short-term exposure (Wrighton and Thummel 2000). St John's wort also affects CYP2D6, CYP2C19, CYP2C9, and the P-glycoprotein (P-gp) transporter (Mannel 2004; Ott et al. 2010).

In 10 patients on docetaxel, the addition of St. John's wort caused the AUC to decrease from $3{,}035 \pm 756$ to $2{,}682 \pm 717$ ng ($P = .045$), and the frequency of toxicities was diminished (Goey et al. 2014). St. John's wort affects the clearance of imatinib. In normal volunteers taking both agents, St. John's wort administered with imatinib at 400 mg increased imatinib clearance by 43 % (Barnes et al. 2001). Many drugs in oncology that are metabolized by the CYP3A4 isoform can show an increase in clearance and a reduction in efficacy or in side effects. Dosing of the antineoplastic drug may need to be increased to maintain effectiveness.

The use of St. John's wort with prescription antidepressants can produce a pharmacodynamic effect—the herb inhibits uptake of dopamine, serotonin, and norepinephrine and increases the potential for serotonin syndrome (Lantz et al. 1999).

In palliative or supportive care, classes of drugs that use the CYP3A4 pathway primarily include the -setron antiemetics such as ondansetron and the NK-1 inhibitor aprepitant.

Other classes of compounds that are relevant in palliative care that can be affected by the CYP3A4 pathway include the azoles and SSRI antidepressants (also impacted on through the 2D6 isoform) (Barnes et al. 2001; Ott et al. 2010).

Recently curcumin from the turmeric plant has attracted attention in oncology. This herbal compound has multiple effects including anti-TNF-α, antiapoptosis. It acts on several drug-metabolizing enzymes—primarily CYP3A4 and CYP1A2—to inhibit them. It may increase the risk of bleeding due to effects on platelet aggregation. In oncology it has inhibited tumor regression in animals treated with cyclophosphamide and the effects of doxorubicin in vitro (Table 11.2) (Somasundaram et al. 2002).

Table 11.2 Selected drug interactions of herbal therapies

	Agent	Clinical effect	References
St. John's wort			
Oncology	Irinotecan	Decreases level	Goey et al. (2013)
	Imatinib		
	Docetaxel Cyclosporine		Rahimi and Abdollahi (2012)
	Hormonal—anastrozole	Decreases effect	Wrighton and Thummel (2000)
Palliative care	-setron antiemetics	Decreases level	
	SSRI antidepressants—paroxetine, sertraline, fluoxetine	Decreases level Increases pharmacodynamic effect	Barnes et al. (2001), Mannel (2004), Lantz et al. (1999)
Garlic			
Oncology	Irinotecan, imatinib, docetaxel	None	Goey et al. (2013)
Milk thistle			
Oncology	Irinotecan, imatinib, docetaxel	None	
Echinacea			
Oncology	Etoposide—worsens thrombocytopenia	Increases level of drug	Goey et al. (2013)
	Cyclosporine	Decreases effectiveness of drug	Bossaer and Odle (2012)
Curcumin			
Oncology	Cyclophosphamide Doxorubicin	Loss of effectiveness in nonhuman systems	Somasundaram et al. (2002)

11.7 Drug Interactions: Opioids

Several of the major opioids used in both palliative care and oncology are cleared by the CYP P450 system, including the CYP3A4 and CYP2D6 isoforms (Blower et al. 2005). Many of these drugs have a narrow therapeutic range, making drug interactions more likely to occur clinically (Overholser and Foster 2011). A recent effort to correlate single-nucleotide mutations with opioid dose did not reveal any specific pattern (Klepstad et al. 2010).

Codeine is a prodrug that is first metabolized to morphine by the CYP2D6 pathway. Drugs such as azoles that inhibit this conversion may reduce its effectiveness (Kharasch 2000). In the setting of poor metabolizers, changes may be less than in those with extensive metabolism. Somatostatin analogs may decrease codeine clearance by acting on CYP2D6 (Kharasch 2000).

Morphine is metabolized predominately by glucuronidation. In vitro interactions with benzodiazepines and the tricyclic antidepressants have been seen (Kharasch 2000). Potential pharmacodynamic interactions with other opioids can be seen. Another class III opioid—hydromorphone—is also cleared by this pathway. Drug interactions involving the CYP system are not likely (Hughes et al. 2012).

Two other drugs that are metabolized by the CYP2D6 pathway in part are hydrocodone and oxycodone. Clinically significant interactions related to alteration of CYP2D6 have not been reported (Overholser and Foster 2011). Recently, however, clinically significant interactions with inhibitors of the CYP3A4 pathway have been reported including a reduction in dosing of oxycodone in patients on protease inhibitors, grapefruit juice, and azole antifungals (Hagelberg et al. 2011). Immunosuppressives such as cyclosporine have also been reported to have a drug interaction with oxycodone (Lill et al. 2000).

Both methadone and fentanyl are cleared by the CYP3A4 pathway. Inhibitors of this pathway include antibiotics such as erythromycin and quinolone antibiotics such as ciprofloxacin, cardiac meds such as verapamil and amiodarone, azole antifungals such as itraconazole and ketoconazole, and the SSRI antidepressants such as fluoxetine and fluvoxamine (Malone et al. 2004).

However, in the case of fentanyl, clinical cases had not been reported in a review by Kharasch—this may be due to the dependency on hepatic blood flow rather than intrinsic clearance (Kharasch 2000). Patients on anticonvulsants such as phenytoin, carbamazepine, and valproic acid require additional fentanyl following surgery—the mechanism is not clear (Kharasch 2000). Fentanyl is a synthetic phenylpiperidine opioid. Others in this group include alfentanil and meperidine. These agents are proserotonergics. Use with other drugs such as antidepressants that increase serotonin increases the potential for serotonin syndrome.

Methadone is metabolized predominately by CYP3A4 with contributions from other isoforms including CYP2D6. Drugs that are strong inhibitors of CYP3A4 or moderate inhibitors of several CYP isoforms may give rise to significant drug interactions. Phyu reported three cases of acute delirium on a palliative care unit where ketoconazole and sertraline were coadministered (Phyu et al. 2009). Methadone can cause prolongation of the QT interval (repolarization time) electrophysiologically and, in the most extreme example, torsades de pointes. Other arrhythmias have also been seen and fatalities can occur (Finlayson et al. 2004). Prolongation results from an action on the potassium channels in the conduction pathway of the myocardium, in particular the HERG (human ether-a-go-go related gene) channel that has 1,159 amino acids (Finlayson et al. 2004). A recent review of the FDA database showed that the frequency of this side effect was related to several factors such as female gender (Pearson and Woosley 2005). It is also seen in settings where methadone levels are high due to inhibition of metabolism by strong inhibitors of CYP3A4 such as azoles and protease inhibitors. In the series from the FDA, azithromycin and ondansetron were also associated with this finding (Pearson and Woosley 2005).

Tramadol is metabolized by both CYP2D6 and CYP3A4 isoforms. Drugs that inhibit CYP2D6, such as the strong inhibitor paroxetine, may decrease the effect of tramadol; weaker inhibitors such as escitalopram may have no effect. Drugs that inhibit CYP3A4 may slow clearance—azoles, protease inhibitors, and SSRIs (Overholser and Foster 2011).

Meperidine is not widely used anymore except for rigors experienced with infusions of drugs used to treat fungal infection in bone marrow transplant patients and patients with hematologic malignancies. It can interact with monoamine oxidase inhibitors which slow the elimination of meperidine. The concurrent use causes central nervous system excitation by a pharmacodynamic effect. A case report of serotonin syndrome with meperidine and linezolid has recently been published (Das et al. 2008).

The use of opioids with surgery for cancer has been investigated for a role of opioids in causing cancer recurrence. To date, the evidence is primarily retrospective and from in vitro effects of opioids on the immune system and other aspects of host defense (Ash and Buggy 2013).

11.8 Antipyretics

The most commonly used antipyretic in palliative care is acetaminophen. There is increasing recognition of the interactions of this drug with a large group of other drugs. Acetaminophen is metabolized by CYP1A2 and 2E1 but is also a substrate for UGT1A1, the enzyme involved in clearance of irinotecan—no interactions have been reported. Another potential interaction can occur in stem cell transplant patients when high-dose busulfan is given. The mechanism may be competition for glutathione causing higher than expected levels of busulfan (Glotzbecker et al. 2012).

11.9 Anti-inflammatories

Drugs used in palliative or supportive care that are used adjuvantly in the management of bone pain include the nonsteroidal anti-inflammatory agents. Loss of platelet adhesiveness, gastritis, and bleeding limit the use of these drugs in oncology patients on active treatment. While the newer Cox-2 inhibitors may cause these effects slightly less often, they have been associated with a higher incidence of cardiac side effects (McGettigan and Henry 2006).

At end of life, corticosteroids are used for a variety of reasons including their anti-inflammatory effects (Frechen et al. 2012). Steroids are strong inducers of CYP3A4 and the P-glycoprotein pathway. Potential interactions with drugs that use this pathway include the immunosuppressants used in bone marrow transplantation such as tacrolimus and cyclosporine (Glotzbecker et al. 2012).

11.10 Antidepressants

Many patients seen by the palliative care practitioner will have already been started on an antidepressant. In a palliative care or oncology setting, the frequency of major depression was 21 %; however, 40 % of patients may have some form of mood disorder (Mitchell et al. 2011). The different classes of antidepressants used in palliative care have been recently reviewed (Rhondali et al. 2012).

In a recent retrospective review of 2,430 women using selective serotonin reuptake inhibitors (SSRIs) while on tamoxifen as an adjuvant for breast cancer, paroxetine was found to reduce the effectiveness of tamoxifen by inhibiting CYP2D6 and not permitting conversion to endoxifen, the active compound. It is estimated that for every 7 women treated with the combination of these two drugs, 1 woman would die from breast cancer (Kelly et al. 2010). Other SSRIs did not impact negatively, including venlafaxine which is used to treat hot flashes as well as depression. Second-generation antidepressants differ in their potential for pharmacokinetic drug interactions. Fluoxetine and paroxetine are potent inhibitors of CYP2D6 which is involved in the metabolism of several opioids; fluvoxamine markedly inhibits CYP1A2 and CYP2C19, and nefazodone (limited availability in the United States) is a strong inhibitor of CYP3A4 (Spina et al. 2008). Duloxetine and bupropion are moderate inhibitors of CYP2D6, and sertraline may cause significant inhibition of this isoform, but only at high doses. Citalopram, escitalopram, venlafaxine, mirtazapine, and reboxetine are weak or negligible inhibitors of CYP isoforms in vitro and are less likely than others to interact with coadministered medications (Spina et al. 2008).

A pharmacodynamic effect can be seen when switching from an SSRI to another class of antidepressant if both block serotonin uptake. Serotonin syndrome can occur unless there is a sufficient interval between the two drugs. In situations where two classes of antidepressants are being used, there is also increased potential for serotonin syndrome. When tricyclic antidepressants and the SSRI antidepressants are used concurrently, there may be prolongation of the QT interval, especially if both are used at full dose (Ponti et al. 2002).

Fluoxetine and paroxetine (inducers of CYP3A4) and St. John's wort (inducer of both CYP3A4 and P-glycoprotein) may affect the absorption of oral drugs such as imatinib used in chronic myelogenous leukemia and intravenous drugs such as irinotecan and docetaxel (Caraci et al. 2011).

Mirtazapine and citalopram are two newer antidepressants that have become widely used. Citalopram (metabolized by the CYP3A4 isoform) has antianxiety effects as well. It can cause prolongation of the QT interval when used in conjunction with the antifungals ketoconazole and the newer azole—posaconazole; because ketoconazole strongly inhibits CYP3A4, there is increased potential for citalopram side effects. Another drug, arsenic trioxide, used in acute promyelocytic leukemia (Prod Info Celexa® oral tablets, solution, 2012), when used in conjunction with citalopram can cause prolongation of the QT interval as well.

Mirtazapine when used with fentanyl can increase the risk of serotonergic side effects. If used with clonidine, decreased antihypertensive effects may occur with rapid heat beat. The mechanism is due to antagonism at the alpha-2 receptor.

11.11 Antiemetics

Antiemetics are frequently used in both palliative care and oncology either to prevent or treat nausea and vomiting. Commonly, several classes of drugs are used concurrently in oncology. Among the drugs frequently used in combination are an NK-1 inhibitor such as aprepitant, a steroid such as dexamethasone, and a 5-HT3 blocker, ondansetron. In palliative care, often a phenothiazine or ondansetron is used as a single agent.

Phenothiazines have as their main side effect the development of extrapyramidal side effects—facial contortions, rhythmic movements of the tongue, and dystonia. Other drugs that are used in palliative care and oncology such as metoclopramide may have additive effects and should be used with caution. Phenothiazines also cause sedation and when given with opioids can have a combined pharmacodynamic effect. More recently phenothiazines have been noted to prolong the QT interval (Ponti et al. 2002).

Dexamethasone is often used in combinations of antiemetics in oncology. It is a strong inducer of the CYP3A system, and the potential for lowered effectiveness of oncology drugs or other drugs used in palliative care exists; however, in the context of antiemesis, the drug is generally given for only a few days. Since induction usually requires a more prolonged exposure, it is less likely to play a role in this setting (Malone et al. 2004).

The newer 5-HT3 receptor antagonists play a major role in oncology in reducing vomiting from strong emetogens (Chevallier 1993). These drugs vary in their ability to prevent nausea and vomiting or in their half-life or in their side effects. Dolasetron causes prolongation of the QT and is not used. On the other hand, ondansetron also causes prolongation but is in widespread use for nausea and vomiting (Ponti et al. 2002). Palonosetron, a second-generation -setron, is superior to ondansetron in the prevention of chemotherapy-induced nausea and vomiting. Granisetron has a longer half-life and is used for delayed nausea and vomiting.

One of the major side effects of drugs used with ondansetron may be prolongation of the QT interval and the potential for serious arrhythmias. Among the drugs that cause this are newer protease inhibitors by a pharmacodynamic effect; posaconazole by inhibiting CYP3A4; antidepressants, such as the tricyclics, and SSRIs by an additive pharmacodynamic effect; and droperidol, another type of antiemetic. Other drugs that are also used with ondansetron in the supportive care setting include cyclobenzaprine and quinolone antibiotics—both these groups of drugs also prolong the QT interval (Ponti et al. 2002).

Recently, the antipsychotic olanzapine has been shown superior to the NK-1 inhibitor in the prevention of chemotherapy-induced emesis (Navari et al. 2011). The drug is now beginning to be used in the palliative care setting as well. The major drug interaction is a pharmacodynamic one of QT prolongation (Ponti et al. 2002; Navari et al. 2011).

11.12 Hormones

Hormones are used most often in oncology in the management of breast cancer and prostate cancer. Because these are oral agents and are generally well tolerated, patients may continue to receive these until late in their illness course increasing the likelihood that the palliative care practitioner may be involved as well in care while the patient is still on these drugs. As discussed in Sect. 11.10, tamoxifen requires conversion to the active form, endoxifen, via the CYP2D6 system. The use of SSRIs as antidepressants has been shown to decrease the level and potentially increase breast cancer recurrences (Jin et al. 2005; Kelly et al. 2010). A known adverse event of tamoxifen is thrombosis and frequently warfarin is used. Theoretical concerns arise because tamoxifen may inhibit the S isomer of CYP2C9, the isoform that metabolizes warfarin (Givens et al. 2009).

11.13 Other Drugs

Haloperidol is used in palliative care for the management of agitated delirium, which is often an event at end of life. This drug can cause sedation but most importantly can give rise to QT prolongation especially when given intravenously. Other drugs such as methadone or antibiotics such as erythromycin may give an additive effect.

11.14 Newer Agents

11.14.1 Tyrosine Kinase Inhibitors

In recent years, numerous tyrosine kinase inhibitors (TKIs) have been approved for cancer treatment. Unlike traditional chemotherapeutic agents, TKIs are specifically designed to target molecular pathways that are altered in certain types of tumors, which allows for a higher level of selectivity. Many of these agents also differ from traditional chemotherapeutic agents by being administered orally, thus creating increased opportunities for drug interactions (Table 11.3) (Pajares et al. 2012; Di Gion et al. 2011).

11.14.1.1 Multi-Targeted TKIs

Sunitinib is a multi-targeted TKI indicated for the treatment of gastrointestinal stromal tumors (GIST), advanced renal cell carcinoma (RCC), and progressive, well-differentiated pancreatic neuroendocrine tumors (pNET) (Sutent®. [package insert]. Pfizer Labs, New York, New York; 2013). Though no absorption interactions have been reported, sunitinib is a substrate of CYP3A4 and therefore has several relevant drug interactions in palliative care (Bilbao-Meseguer et al. 2014). Induction of CYP3A4 by steroids such as dexamethasone can lead to decreased concentrations of sunitinib, whereas inhibition of CYP3A4 by agent such as aprepitant can lead to increased exposure to sunitinib. Sunitinib also demonstrates a dose-dependent effect on the QT interval (Bello et al. 2009). Special caution must be taken when administering sunitinib in conjunction with 5-HT$_3$ receptor antagonists as both agents can prolong the QTc when used alone, and sunitinib can increase the exposure to these agents by inhibiting PGP.

Another multi-targeted TKI, sorafenib, is indicated for the treatment of advanced RCC and unresectable hepatocellular carcinoma (HCC) (Iyer et al. 2010) Nexavar®. [package insert]. Bayer HealthCare Pharmaceuticals Inc., Wayne, NJ;

Table 11.3 Effect of food and pH on absorption of TKIs

Target	Drug	Food impact	pH impact
Multiple kinases	Sunitinib	None	None
	Sorafenib	↓ Absorption	↓ Absorption at alkaline pH
	Vandetanib	None	None
BCR-ABL	Imatinib	None	None
	Nilotinib	↑ Absorption	↓ Absorption at alkaline pH
	Dasatinib	None	↓ Absorption at alkaline pH
	Bosutinib	↑ Absorption	↓ Absorption at alkaline pH
	Ponatinib	None	↓ Absorption at alkaline pH
HER2	Lapatinib	↑ Absorption	None
EGFR	Erlotinib	↑ Absorption	↓ Absorption at alkaline pH?
	Afatinib	↓ Absorption	None
VEGF	Axitinib	None	None
	Pazopanib	↑ Absorption	↓ Absorption at alkaline pH
ALK	Crizotinib	None	None
BRAF	Vemurafenib	None	None
	Dabrafenib	↓ Absorption	↓ Absorption at alkaline pH
MEK	Trametinib	↓ Absorption	None

2010. Though the package insert reports a 30 % reduction in absorption when taken with a high-fat meal, studies evaluating the effect of food on sorafenib concentrations have not provided consistent results. A moderate-fat diet did not decrease absorption (Strumberg et al. 2007). Administration with a high-fat diet caused a decrease in absorption by 29 % (Rini 2006). As a result, it is recommended that sorafenib be administered without food. Sorafenib is metabolized by CYP3A4 and UGT1A9. There is a case report of increased sorafenib exposure and resultant mucositis as a result of coadministration of a steroid (CYP3A4 inducer) (Noda et al. 2013).

The combination of sorafenib and docetaxel has been investigated for advanced, refractory solid tumors (Awada et al. 2012). In a Phase I study, sorafenib was found to significantly alter the pharmacokinetics of docetaxel, leading to an increased incidence of dermatologic adverse drug events (ADEs). As this treatment was used in patients with advanced refractory disease, the interaction becomes extremely relevant in the palliative care arena. Caution is recommended when administering these two agents together with dose reductions in the event of dermatologic ADEs.

Vandetanib is a multi-kinase inhibitor indicated for the treatment of symptomatic or progressive medullary thyroid cancer (Caprelsa®. [package insert]. AztraZeneca Pharmaceuticals LP, Wilmington, DE; 2011). QTc prolongation is a major ADE of vandetanib and has even necessitated the creation of a REMS program. A meta-analysis of patients receiving vandetanib demonstrated that the risk of QTc prolongation was highest in patients being treated for thyroid cancer, as well as for patients being treated for a longer duration (Zang et al. 2012). As such, concomitant use of QTc-prolonging agents should be avoided with vandetanib.

11.14.1.2 BCR-ABL TKIs

There are currently five different TKIs that have activity against BCR-ABL including imatinib, nilotinib, dasatinib, bosutinib, and ponatinib (Tasigna®. [package insert]. Novartis Pharmaceuticals Corporation, East Hanover, NJ; 2014, Sprycel®. [package insert]. Bristol-Myers Squibb, Princeton, NJ; 2013, Bosulif®. [package insert]. Pfizer Labs, New York, New York; 2012, Iclusig®. [package insert]. Ariad Pharmaceuticals, Inc., Cambridge, MA; 2012, (Gleevec®. [package insert]. Novartis Pharmaceuticals Corporation, East Hanover, NJ; 2013). Though these agents are all BCR-ABL TKIs, they differ greatly in their pharmacokinetic profiles. While food does not have a clinically relevant impact on the absorption of imatinib, dasatinib, or ponatinib, it can have a large impact on the absorption of nilotinib and bosutinib. Administering nilotinib with a high-fat meal has been shown to increase the absorption significantly (50 % or more), which is concerning because nilotinib also prolongs ventricular repolarization in a concentration-dependent manner (Tanaka et al. 2010). As such, nilotinib is recommended to be given on an empty stomach. The absorption of bosutinib has also been shown to increase significantly with a high-fat meal, as demonstrated in a Phase I trial in which patients that took bosutinib with food had an area under the curve (AUC) over twice as high as those that fasted (Abbas et al. 2012). Since bosutinib is also well tolerated with the increased absorption, it is recommended to give bosutinib with food.

On the whole, the BCR-ABL TKIs require acidic conditions for absorption, and as such administration with acid-suppressive therapy should generally be avoided. For example, the exposure to dasatinib has been shown to decrease significantly when administered concomitantly with H_2 receptor antagonists and antacids (Matsuoka et al. 2012; Eley et al. 2009). In contrast, the absorption of imatinib has not been shown to be impacted by the administration of either antacids or H_2-receptor antagonists (Sparano et al. 2009; Egorin et al. 2009; Tawbi et al. 2014).

Imatinib has been shown to be a viable treatment option for glioblastoma (GBM) when used in combination with hydroxyurea (Pursche et al. 2008). Concomitant administration of enzyme-inducing antiepileptic drugs (EIAEDs), such as phenytoin and carbamazepine, or non-EIAEDs, such as valproic acid and levetiracetam, in GBM patients is a common supportive care therapy used in patients with brain tumors to prevent seizure activity. When the effects of EIAEDs and non-EIAEDs on the serum trough levels of imatinib were compared, it was found that EIAEDs significantly decreased the serum levels of imatinib. This reduction in serum concentration can be avoided by either switching to a non-EIAED or increasing the dose of imatinib (Table 11.4).

11.14.1.3 EGFR TKIs

Both erlotinib and afatinib target the epidermal growth factor receptor (EGFR) tyrosine kinase (Tarceva®. [package insert]. OSI Pharmaceuticals, Inc., Melville, NY; 2010, Gilotrif®. [package insert]. Boehringer Ingelheim Pharmaceuticals, Inc., Ridgefield, CT; 2013). While neither afatinib nor erlotinib is recommended to be given concomitantly with food, the effects of food on the absorption of the two agents are very different. Concomitant administration of erlotinib with meals

Table 11.4 Manufacturer recommended management of CYP interactions

Drug	Enzyme	Dose modifications recommended with concomitant enzyme inhibitors or inducers	
Sunitinib	CYP3A4	Strong inhibitor	Consider dose ↓
		Strong inducer	Consider dose ↑
Sorafenib	CYP3A4	Any inhibitor	No dose adjustment
		Strong inducer	Consider dose ↑
Imatinib	CYP3A4	Strong inhibitor	Caution recommended
		Strong inducer	↑ Dose by 50 %
Nilotinib	CYP3A4	Strong inhibitor	↓ Dose (indication specific)
		Strong inducer	Avoid use
Dasatinib	CYP3A4	Strong inhibitor	↓ Dose (starting dose specific)
		Strong inducer	Consider dose ↑
Bosutinib	CYP3A4	Strong/moderate inhibitor	Avoid use
		Strong/moderate inducer	Avoid use
Ponatinib	CYP3A4	Strong inhibitor	↓ Dose to 30 mg daily
		Strong inducer	Avoid use
Erlotinib	CYP3A4	Strong inhibitor	Consider dose ↓
		Strong inducer	↑ Dose
Afatinib	PGP	Strong inhibitor	↓ Dose by 10 mg
		Strong inducer	↑ Dose by 10 mg
Pazopanib	CYP3A4	Strong inhibitor	↓ Dose to 400 mg
		Strong inducer	Avoid use
CYP3A4/5	Axitinib	Strong inhibitor	↓ Dose by 50 %
		Strong inducer	Avoid use
CYP3A4	Lapatinib	Strong inhibitor	↓ Dose to 500 mg/day
		Strong inducer	↑ Dose (gradual titration)
CYP3A	Crizotinib	Strong inhibitor	Avoid use
		Strong inducer	Avoid use
CYP3A4	Vandetanib	Strong inhibitor	No dose adjustment
		Strong inducer	Avoid use
CYP3A4	Vemurafenib	Strong inhibitor	Avoid use
		Strong inducer	Avoid use
CYP3A4 CYP2C8	Dabrafenib	Strong inhibitor	Avoid use
		Strong inducer	Avoid use
None reported	Trametinib	–	–
		–	–

significantly increases absorption, while concomitant administration of food with afatinib has been shown to significantly decrease absorption and systemic exposure (Ling et al. 2008; Freiwald et al. 2014).

The effect of concomitant acid-suppressive agents is also significantly different between the two agents. Whereas no effect on absorption has been reported with afatinib, the effect of pH on the absorption of erlotinib is questionable. Though the package insert reports a decrease in the absorption of erlotinib by 46 and 33 % when administered concomitantly with a PPI and H2RA, respectively, additional studies have reported no clinically significant impact on drug levels or outcomes (Hilton et al. 2013; Duong and Leung 2011). Individualization of dose, based on potential benefit and risk, may be needed.

A unique interaction that can be seen with erlotinib therapy involves the impact of cigarette smoking on erlotinib pharmacokinetics. Cigarette smoking, which is relatively common in patients with NSCLC, induces CYP1A1 and CYP1A2. A study in NSCLC patients demonstrated that the maximum tolerated dose (MTD) in current smokers was twice as high as the MTD in nonsmokers, suggesting that cigarette smoking induces the metabolism and clearance of erlotinib (Hughes et al. 2009). As such, higher doses of erlotinib need to be considered in patients that continue to smoke while on therapy.

11.14.1.4 VEGF TKIs

Axitinib and pazopanib are both TKIs that target vascular endothelial growth factor (VEGF) and indicated for the treatment of renal cell carcinoma (RCC), though pazopanib is also indicated for the treatment of advanced soft tissue sarcoma (Inlyta®. [package insert]. Pfizer Labs, New York, New York; 2012, Votrient®. [package insert]. GlaxoSmithKline, Research Triangle Park, NC; 2013). Concomitant administration of axitinib with food does not have a clinically meaningful impact on the absorption, while concomitant administration of pazopanib with food results in a twofold increase in serum concentrations (Pithavala et al. 2012; Heath et al. 2010).

Though in vitro data suggests that pazopanib inhibits many CYP enzymes, a pharmacokinetic study using CYP-specific probe drugs demonstrated that pazopanib is a weak inhibitor of CYP3A4 and CYP2D6 with no effect on CYP1A2, CYP2C9, or CYP2C19 (Goh et al. 2010). Of interest in the palliative care setting, the CYP3A4-specific probe that was utilized was midazolam, suggesting that pazopanib has the potential to decrease the clearance of midazolam. Clinically meaningful interactions as a result of CYP enzyme inhibition/induction by axitinib have not been demonstrated (Chen et al. 2013).

11.14.1.5 HER2 TKI

Lapatinib is indicated for the treatment of HER2-positive advanced or metastatic breast cancer (Tykerb®. [package insert]. GlaxoSmithKline, Research Triangle Park, NC; 2013). It has been well established that absorption is significantly improved with concomitant food, as well as with twice-daily dosing as compared to once-daily dosing (Koch et al. 2009; Burris et al. 2009; Devriese et al. 2013). Lapatinib has also been shown to have a concentration-dependent impact on the QTc, suggesting that agents that increase serum concentrations of lapatinib may also increase the risk of QTc prolongation (Lee et al. 2010).

Though not commonly used in the treatment of gastrointestinal cancers, lapatinib has been studied in combination with FOLFIRI in patients with a range of advanced gastrointestinal cancers (Midgley et al. 2007). In this Phase I study, concomitant administration of lapatinib and irinotecan resulted in a 41 % increase in exposure to the active metabolite of irinotecan, SN-38. This action could lead to increased toxicities (i.e., diarrhea, myelosuppression) clinically. In vitro, lapatinib and SN-38 work synergistically to inhibit cell proliferation in colon and gastric cancers (LaBonte et al. 2009).

11.14.1.6 ALK TKI

Crizotinib is an anaplastic lymphoma kinase (ALK) inhibitor that is indicated for the treatment of patients with ALK-positive metastatic NSCLC (Xalkori®. [package insert]. Pfizer Labs, New York, New York; 2011). Crizotinib can cause QTc prolongation, and as such caution should be exercised with concomitant QTc-prolonging agents (Nickens et al. 2010). In addition, crizotinib has been shown to cause profound asymptomatic bradycardia (Ou et al. 2011). As a result, concomitant medications that slow the heart rate should be used with caution in patients receiving crizotinib.

11.14.1.7 BRAF TKIs

Both vemurafenib and dabrafenib are approved for the treatment of unresectable or metastatic melanoma with the BRAF V600E mutation; however, they differ greatly in their pharmacokinetic profiles (Zelboraf®. [package insert]. Genentech USA, Inc., South San Francisco, CA; 2011, (Tafinlar®. [package insert]. GlaxoSmithKline, Research Triangle Park, NC; 2013). Though the absorption of a single dose of vemurafenib has been shown to increase significantly when administered with a high-fat meal, there is no effect on the terminal half-life, and as such it is difficult to determine the impact of high-fat meals on continuous dosing (Ribas et al. 2014). As a result, the package insert does not stipulate whether vemurafenib should be given with food. In contrast, the absorption of dabrafenib has been shown to be greater in the absence of food (Ouellet et al. 2013). As such, the package insert recommends administering dabrafenib on an empty stomach (Tafinlar®. [package insert]. GlaxoSmithKline, Research Triangle Park, NC; 2013). Finally, vemurafenib is associated with a concentration-dependent QTc interval prolongation, whereas such an impact has not been shown with dabrafenib (Iddawela et al. 2013).

There has been great interest in the combination treatment of ipilimumab plus vemurafenib, since these agents have different mechanisms of action and both have been shown to improve overall survival in metastatic melanoma patients. A Phase I study that was conducted to evaluate the safety of concurrent vemurafenib and ipilimumab administration demonstrated increased rates of hepatic adverse events, including increased aminotransferase and total bilirubin levels (Ribas et al. 2013). All adverse events were asymptomatic and reversible with corticosteroids; however, the study demonstrated the increased risk of hepatic injury with concomitant use of ipilimumab and vemurafenib. No data on the combination of ipilimumab and dabrafenib has been published.

11.14.1.8 MEK TKI

Trametinib is indicated for the treatment of unresectable or metastatic melanoma with BRAF V600E or V600K mutations (Mekinist®. [package insert]. GlaxoSmithKline, Research Triangle Park, NC; 2013). Food has been shown to delay both the rate and absorption of trametinib, and as such it is recommended to be given on an empty stomach (Cox et al. 2013). Trametinib is not a substrate of the CYP enzymes or efflux transporters, nor is trametinib an inhibitor of the CYP enzymes. Though trametinib is an inducer of 3A4 in vitro, the package insert alludes to data that demonstrates no significant impact of trametinib on the serum concentration of everolimus.

11.14.2 Monoclonal Antibodies

The elimination of monoclonal antibodies (mAbs) is largely mediated via catabolic processes such as target binding, internalization, and proteolysis. Small molecules, in contrast, are largely eliminated through non-catabolic pathways such as hepatic metabolism, renal excretion, and biliary excretion. As a result of the lack of competition for elimination pathways, there is a lower likelihood of direct drug interactions between mAbs and small molecules (Zhou and Mascelli 2011; Seitz and Zhou 2007; Mahmood and Green 2007).

Even though mAbs and small molecules do not compete for the same elimination pathways, there are several ways in which drug interactions can occur (Zhou and Mascelli 2011). Though mAbs do not have a direct effect on hepatic clearance pathways, there is potential for an indirect effect by targeting certain cytokines that modulate CYP450 enzymes. One example of such an interaction has been documented with the IL-2-targeting mAb basiliximab (Sifontis et al. 2002). It was found that concomitant administration of basiliximab and cyclosporine (CSA) in renal transplant patients resulted in significantly higher trough levels of CSA. This interaction was postulated to be a result of cytokine-induced inhibition of CYP3A4 metabolism. Though this example occurred in renal transplant patients, concern for cytokine release is present in oncology patients receiving mAbs and in bone marrow transplant patients experiencing graft-versus-host disease (GVHD). Just as mAbs are capable of indirectly impacting the clearance of small molecules, small molecule agents have the potential to impact the clearance of mAbs. The best characterized example of such a potential interaction occurs between paclitaxel, a small molecule anti-microtubule agent, and trastuzumab, an anti-HER2 mAb. Though the results of a nonhuman primate study demonstrated a twofold decrease in trastuzumab clearance and a 1.5-fold increase in trastuzumab serum concentrations, these results have not been consistently demonstrated in subsequent studies done in humans (Table 11.5) (Leyland-Jones et al. 2003).

In addition to pharmacokinetic interactions with mAbs, the potential for pharmacodynamic interactions exists as well. One such example is the potential interaction between ipilimumab and corticosteroids. Ipilimumab is an anti-CTLA-4 mAb used in the treatment of metastatic melanoma that results in prolonged T-cell activation and proliferation. As such, immune-related adverse events (irAEs) are relatively common and are routinely managed with corticosteroids. However, since the antitumor effects of ipilimumab are also dependent on these immune effects, the impact of systemic corticosteroids on the antitumor effect of ipilimumab has been called into question. An analysis of patients who received ipilimumab and subsequent systemic corticosteroids suggests that systemic corticosteroids do not appear to impact the clinical activity of ipilimumab (Amin et al. 2009; Harmankaya et al. 2011). This potential interaction is extremely relevant to supportive care as it illustrates a scenario in which management of an adverse effect could lead to decreased effectiveness of the primary therapy.

11.14.3 Sonic Hedgehog Inhibitor

Vismodegib is a first-in-class selective inhibitor of the Hedgehog pathway by binding to Smoothened, a transmembrane protein involved in Hedgehog signal transduction (Erivedge®. [package insert]. Genentech, Inc., South San Francisco, CA;

Table 11.5 FDA-approved monoclonal antibodies used in oncology 2014

Generic name (brand)	Target
Ado-trastuzumab emtansine (Kadcyla®)	HER2
Alemtuzumab (Campath®)	CD52
Basiliximab (Simulect®)	IL-2
Bevacizumab (Avastin®)	VEGF
Brentuximab vedotin (Adcetris®)	CD30
Cetuximab (Erbitux®)	EGFR
Ibritumomab tiuxetan (Zevalin®)	CD20
Ipilimumab (Yervoy®)	CTLA-4
Obinutuzumab (Gazyva®)	CD20
Ofatumumab (Arzerra®)	CD20
Panitumumab (Vectibix®)	EGFR
Pertuzumab (Perjeta®)	HER2
Rituximab (Rituxan®)	CD20
Tositumomab (Bexxar®)	CD20
Trastuzumab (Herceptin®)	HER2

2012). Vismodegib is indicated for the treatment of adults with metastatic basal cell carcinoma. The package insert recommends administering vismodegib either with or without food, as there appears to be no effect of food on the absorption of vismodegib. Though there is data demonstrating that the administration of vismodegib with a high-fat meal increases the absorption of a single dose, there is no pharmacokinetic difference seen at steady state (Sharma et al. 2013).

Though vismodegib is primarily excreted as an unchanged drug, several minor metabolites are produced by CYP enzymes including CYP2C9 and CYP3A4. Despite being a substrate of these CYP enzymes, however, inhibition of these enzymes is not thought to affect systemic exposure to vismodegib. In addition, the effect of vismodegib on systemic exposure to agents metabolized by CYP2C8 (rosiglitazone) and CYP3A4 (oral contraceptives) has been shown to be negligible (LoRusso et al. 2013). CYP interactions with vismodegib are not likely to be clinically relevant.

11.14.4 MTOR Inhibitors

Mammalian target of rapamycin (mTOR) has been described as a master switch of cellular catabolism and anabolism, thereby determining whether cells grow and proliferate (Faivre et al. 2006). This ability, in conjunction with the ability to regulate apoptotic cell death, has made mTOR a very attractive target. Sirolimus is used in the prevention of GVHD in bone marrow transplant patients, whereas temsirolimus and everolimus are approved for the treatment of renal cell carcinoma (RCC) Rapamune®: [package insert]. Wyeth Pharmaceuticals, Inc., Philadelphia, PA; 2012, Afinitor®. [package insert]. Novartis Pharmaceuticals Corporation, East Hanover, NJ; 2014, Torisel®. [package insert]. Wyeth, Pharmaceuticals, Inc., Philadelphia, PA; 2007.

Sirolimus is frequently given in conjunction with a calcineurin inhibitor for the prevention of GVHD. However, caution must be taken when this combination is used due to the increased risk of the development of thrombotic microangiopathy (TMA) (Fortin et al. 2004). The mechanism behind this increased risk is thought to be due to the fact that calcineurin inhibitors increase the production of thromboxane A_2, decrease production of prostacyclin, and damage renal endothelial cells while sirolimus enhances platelet activation and aggregation (Shayani et al. 2013). Increased incidence of posttransplant TMA has been shown to be associated with higher sirolimus serum levels, and as such the dosage of sirolimus must be carefully monitored and adjusted if used in combination with a calcineurin inhibitor. A similar increased incidence of TMA has been demonstrated with everolimus and tacrolimus (Platzbecker et al. 2009).

Temsirolimus and everolimus are both indicated for the treatment of RCC, though there are potential downfalls to concomitant administration of either agent with sunitinib, another agent indicated for the treatment of RCC. Phase I studies have investigated the use of both agents in combination with sunitinib with the hope that inhibiting multiple oncogenic signaling pathways would improve the efficacy and abrogate resistance (Molina et al. 2012; Patel et al. 2009). However, the combination of

Table 11.6 Recommended management of CYP interactions

Drug	Enzyme	Dose modifications recommended with concomitant enzyme inhibitors or inducers	
Sirolimus	CYP3A4	Strong inhibitor(s)	Avoid use
		Moderate inhibitor(s)	Exercise caution
		Strong inducer(s)	Avoid use
		Moderate inducer(s)	Exercise caution
	PGP	Strong inhibitor(s)	Avoid use
		Moderate inhibitor(s)	Exercise caution
		Strong inducer(s)	Avoid use
		Moderate inducer(s)	Exercise caution
Everolimus	CYP3A4	Strong inhibitor(s)	Avoid use
		Moderate inhibitor(s)	Consider dose decrease
		Strong inducer(s)	Avoid use
		Moderate inducer(s)	Consider dose increase
	PGP	Strong inhibitor(s)	Avoid use
		Moderate inhibitor(s)	Consider dose decrease
		Strong inducer(s)	Avoid use
		Moderate inducer(s)	Consider dose increase
Temsirolimus	CYP3A4	Strong inhibitor(s)	Reduce dose to 12.5 mg/week
		Strong inducer(s)	Increase dose to 50 mg/week

temsirolimus with sunitinib was found to increase the incidence of dose-limiting toxicities (DLTs) including rash, thrombocytopenia, diarrhea, and asthenia (Patel et al. 2009). As a result, it is not recommended to give temsirolimus in combination with sunitinib. The combination of everolimus with sunitinib was also shown to increase the incidence of DLTs; however, patients did tolerate chronic combination therapy at a reduced dose of everolimus (Table 11.6) (Molina et al. 2012).

11.14.5 Vaccines

Anticancer vaccines represent a heterogeneous group of biologic agents that are administered to cancer patients with the intent of strengthening the patients' immune response to eradicate cancer cells (Hoos et al. 2007). The first anticancer vaccine to be FDA approved was Sipuleucel-T, which is composed of autologous mononuclear cells incubated with a fusion protein (Hammerstrom et al. 2011) (Provenge®. [package insert]. Dendreon Corporation, Seattle, WA; 2011). The fusion protein is comprised of prostatic acid phosphatase linked to granulocyte-macrophage colony-stimulating factor, which is intended to induce an immune response against the tumor antigen. Since the action of Sipuleucel-T is dependent on stimulating the immune system, concomitant chemotherapy or immunosuppressive agents have the potential to alter efficacy. The appropriateness of concomitant systemic chemotherapy or immunosuppressants (such as corticosteroids) needs to be assessed on an individual patient basis. Palliative care may be involved with patients on Sipuleucel-T which is currently indicated for the treatment of advanced prostate cancer, where steroids are given for multiple indications. Various other anticancer vaccines are under clinical investigation. When attempting to assess these vaccines for drug interaction potential, conventional pharmacokinetic measurements are often of limited use (Hoos et al. 2007).

Conclusion

As palliative care has moved into the outpatient practice, there is the potential for a dramatic increase in potential drug interactions, especially with newer oral agents.

References

Abbas R, Hug BA, Leister C, Gaaloul ME, Chalon S, Sonnichsen D (2012) A phase I ascending single-dose study of the safety, tolerability, and pharmacokinetics of bosutinib (SKI-606) in healthy adult subjects. Cancer Chemother Pharmacol 69(1):221–227. doi:10.1007/s00280-011-1688-7

Admassie E, Melese T, Mequanent W, Hailu W, Srikanth BA (2013) Extent of poly-pharmacy, occurrence and associated factors of drug-drug interaction and potential adverse drug reactions in Gondar Teaching Referral Hospital, North West Ethiopia. J Adv Pharm Technol Res 4(4):183–189. doi:10.4103/2231-4040.121412

Amin A, DePril V, Hamid O, Wolchock J, Maio M, Neyns B, Chin K, Ibrahim R, Hoos A, O'Day S (2009) Evaluation of the effect of systemic corticosteroids for the treatment of immune-related adverse events (irAEs) on the development or maintenance of ipilimumab clinical activity. J Clin Oncol 27:15s (suppl; abstr 9037)

Ash SA, Buggy DJ (2013) Does regional anaesthesia and analgesia or opioid analgesia influence recurrence after primary cancer surgery? An update of available evidence. Best Pract Res Clin Anaesthesiol 27(4):441–456. doi:10.1016/j.bpa.2013.10.005

Awada A, Hendlisz A, Christensen O, Lathia CD, Bartholomeus S, Lebrun F, de Valeriola D, Brendel E, Radtke M, Delaunoit T, Piccart-Gebhart M, Gil T (2012) Phase I trial to investigate the safety, pharmacokinetics and efficacy of sorafenib combined with docetaxel in patients with advanced refractory solid tumours. Eur J Cancer 48(4):465–474, doi:www.http://dx.doi.org/10.1016/j.ejca.2011.12.026

Barnes J, Anderson LA, Phillipson JD (2001) St John's wort (Hypericum perforatum L.): a review of its chemistry, pharmacology and clinical properties. J Pharm Pharmacol 53(5):583–600

Beijnen JH, Schellens JH (2004) Drug interactions in oncology. Lancet Oncol 5(8):489–496. doi:10.1016/S1470-2045(04)01528-1

Bello CL, Mulay M, Huang X, Patyna S, Dinolfo M, Levine S, Van Vugt A, Toh M, Baum C, Rosen L (2009) Electrocardiographic characterization of the QTc interval in patients with advanced solid tumors: pharmacokinetic-pharmacodynamic evaluation of sunitinib. Clin Cancer Res 15(22):7045–7052. doi:10.1158/1078-0432.CCR-09-1521

Bernard S, Neville KA, Nguyen AT, Flockhart DA (2006) Interethnic differences in genetic polymorphisms of CYP2D6 in the U.S. population: clinical implications. Oncologist 11(2):126–135. doi:10.1634/theoncologist.11-2-126

Bilbao-Meseguer I, Jose BS, Lopez-Gimenez LR, Gil MA, Serrano L, Castano M, Sautua S, Basagoiti AD, Belaustegui A, Baza B, Baskaran Z, Bustinza A (2014) Drug interactions with sunitinib. J Oncol Pharm Pract. doi:10.1177/1078155213516158

Blower P, de Wit R, Goodin S, Aapro M (2005) Drug-drug interactions in oncology: why are they important and can they be minimized? Crit Rev Oncol Hematol 55(2):117–142. doi:10.1016/j.critrevonc.2005.03.007

Bossaer JB, Odle BL (2012) Probable etoposide interaction with Echinacea. Journal of dietary supplements 9(2):90–95. doi:10.3109/19390211.2012.682643

Buajordet I, Ebbesen J, Erikssen J, Brors O, Hilberg T (2001) Fatal adverse drug events: the paradox of drug treatment. J Intern Med 250(4):327–341

Burris HA 3rd, Taylor CW, Jones SF, Koch KM, Versola MJ, Arya N, Fleming RA, Smith DA, Pandite L, Spector N, Wilding G (2009) A phase I and pharmacokinetic study of oral lapatinib administered once or twice daily in patients with solid malignancies. Clin Cancer Res 15(21):6702–6708. doi:10.1158/1078-0432.CCR-09-0369

Caraco J, Sheller J, Wood AJJ (1996) Pharmacogenetic determination of the effects of codeine and prediction of drug interactions. J of Pharmacology and Exp Ther 278:1165–1174

Caruso F, Mehlisch DR, Minn FL, Daniels SE, Memarich AN, Conforto ME (1998) Synergistic analgesic interaction of morphine with dextromethorphan, an NMDA receptor antagonist in oral surgery. Clin Pharm and Therapeutics 63(2):139, Abstract PI–110

Caraci F, Crupi R, Drago F, Spina E (2011) Metabolic drug interactions between antidepressants and anticancer drugs: focus on selective serotonin reuptake inhibitors and hypericum extract. Curr Drug Metab 12(6):570–577

Chen Y, Tortorici MA, Garrett M, Hee B, Klamerus KJ, Pithavala YK (2013) Clinical pharmacology of axitinib. Clin Pharmacokinet 52(9):713–725. doi:10.1007/s40262-013-0068-3

Chevallier B (1993) The control of acute cisplatin-induced emesis – a comparative study of granisetron and a combination regimen of high-dose metoclopramide and dexamethasone. Br J Cancer 68(1):176–180

Cox DS, Papadopoulos K, Fang L, Bauman J, LoRusso P, Tolcher A, Patnaik A, Pendry C, Orford K, Ouellet D (2013) Evaluation of the effects of food on the single-dose pharmacokinetics of trametinib, a first-in-class MEK inhibitor, in patients with cancer. J Clin Pharmacol 53(9):946–954. doi:10.1002/jcph.115

Das PK, Warkentin DI, Hewko R, Forrest DL (2008) Serotonin syndrome after concomitant treatment with linezolid and meperidine. Clin Infect Dis 46(2):264–265. doi:10.1086/524671

Devriese LA, Koch KM, Mergui-Roelvink M, Matthys GM, Ma WW, Robidoux A, Stephenson JJ, Chu QS, Orford KW, Cartee L, Botbyl J, Arya N, Schellens JH (2013) Effects of low-fat and high-fat meals on steady-state pharmacokinetics of lapatinib in patients with advanced solid tumours. Invest New Drugs. doi:10.1007/s10637-013-0055-4

Di Gion P, Kanefendt F, Lindauer A, Scheffler M, Doroshyenko O, Fuhr U, Wolf J, Jaehde U (2011) Clinical pharmacokinetics of tyrosine kinase inhibitors: focus on pyrimidines, pyridines and pyrroles. Clin Pharmacokinet 50(9):551–603

Duong S, Leung M (2011) Should the concomitant use of erlotinib and acid-reducing agents be avoided? The drug interaction between erlotinib and acid-reducing agents. J Oncol Pharm Pract 17(4):448–452. doi:10.1177/1078155210381794

Egorin MJ, Shah DD, Christner SM, Yerk MA, Komazec KA, Appleman LR, Redner RL, Miller BM, Beumer JH (2009) Effect of a proton pump inhibitor on the pharmacokinetics of imatinib. Br J Clin Pharmacol 68(3):370–374. doi:10.1111/j.1365-2125.2009.03466.x

Eley T, Luo F, Agrawal S, Sanil A, Manning J, Li T, Blackwood-Chirchir A, Bertz R (2009) Phase I study of the effect of gastric acid pH modulators on the bioavailability of oral dasatinib in healthy subjects. J Clin Pharmacol 49:700–709

Engdal S, Steinsbekk A, Klepp O, Nilsen OG (2008) Herbal use among cancer patients during palliative or curative chemotherapy treatment in Norway. Support Care Cancer 16(7): 763–769

Fainsinger R, Bruera E, Watanabe S (1995) Commonly prescribed medications in advanced cancer patients. In: 6th Canadian palliative care conference, Halifax, 15–17 Oct 1995

Faivre S, Kroemer G, Raymond E (2006) Current development of mTOR inhibitors as anticancer agents. Nat Rev Drug Discov 5(8):671–688. doi:10.1038/nrd2062

Finlayson K, Witchel HJ, McCulloch J, Sharkey J (2004) Acquired QT interval prolongation and HERG: implications for drug discovery and development. Eur J Pharmacol 500(1–3):129–142. doi:10.1016/j.ejphar.2004.07.019

Fortin MC, Raymond MA, Madore F, Fugere JA, Paquet M, St-Louis G, Hebert MJ (2004) Increased risk of thrombotic microangiopathy in patients receiving a cyclosporin-sirolimus combination. Am J Transplant 4(6):946–952. doi:10.1111/j.1600-6143.2004.00428.x

Frechen S, Zoeller A, Ruberg K, Voltz R, Gaertner J (2012) Drug interactions in dying patients: a retrospective analysis of hospice inpatients in Germany. Drug Safety 35(9):745–758. doi:10.2165/11631280-000000000-00000

Freiwald M, Schmid U, Fleury A, Wind S, Stopfer P, Staab A (2014) Population pharmacokinetics of afatinib, an irreversible ErbB family blocker, in patients with various solid tumors. Cancer Chemother Pharmacol. doi:10.1007/s00280-014-2403-2

Gaertner J, Ruberg K, Schlesiger G, Frechen S, Voltz R (2012) Drug interactions in palliative care-it's more than cytochrome P450. Palliative Medicine 26(6):813–825

Givens CB, Bullock LN, Franks AS (2009) Safety of concomitant tamoxifen and warfarin. Ann Pharmacother 43(11):1867–1871. doi:10.1345/aph.1M176

Glotzbecker B, Duncan C, Alyea E 3rd, Campbell B, Soiffer R (2012) Important drug interactions in hematopoietic stem cell transplantation: what every physician should know. Biol Blood Marrow Transplant 18(7):989–1006. doi:10.1016/j.bbmt.2011.11.029

Goey AK, Mooiman KD, Beijnen JH, Schellens JH, Meijerman I (2013) Relevance of in vitro and clinical data for predicting CYP3A4-mediated herb-drug interactions in cancer patients. Cancer treatment reviews 39(7):773–783. doi:10.1016/j.ctrv.2012.12.008

Goey AK, Meijerman I, Rosing H, Marchetti S, Mergui-Roelvink M, Keessen M, Burgers JA, Beijnen JH, Schellens JH (2014) The effect of St John's wort on the pharmacokinetics of docetaxel. Clin Pharmacokinet 53(1):103–110. doi:10.1007/s40262-013-0102-5

Goh BC, Reddy NJ, Dandamudi UB, Laubscher KH, Peckham T, Hodge JP, Suttle AB, Arumugham T, Xu Y, Xu CF, Lager J, Dar MM, Lewis LD (2010) An evaluation of the drug interaction potential of pazopanib, an oral vascular endothelial growth factor receptor tyrosine kinase inhibitor, using a modified Cooperstown 5+1 cocktail in patients with advanced solid tumors. Clin Pharmacol Ther 88(5):652–659. doi:10.1038/clpt.2010.158

Gratus C, Damery S, Wilson S, Warmington S, Routledge P, Grieve R, Steven N, Jones J, Greenfield S (2009) The use of herbal medicines by people with cancer in the UK: a systematic review of the literature. QJM 102(12):831–842. doi:10.1093/qjmed/hcp137

Hagelberg NM, Nieminen TH, Saari TI, Neuvonen M, Neuvonen PJ, Laine K, Olkkola KT (2011) Interaction of oxycodone and voriconazole-a case series of patients with cancer pain supports the findings of randomised controlled studies with healthy subjects. Eur J Clin Pharmacol 67(8):863–864. doi:10.1007/s00228-010-0969-0

Hammerstrom AE, Cauley DH, Atkinson BJ, Sharma P (2011) Cancer immunotherapy: sipuleucel-T and beyond. Pharmacotherapy 31(8):813–828. doi:10.1592/phco.31.8.813

Hansten PD, Horn JR, Hazlet TK (2001) ORCA: OpeRational ClassificAtion of drug interactions. J Am Pharm Assoc (Washington, DC: 1996) 41(2):161–165

Harmankaya K, Erasim C, Koelblinger C, Ibrahim R, Hoos A, Pehamberger H, Binder M (2011) Continuous systemic corticosteroids do not affect the ongoing regression of metastatic melanoma for more than two years following ipilimumab therapy. Med Oncol 28(4):1140–1144. doi:10.1007/s12032-010-9606-0

Heath EI, Chiorean EG, Sweeney CJ, Hodge JP, Lager JJ, Forman K, Malburg L, Arumugham T, Dar MM, Suttle AB, Gainer SD, LoRusso P (2010) A phase I study of the pharmacokinetic and safety profiles of oral pazopanib with a high-fat or low-fat meal in patients with advanced solid tumors. Clin Pharmacol Ther 88(6):818–823. doi:10.1038/clpt.2010.199

Hewish M, Miller R, Forster M, Smith I (2009) Severe synergistic toxicity from docetaxel in a patient treated concurrently with protease inhibitors as part of HIV post-exposure prophylaxis: a case report. J Med Case Reports 3(1):8866

Hilton JF, Tu D, Seymour L, Shepherd FA, Bradbury PA (2013) An evaluation of the possible interaction of gastric acid suppressing medication and the EGFR tyrosine kinase inhibitor erlotinib. Lung Cancer 82(1):136–142. doi:10.1016/j.lungcan.2013.06.008

Hines LE, Murphy JE (2011) Potentially harmful drug-drug interactions in the elderly: a review. Am J Geriatr Pharmacother 9(6):364–377. doi:10.1016/j.amjopharm.2011.10.004

Hoos A, Parmiani G, Hege K, Sznol M, Loibner H, Eggermont A, Urba W, Blumenstein B, Sacks N, Keilholz U, Nichol G, Group ftCVCTW (2007) A clinical development paradigm for cancer vaccines and related biologics. J Immunother 30(1):1–15. doi:10.1097/1001. cji.0000211341.0000288835.ae

Hughes AN, O'Brien ME, Petty WJ, Chick JB, Rankin E, Woll PJ, Dunlop D, Nicolson M, Boinpally R, Wolf J, Price A (2009) Overcoming CYP1A1/1A2 mediated induction of metabolism by escalating erlotinib dose in current smokers. J Clin Oncol 27(8):1220–1226. doi:10.1200/JCO.2008.19.3995

Hughes MM, Atayee RS, Best BM, Pesce AJ (2012) Observations on the metabolism of morphine to hydromorphone in pain patients. J Anal Toxicol 36(4):250–256. doi:10.1093/jat/bks021

Hui D, Elsayem A, De la Cruz M, Berger A, Zhukovsky DS, Palla S, Evans A, Fadul N, Palmer JL, Bruera E (2010) Availability and integration of palliative care at US cancer centers. JAMA 303(11):1054–1061. doi:10.1001/jama.2010.258

Iyer R, Fetterly G, Lugade A, Thanavala Y (2010) Sorafenib: a clinical and pharmacologic review. Expert opinion on pharmacotherapy 11(11):1943–1955. doi:10.1517/14656566.2010.496453

Iddawela M, Crook S, George L, Lakkaraju A, Nanayakkara N, Hunt R, Adam W (2013) Safety and efficacy of vemurafenib in end stage renal failure. BMC Cancer 13:581

Jin Y, Desta Z, Stearns V, Ward B, Ho H, Lee KH, Skaar T, Storniolo AM, Li L, Araba A, Blanchard R, Nguyen A, Ullmer L, Hayden J, Lemler S, Weinshilboum RM, Rae JM, Hayes DF, Flockhart DA (2005) CYP2D6 genotype, antidepressant use, and tamoxifen metabolism during adjuvant breast cancer treatment. J Natl Cancer Inst 97(1):30–39. doi:10.1093/jnci/dji005

Juurlink DN, Mamdani M, Kopp A, Laupacis A, Redelmeier DA (2003) Drug-drug interactions among elderly patients hospitalized for drug toxicity. JAMA 289(13):1652–1658. doi:10.1001/jama.289.13.1652

Kelly CM, Juurlink DN, Gomes T, Duong-Hua M, Pritchard KI, Austin PC, Paszat LF (2010) Selective serotonin reuptake inhibitors and breast cancer mortality in women receiving tamoxifen: a population based cohort study. BMJ 340:c693. doi:10.1136/bmj.c693

Kharasch E (2000) Opioid analgesics. In: Levy R, Thummel KE, Trager WF et al (eds) Metabolic drug interactions. Lippincott Williams and Wilkins, Philadelphia, pp 297–319

Klepstad P, Fladvad T, Skorpen F, Bjordal K, Caraceni A, Dale O, Davies A, Kloke M, Lundstrom S, Maltoni M, Radbruch L, Sabatowski R, Sigurdadottir V, Strasser F, Fayers P, Kaasa S (2010) The European Pharmacogenetic Opioid Study (EPOS): influence from genetic variability on opioid use in 2209 cancer pain patients. Palliat Med 24(4):S5

Koch KM, Reddy NJ, Cohen RB, Lewis NL, Whitehead B, Mackay K, Stead A, Beelen AP, Lewis LD (2009) Effects of food on the relative bioavailability of lapatinib in cancer patients. J Clin Oncol 27(8):1191–1196. doi:10.1200/JCO.2008.18.3285

LaBonte MJ, Manegold PC, Wilson PM, Fazzone W, Louie SG, Lenz HJ, Ladner RD (2009) The dual EGFR/HER-2 tyrosine kinase inhibitor lapatinib sensitizes colon and gastric cancer cells to the irinotecan active metabolite SN-38. Int J Cancer 125(12):2957–2969. doi:10.1002/ijc.24658

Langler A, Boeker R, Kameda G, Seifert G, Edelhauser F, Ostermann T (2013) Attitudes and beliefs of paediatric oncologists regarding complementary and alternative therapies. Complement Ther Med 21(Suppl 1):S10–S19. doi:10.1016/j.ctim.2012.02.006

Lantz MS, Buchalter E, Giambanco V (1999) St. John's wort and antidepressant drug interactions in the elderly. J Geriatr Psychiatry Neurol 12(1):7–10

Lee H, Kim E, Hyun S, Park S, Kim K (2010) Electrophysiological effects of the anti-cancer drug lapatinib on cardiac repolarization. Basic Clin Pharmacol Toxicol 107:614–618

Leyland-Jones B, Gelmon K, Ayoub JP, Arnold A, Verma S, Dias R, Ghahramani P (2003) Pharmacokinetics, safety, and efficacy of trastuzumab administered every three weeks in combination with paclitaxel. J Clin Oncol 21(21):3965–3971. doi:10.1200/jco.2003.12.109

Lill J, Bauer LA, Horn JR, Hansten PD (2000) Cyclosporine-drug interactions and the influence of patient age. Am J Health Syst Pharm 57(17):1579–1584

Ling J, Fettner S, Lum BL, Riek M, Rakhit A (2008) Effect of food on the pharmacokinetics of erlotinib, an orally active epidermal growth factor receptor tyrosine-kinase inhibitor, in healthy individuals. Anticancer Drugs 19:209–216

LoRusso PM, Piha-Paul SA, Mita M, Colevas AD, Malhi V, Colburn D, Yin M, Low JA, Graham RA (2013) Co-administration of vismodegib with rosiglitazone or combined oral contraceptive in patients with locally advanced or metastatic solid tumors: a pharmacokinetic assessment of drug-drug interaction potential. Cancer Chemother Pharmacol 71(1):193–202. doi:10.1007/s00280-012-1996-6

Mahmood I, Green MD (2007) Drug interaction studies of therapeutic proteins or monoclonal antibodies. J Clin Pharmacol 47(12):1540–1554. doi:10.1177/0091270007308616

Malone DC, Abarca J, Hansten PD, Grizzle AJ, Armstrong EP, Van Bergen RC, Duncan-Edgar BS, Solomon SL, Lipton RB (2004) Identification of serious drug-drug interactions: results of the partnership to prevent drug-drug interactions. J Am Pharm Assoc 44(2):142–151

Mannel M (2004) Drug interactions with St John's wort: mechanisms and clinical implications. Drug Safety 27(11):773–797

Matsuoka A, Takahashi N, Miura M, Niioka T, Kawakami K, Matsunaga T, Sawada K (2012) H2-receptor antagonist influences dasatinib pharmacokinetics in a patient with Philadelphia-positive acute lymphoblastic leukemia. Cancer Chemother Pharmacol 70(2):351–352. doi:10.1007/s00280-012-1900-4

McGettigan P, Henry D (2006) Cardiovascular risk and inhibition of cyclooxygenase: a systematic review of the observational studies of selective and nonselective inhibitors of cyclooxygenase 2. JAMA 296(13):1633–1644. doi:10.1001/jama.296.13.jrv60011

Midgley RS, Kerr DJ, Flaherty KT, Stevenson JP, Pratap SE, Koch KM, Smith DA, Versola M, Fleming RA, Ward C, O'Dwyer PJ, Middleton MR (2007) A phase I and pharmacokinetic study of lapatinib in combination with infusional 5-fluorouracil, leucovorin and irinotecan. Ann Oncol 18(12):2025–2029. doi:10.1093/annonc/mdm366

Mitchell AJ, Chan M, Bhatti H, Halton M, Grassi L, Johansen C, Meader N (2011) Prevalence of depression, anxiety, and adjustment disorder in oncological, haematological, and palliative-care settings: a meta-analysis of 94 interview-based studies. Lancet Oncol 12(2):160–174. doi:10.1016/s1470-2045(11)70002-x

Molina AM, Feldman DR, Voss MH, Ginsberg MS, Baum MS, Brocks DR, Fischer PM, Trinos MJ, Patil S, Motzer RJ (2012) Phase 1 trial of everolimus plus sunitinib in patients with metastatic renal cell carcinoma. Cancer 118(7):1868–1876. doi:10.1002/cncr.26429

Navari RM, Gray SE, Kerr AC (2011) Olanzapine versus aprepitant for the prevention of chemotherapy-induced nausea and vomiting: a randomized phase III trial. J Support Oncol 9(5):188–195. doi:10.1016/j.suponc.2011.05.002

Nickens D, Tan W, Wilner K (2010) Pharmacokinetic/pharmacodynamic evaluation of the concentration-QTc relationship of crizotinib (PF-02341066), an anaplastic lymphoma kinase and c-MET/hepatocyte growth factor receptor dual inhibitor administered orally to patients with advanced cancer. In: Poster presented at the 101st annual meeting of the American Association for Cancer Research, Washington, DC

Noda S, Shioya M, Hira D, Fujiyama Y, Morita SY, Terada T (2013) Pharmacokinetic interaction between sorafenib and prednisolone in a patient with hepatocellular carcinoma. Cancer Chemother Pharmacol 72(1):269–272. doi:10.1007/s00280-013-2187-9

Ott M, Huls M, Cornelius MG, Fricker G (2010) St. John's Wort constituents modulate P-glycoprotein transport activity at the blood-brain barrier. Pharm Res 27(5):811–822. doi:10.1007/s11095-010-0074-1

Ou SH, Azada M, Dy J, Stiber JA (2011) Asymptomatic profound sinus bradycardia (heart rate ≤45) in non-small cell lung cancer patients treated with crizotinib. J Thorac Oncol 6(12):2135–2137. doi:10.1097/JTO.0b013e3182307e06

Ouellet D, Grossmann KF, Limentani G, Nebot N, Lan K, Knowles L, Gordon MS, Sharma S, Infante JR, Lorusso PM, Pande G, Krachey EC, Blackman SC, Carson SW (2013) Effects of particle size, food, and capsule shell composition on the oral bioavailability of dabrafenib, a BRAF inhibitor, in patients with BRAF mutation-positive tumors. J Pharm Sci 102(9):3100–3109. doi:10.1002/jps.23519

Overholser BR, Foster DR (2011) Opioid pharmacokinetic drug-drug interactions. Am J Manag Care 17(Suppl 11):S276–S287

Pajares B, Torres E, Trigo JM, Saez MI, Ribelles N, Jimenez B, Alba E (2012) Tyrosine kinase inhibitors and drug interactions: a review with practical recommendations. Clin Transl Oncol 14(2):94–101. doi:10.1007/s12094-012-0767-5

Patel PH, Senico PL, Curiel RE, Motzer RJ (2009) Phase I study combining treatment with temsirolimus and sunitinib malate in patients with advanced renal cell carcinoma. Clin Genitourin Cancer 7(1):24–27. doi:10.3816/CGC.2009.n.004

Pearson EC, Woosley RL (2005) QT prolongation and torsades de pointes among methadone users: reports to the FDA spontaneous reporting system. Pharmacoepidemiol Drug Saf 14(11):747–753. doi:10.1002/pds.1112

Peng B, Lloyd P, Schran H (2005) Clinical pharmacokinetics of imatinib. Clin Pharmacokinet 44(9):879–894

Phyu K, Chau D, Shumaker N, Donepudi S (2009) Drug-drug interaction with methadone. J Support Oncol 7(5):202

Pithavala YK, Chen Y, Toh M, Selaru P, LaBadie RR, Garrett M, Hee B, Mount J, Ni G, Klamerus KJ, Tortorici MA (2012) Evaluation of the effect of food on the pharmacokinetics of axitinib in healthy volunteers. Cancer Chemother Pharmacol 70(1):103–112. doi:10.1007/s00280-012-1888-9

Platzbecker U, von Bonin M, Goekkurt E, Radke J, Binder M, Kiani A, Stoehlmacher J, Schetelig J, Thiede C, Ehninger G, Bornhauser M (2009) Graft-versus-host disease prophylaxis with everolimus and tacrolimus is associated with a high incidence of sinusoidal obstruction syndrome and microangiopathy: results of the EVTAC trial. Biol Blood Marrow Transplant 15(1):101–108. doi:10.1016/j.bbmt.2008.11.004

Ponti FD, Poluzzi E, Cavalli A, Recanatini M, Montanaro N (2002) Safety of non-antiarrhythmic drugs that prolong the QT interval or induce torsade de pointes: an overview. Drug Saf 25(4):263–286

Pronsky ZC, Crowe J (2014) Food medication interactions. Food Medication Interactions, Birchrunville, PA, USA

Pursche S, Schleyer E, von Bonin M, Ehninger G, Mustafa Said S, Prondzinsky R, Illmer T, Wang Y, Hosius C, Nikolova Z (2008) Influence of enzyme-inducing antiepileptic drugs on trough level of imatinib in glioblastoma patients. Curr Clin Pharmacol 3:198–203

Rahimi R, Abdollahi M (2012) An update on the ability of St. John's wort to affect the metabolism of other drugs. Expert opinion on drug metabolism and toxicology 8(6):691–708. doi:10.1517/17425255.2012.680886

Rhondali W, Reich M, Filbet M (2012) A brief review on the use of antidepressants in palliative care. Eur J Hosp Pharm Sci Pract 19(1):41–44. doi:10.1136/ejhpharm-2011-000024

Ribas A, Hodi FS, Callahan M, Konto C, Wolchok J (2013) Hepatotoxicity with combination of vemurafenib and ipilimumab. N Engl J Med 368(14):1365–1366. doi:10.1056/NEJMc1302338

Ribas A, Zhang W, Chang I, Shirai K, Ernstoff MS, Daud A, Cowey CL, Daniels G, Seja E, O'Laco E, Glaspy JA, Chmielowski B, Hill T, Joe AK, Grippo JF (2014) The effects of a high-fat meal on single-dose vemurafenib pharmacokinetics. J Clin Pharmacol 54(4):368–374. doi:10.1002/jcph.255

Riechelmann RP, Del Giglio A (2009) Drug interactions in oncology: how common are they? Ann Oncol 20(12):1907–1912. doi:10.1093/annonc/mdp369

Riechelmann RP, Tannock IF, Wang L, Saad ED, Taback NA, Krzyzanowska MK (2007) Potential drug interactions and duplicate prescriptions among cancer patients. J Natl Cancer Inst 99(8):592–600. doi:10.1093/jnci/djk130

Riechelmann RP, Zimmermann C, Chin SN, Wang L, O'Carroll A, Zarinehbaf S, Krzyzanowska MK (2008) Potential drug interactions in cancer patients receiving supportive care exclusively. J Pain Symptom Manage 35(5):535–543. doi:10.1016/j.jpainsymman.2007.06.009

Rini BI (2006) Sorafenib. Expert Opin Pharmacother 7(4):453–461. doi:10.1517/14656566.7.4.453

Seitz K, Zhou H (2007) Pharmacokinetic drug-drug interaction potentials for therapeutic monoclonal antibodies: reality check. J Clin Pharmacol 47(9):1104–1118. doi:10.1177/0091270007306958

Sharma MR, Karrison TG, Kell B, Wu K, Turcich M, Geary D, Kang SP, Takebe N, Graham RA, Maitland ML, Schilsky RL, Ratain MJ, Cohen EE (2013) Evaluation of food effect on pharmacokinetics of vismodegib in advanced solid tumor patients. Clin Cancer Res 19(11):3059–3067. doi:10.1158/1078-0432.CCR-12-3829

Shayani S, Palmer J, Stiller T, Liu X, Thomas SH, Khuu T, Parker PM, Khaled SK, Forman SJ, Nakamura R (2013) Thrombotic microangiopathy associated with sirolimus level after allogeneic hematopoietic cell transplantation with tacrolimus/sirolimus-based graft-versus-host disease prophylaxis. Biol Blood Marrow Transplant 19(2):298–304. doi:10.1016/j.bbmt.2012.10.006

Sifontis NM, Benedetti E, Vasquez EM (2002) Clinically significant drug interaction between basiliximab and tacrolimus in renal transplant recipients. Transplant Proc 34(5):1730–1732

Sinclair J (1973) Dextromethorphan-monoamine oxidase inhibitor interaction in rabbits. J Pharm and Pharmac 25:803–808

Somasundaram S, Edmund NA, Moore DT, Small GW, Shi YY, Orlowski RZ (2002) Dietary curcumin inhibits chemotherapy-induced apoptosis in models of human breast cancer. Cancer Res 62(13):3868–3875

Sonpavde G, Hutson TE (2007) Pazopanib: a novel multitargeted tyrosine kinase inhibitor. Curr Oncol Rep 9(2):115–119

Sparano BA, Egorin MJ, Parise RA, Walters J, Komazec KA, Redner RL, Beumer JH (2009) Effect of antacid on imatinib absorption. Cancer Chemother Pharmacol 63(3):525–528. doi:10.1007/s00280-008-0778-7

Spina E, Santoro V, D'Arrigo C (2008) Clinically relevant pharmacokinetic drug interactions with second-generation antidepressants: an update. Clin Ther 30(7):1206–1227. doi:10.1016/j.clinthera.2008.07.009

Strumberg D, Clark JW, Awada A, Moore MJ, Richly H, Hendlisz A, Hirte HW, Eder JP, Lenz HJ, Schwartz B (2007) Safety, pharmacokinetics, and preliminary antitumor activity of sorafenib: a review of four phase I trials in patients with advanced refractory solid tumors. Oncologist 12(4):426–437. doi:10.1634/theoncologist.12-4-426

Tanaka C, Yin OQ, Sethuraman V, Smith T, Wang X, Grouss K, Kantarjian H, Giles F, Ottmann OG, Galitz L, Schran H (2010) Clinical pharmacokinetics of the BCR-ABL tyrosine kinase inhibitor nilotinib. Clin Pharmacol Ther 87(2):197–203. doi:10.1038/clpt.2009.208

Tavakoli-Ardakani M, Kazemian K, Salamzedeh J, Mehdizadeh M (2013) Potential of drug interactions among hospitalized cancer patients in a developing country. Iran J Pharm Res 12(Supplement):175–182

Tawbi H, Christner SM, Lin Y, Johnson M, Mowrey ET, Cherrin C, Chu E, Lee JJ, Puhalla S, Stoller R, Appleman LR, Miller BM, Beumer JH (2014) Calcium carbonate does not affect imatinib pharmacokinetics in healthy volunteers. Cancer Chemother Pharmacol 73(1):207–211. doi:10.1007/s00280-013-2337-0

Tawbi HA, Tran AL, Christner SM, Lin Y, Johnson M, Mowrey E, Appleman LR, Stoller R, Miller BM, Egorin MJ, Beumer JH (2013) Calcium carbonate does not affect nilotinib pharmacokinetics in healthy volunteers. Cancer Chemother Pharmacol 72(5):1143–1147. doi:10.1007/s00280-013-2283-x

Wilkinson GR (2005) Drug metabolism and variability among patients in drug response. N Engl J Med 352(21):2211–2221. doi:10.1056/NEJMra032424

Wrighton SA, Thummel KE (2000) CYP3A. In: Levy R, Thummel KE, Trager WF et al (eds) Metabolic drug interactions. Lippincott Williams and Wilkins, Philadelphia, pp 115–133

Zang J, Wu S, Tang L, Xu X, Bai J, Ding C, Chang Y, Yue L, Kang E, He J (2012) Incidence and risk of QTc interval prolongation among cancer patients treated with vandetanib: a systematic review and meta-analysis. PLoS One 7(2):e30353

Zeller T, Muenstedt K, Stoll C, Schweder J, Senf B, Ruckhaeberle E, Becker S, Serve H, Huebner J (2013) Potential interactions of complementary and alternative medicine with cancer therapy in outpatients with gynecological cancer in a comprehensive cancer center. J Cancer Res Clin Oncol 139(3):357–365

Zhou H, Mascelli MA (2011) Mechanisms of monoclonal antibody-drug interactions. Annu Rev Pharmacol Toxicol 51:359–372. doi:10.1146/annurev-pharmtox-010510-100510

Outpatient and Inpatient Structures: What Does It Need to Integrate Palliative Care Services?

Birgit Jaspers and Friedemann Nauck

Contents

12.1   Introduction

How to organise comprehensive cancer care from the onset of metastatic disease to the end of life is debated. Arguments exist for full integration of palliative services into general oncology care, and some studies have shown that oncologists having insight and knowledge about palliative care result in improved collaboration and early referral (Kaasa 2013). There is strong evidence underscoring the importance of integrating palliative care across the trajectory of cancer (Shin and Temel 2013; Bakitas et al. 2009; Alt-Epping et al. 2012). Recommendations for such integration have been made by oncological societies, among others, the American Society of Clinical

B. Jaspers, DMSc (✉)
Department of Palliative Medicine, University Medical Center, Göttingen, Germany

Department of Palliative Medicine, University Hospital, Bonn, Germany
e-mail: birgit.jaspers@med.uni-goettingen.de; birgit.jaspers@ukb.uni-bonn.de

F. Nauck, MD
Department of Palliative Medicine, University Medical Center, Göttingen, Germany
e-mail: friedemann.nauck@med.uni-goettingen.de

© Springer-Verlag Berlin Heidelberg 2015
B. Alt-Epping, F. Nauck (eds.), *Palliative Care in Oncology*,
DOI 10.1007/978-3-662-46202-7_12

Oncology (Smith et al. 2012), and by authors of comprehensive review articles on this matter (Gaertner et al. 2013; Greer et al. 2013). These include triangular cooperation between cancer specialists, primary care services and specialist palliative care teams; communication, congruity and continuity of care; and coordination, cooperation contracts and collegiality. A qualitative study among oncologists showed that they believed that integrating palliative care enhanced patient care, complemented their own practice and enabled them to 'share the load' (Bakitas et al. 2013).

How this integration can be tackled depends not only on the willingness of providers of oncology and palliative care but also, among others, on

- The national and perhaps regional organisation of palliative care in the respective country
- Its integration in the healthcare system
- Access and availability of palliative care services
- Financial, educational and cultural issues

12.2 Information on the Organisation of Palliative Care Across Countries

The organisation of palliative care varies across countries. Quite recent information can be found in the Atlas of Palliative Care in Europe 2013 launched by the European Association for Palliative Care (EAPC), which can be retrieved from the Internet (Centeno et al. 2013). An Atlas of Palliative Care in Latin America was also published (Pastrana et al. 2012). Country reports from the EAPC Task Force Development of Palliative Care in Europe presented on the EAPC website (http://www.eapc-task-force-development.eu/country.php), however, are mostly outdated but may be helpful in case no other information can be found. More current information is provided by the EAPC at http://www.eapcnet.eu/Themes/Organisation/Countryreports.aspx, where publications from various countries are listed. A search in literature databases such as PubMed and on websites of national societies or associations for palliative care/palliative medicine and hospice care can be useful to obtain information about the provision and organisation of palliative care in a particular country, if required.

In many countries, a lot of both general and more specific information on the organisation of palliative care and its integration in oncology is available from papers of national health agencies (e.g. NICE in the UK), textbooks, the so-called grey literature as well as in local scientific magazines published in the respective national language which are not listed in databases such as PubMed. This kind of literature may also be helpful when it comes to the need of access to country-specific information that includes current developments (organisational, legal, practical, etc.), because such matters are hardly and, if, mostly with substantial delay published in English (unless their origin is from English-speaking countries).

An overview of legal regulations in seven countries has been published in 2013 (Van Beek et al. 2013).

Terms that describe palliative care structures, i.e. kinds of services delivering inpatient and outpatient palliative care, such as palliative care unit, home palliative care team, hospice, hospice programme and day clinic, may be used for different concepts of services in different countries. In an attempt to provide some clarification, the EAPC commissioned two papers with suggestions for a common European terminology following a consensus process with the national associations and outlined general requirements for palliative care services and the specific requirements for each service type (Radbruch and Payne 2009, 2010). These papers can also be retrieved from the Internet (http://www.eapcnet.eu/Themes/Organisation/EAPCStandardsNorms.aspx 2014). As of April 2014, translations of these papers are provided in German, Spanish, Romanian, Russian, Polish and Hungarian. Links for download are provided at the EAPC website (http://www.eapcnet.eu/Themes/Organisation/EAPCStandardsNorms/Translations.aspx 2014). Further terms were consented in the framework of an international research project on the state-of-art and quality of palliative care (EUROPALL; homepage: http://www.europall.eu/).

In order to clearly understand the use of organisational terms and concepts in the field of palliative care in a particular country, these overviews may need 'more flesh to the bone' by seeking additional information via the above-mentioned sources.

12.3 Most Common Organisational Terms, Based on the EAPC White Papers (Radbruch and Payne 2009, 2010) and EUROPALL (Ahmedzai 2010)

There are some common structures, but also a wide variety in the structure of service development and care delivery. These differences are at least partly related to different understanding of the underlying concepts and the terms of palliative care. The development of a common terminology has been claimed as a prerequisite for meaningful comparisons, but will also serve to facilitate an international dialogue on the grounds of use of unambiguous terms. Also, the lack of standard definitions in the palliative oncology literature has been claimed, including a clear distinction between specialist palliative care, palliative care, supportive and best supportive care and the impact of the use of different terms on professional carers and patients (Hui et al. 2012; Maciasz et al. 2013; Wedding 2014). Therefore, the organisational terms used in this chapter are clearly assigned to the field of palliative care and based on the EAPC White Papers on standards and norms in palliative care, complemented with terms consented in the EUROPALL project.

12.3.1 Levels of Care

Palliative care can be delivered on different levels. At least two levels should be provided: a palliative care approach and specialist palliative care. This two-step ladder of care levels can be extended to three steps, including general palliative care:

(a) The palliative care approach and basic skills in palliative care would be used in settings and services only occasionally treating patients in need of palliative care.
    It is a way to integrate palliative care methods and procedures in settings not specialised in palliative care. This includes not only pharmacological and

non-pharmacological measures for symptom control, but also communication with patient and family as well as with other healthcare professionals, decision-making and goal setting in accordance with the principles of palliative care.

The palliative care approach should be made available for general practitioners and staff in general hospitals, as well as for nursing services and for nursing home staff. To enable these service providers to use the palliative care approach, palliative care has to be included in the curricula for medical, nursing and other related professionals' basic education. The Council of Europe recommends that all professionals working in healthcare should be confident with the basic palliative care principles and able to put them into practice.

(b) General palliative care is provided by primary care professionals and specialists treating patients with life-threatening diseases who have good basic palliative care skills and knowledge.

Professionals who are involved more frequently in palliative care, such as **oncologists** or geriatric specialists, but do not provide palliative care as the main focus of their work, still may have acquired special education and training in palliative care and may provide additional expertise.

(c) In contrast, specialist palliative care applies to a team of appropriately trained physicians, nurses, social workers, chaplains and others whose expertise is required to optimise quality of life for those with a life-threatening or debilitating chronic illness.

Patients with life-threatening disease, and those important to them, may have complex needs, which may require the input of the specialist palliative care team. Specialist palliative care describes services whose main activity is the provision of palliative care. These services generally care for patients with complex and difficult needs and therefore require a higher level of education, staff and other resources. Specialist palliative care is provided by specialised services for patients with complex problems not adequately covered by other treatment options.

The ladder can also be extended to a fourth level, that of centres of excellence.

(d) Centres of excellence should provide specialist palliative care in a wide variety of settings, including in- and outpatient care, home care and consultation services and should provide academic facilities for research and education. The role of centres of excellence is still under discussion, and the position of such centres in a multilevel approach will depend on that discussion.

12.3.2 Settings and Services

Palliative care units (PCUs) provide specialist inpatient care. It is usually a ward within or adjacent to a hospital, but it can also exist as a stand-alone service. In some countries, palliative care units will be regular units of hospitals, providing crisis intervention for patients with complex symptoms and problems; in other countries,

PCUs can also be freestanding institutions, providing end-of-life care for patients where home care is no longer possible.

A central feature of PCUs is a multiprofessional team with specially trained members from different healthcare professions, completed by voluntary workers.

Essential services should be available 24 h per day and seven days per week. If possible, there should be 24-h telephone advice for healthcare professionals and 24-h telephone support service for known outpatients and their carers. PCUs are supposed to collaborate with various services in the outpatient and inpatient sector. They work in a network with medical centres, hospital units, general practitioners, outpatient nursing services and hospice services, as well as other appropriate services.

The aim of palliative care units is to alleviate disease- and therapy-related discomfort and, if possible, to stabilise the functional status of the patient and offer patient and carers psychological and social support in a way that allows for discharge or transfer to the patients' home or other care settings.

Hospitals, particularly those without a dedicated palliative care unit, may offer *crisis intervention beds* for patients in need of palliative care. A crisis is defined as an episode that produces emotional, mental, physical and behavioural distress or problems (Nauck and Alt-Epping 2008). This short-term help is limited from one session to several weeks with a maximum of 4 weeks in the Netherlands, where these beds are mostly located in academic medical centres. In Germany, these beds are located mostly in hospitals that want to provide a special area for patients in need of specialist inpatient palliative care but were not included in the regional hospital plan for palliative care beds or units. Thus, the provision of these beds depends on the willingness of hospital owners to offer such services, often with substantial financial contribution. The staff for these crisis beds must have undergone training in specialist palliative care; physicians are mostly working in the anaesthesiology or intensive care medicine department and dedicate a certain percentage of their work time to the crisis intervention beds; nurses may be hired to work solely with these patients. Other relevant staff, such as social or religious workers, are working with all patients in such hospitals, if required, and thus also with patients in the crisis intervention area.

An *inpatient hospice* admits patients in their last phase of life, when treatment in a hospital is not necessary and care at home or in a nursing home is not possible. It requires a multiprofessional team that cares for patients and their relatives using a holistic approach. The core team of an inpatient hospice consists of nurses and requires ready access to a trained physician (24/7); an extended team of multiprofessional healthcare specialists and volunteers should be available.

The central aims of an inpatient hospice are the alleviation of symptoms and achievement of the best possible quality of life until death, as well as bereavement support. In many countries, the function of an inpatient hospice is similar to that of a PCU, whereas, in other countries, e.g. Germany, a clear distinction can be observed. In some countries, a hospice, in contrast to a PCU, is a freestanding service with end-of-life care as its main focus of work.

Palliative beds in nursing homes (in the Netherlands also called independent hospices) are equipped with three to ten beds and often affiliated to, or embedded in, a larger nursing home organisation. Daily care is provided by registered nurses supported by volunteers, general practitioners or medical specialists, mostly nursing home physicians.

Hospital palliative care support teams provide specialist palliative care advice and support to other clinical staff, patients, their families and carers in the hospital environment. They are composed of a multiprofessional team with at least one physician and one nurse with specialist palliative care training, offer formal and informal education and liaise with other services in and out of the hospital. Hospital palliative care support teams are also known as hospital supportive care teams or hospital mobile teams. Hospital palliative care support teams, in the first instance, offer support to healthcare professionals in hospital units and polyclinics not specialised in palliative care.

One central aim of a hospital palliative care support team is the alleviation of multiple symptoms of palliative care patients on different hospital wards by mentoring the attending staff and by supporting the patients and their relatives. Furthermore, expertise in palliative medicine and palliative care shall be made available in the respective environments. Comprehensive support and education is offered on pain therapy, symptom control and psychosocial issues. This involves attending to patients on a variety of different wards and providing advice to other clinicians. However, decisions on, and implementation of, therapies and interventions remain the responsibility of the attending medical staff. The hospital palliative care support team contributes at the request of medical and nursing staff, the admitted patient and his relatives. The team is supposed to act in close collaboration with other specialists.

The aims of a hospital palliative care support team are the improvement of care to foster discharge from an acute hospital unit and the facilitation of the transfer between inpatient and outpatient care.

Palliative care support team describes a specialist palliative care team made up of at least one physician and one nurse that provides professional advice and support to professional caregivers in a certain region (as well in hospitals, at home or in other settings).

Home palliative care teams provide multiprofessional specialised palliative care to patients, support to their families and specialist advice to general practitioners, family doctors and nurses, physiotherapists and others, caring for the patient at home. They offer support with a graded approach and have to be available 7 days a week and 24 h a day. The core team of a home palliative care team consists of four to five full-time professionals and comprises physicians and nurses with specialist training, a social worker and administrative staff.

Most often, the home palliative care team has an advisory and mentoring function and offers its expertise in pain therapy, symptom control and psychosocial support. Advice and support by the home palliative care team can also be provided directly to the patient. Less frequently, the home palliative care team may provide 'hands-on', direct care in collaboration with the general practitioner and other primary care workers. In selected cases with highly complex symptoms and problems, the home palliative care team may take over treatment from the general practitioner and the nursing service and provide comprehensive palliative care. The mode of action also depends on the local model of care delivery and the level of involvement of primary carers. The home palliative care team also assists in the transfer between hospital and home.

The 'hospital at home' provides intensive hospital-like care for the patient at home. In some European countries, for example, France or Finland, the 'hospital at home' offers an intensive medical and nursing service that allows patients who would otherwise be admitted to a hospital to stay at home. This implies a type of care that is much more similar to inpatient hospital treatment than to the usual home care. Different organisational models can be found, ranging from an expansion of existing resources within the home environment to the allocation of a specialist team that can cover all demands.

A *volunteer hospice team* offers support and befriending to palliative care patients and their families in times of disease, pain, grief and bereavement. It comprises at least 10–12 specially trained voluntary hospice workers and one professional coordinator.

The volunteer hospice team is part of a comprehensive support network and collaborates closely with other professional services in palliative care. Volunteer hospice teams are vital in contributing to the psychosocial and emotional support of patients, relatives and professionals and foster the maintenance and improvement of patients' and carers' quality of life. The support persists beyond the patient's death and continues in the phase of bereavement.

Day hospices or day-care centres are located in hospitals, hospices, PCUs or the community and especially designed to promote recreational and therapeutic activities among patients in need of palliative care. They are staffed by a multiprofessional team supplemented by voluntary workers. Patients usually spend part of the day in the day-care centre, either each day or once weekly. Day hospices focus on creative living and social care, offering patients the opportunity to participate in various activities during the daytime outside their familiar surroundings.

Formal medical consultations are not usually part of routine day care, but, in some day-care centres, patients may have some treatments, such as a blood transfusion or a course of chemotherapy, while at the centre. Central aims are social and therapeutic care, to avoid social isolation as well as to relieve the burden of care on relatives and carers.

Palliative outpatient clinics offer consultation for patients living at home who are able to visit the clinic. They are an important component of a community palliative care programme. Usually, they are affiliated to specialist PCUs or inpatient hospices. Patients with progressive disease and reduced performance status will often no longer be able to visit the outpatient clinic. Therefore, outpatient clinics should be integrated in regional networks, in order to consult with inpatient services, home palliative care teams or the primary care team.

Tumour boards (or in some countries multidisciplinary clinics) are where specialists from surgery, medical oncology, radiation oncology, radiology, pathology and palliative medicine/palliative care evaluate and discuss patients for whom a multidisciplinary approach is being considered. Depending on country and healthcare regulations, either treating physicians or the patients themselves can request that their care be discussed by a tumour board. The multidisciplinary group will collectively design the best course of action for each patient.

12.4 Organisational Integration of Palliative Care and Oncological Care

As reported in a review by Shin and Temel (2013), the American Society of Clinical Oncology (ASCO) Provisional Clinical Opinion states that patients with metastatic NSCLC should be offered concurrent palliative care along with standard oncology care at initial diagnosis (Smith et al. 2012). Moreover, palliative care should be considered early in the course of disease for any patient with metastatic cancer and high symptom burden, alongside usual oncology care. Furthermore, the National Comprehensive Cancer Network (NCCN) Clinical Practice Guidelines in Oncology for NSCLC recommend that an initial evaluation for all patients with a new diagnosis of NSCLC should include an assessment of supportive care needs and all cancer patients be screened for palliative care needs at their initial visit, at appropriate intervals and as clinically indicated (Shin and Temel 2013; Levy et al. 2012). Whereas some authors describe which actions in considering the delivery of general palliative care can be undertaken by the oncologists themselves, which skills and tools, respectively, are required and how these actions should be performed (Cheng et al. 2013), it is widely recommended that oncologists recognise when to approach specialist palliative services (Shin and Temel 2013; Howie and Peppercorn 2013; Quill and Abernethy 2013; Stavas et al. 2014; Ostgathe et al. 2010). This is particularly important because there is evidence that patients in need of specialist palliative care services may neither report this need without being prompted nor ask for such services (Schenker et al. 2014). Conceptual models for integrating palliative care in oncology are provided by cancer societies and in scientific articles (Bruera and Hui 2012; Cancer Care Ontario 2013; Alt-Epping and Nauck 2010).

An algorithm for the integration of palliative care services (collaboration, referral and transfer), using terms as defined and described above, is presented in Fig. 12.1.

On the basis that the patient is the main responsibility of the treating oncologist or team of oncologists, the inclusion of specialist palliative care services, depending on national/regional resources and availability of services, may be useful as follows:

Symptom Control Symptom control (pain, dyspnoea, nausea and vomiting, delirium, anxiety, depression, appetite, fatigue, oral care, bowel care, malignant wounds)

Oncology practice	Home palliative care team, palliative care unit, palliative outpatient clinic
Oncology department in hospital	Hospital palliative care support teams, palliative care unit, palliative outpatient clinic, tumour board

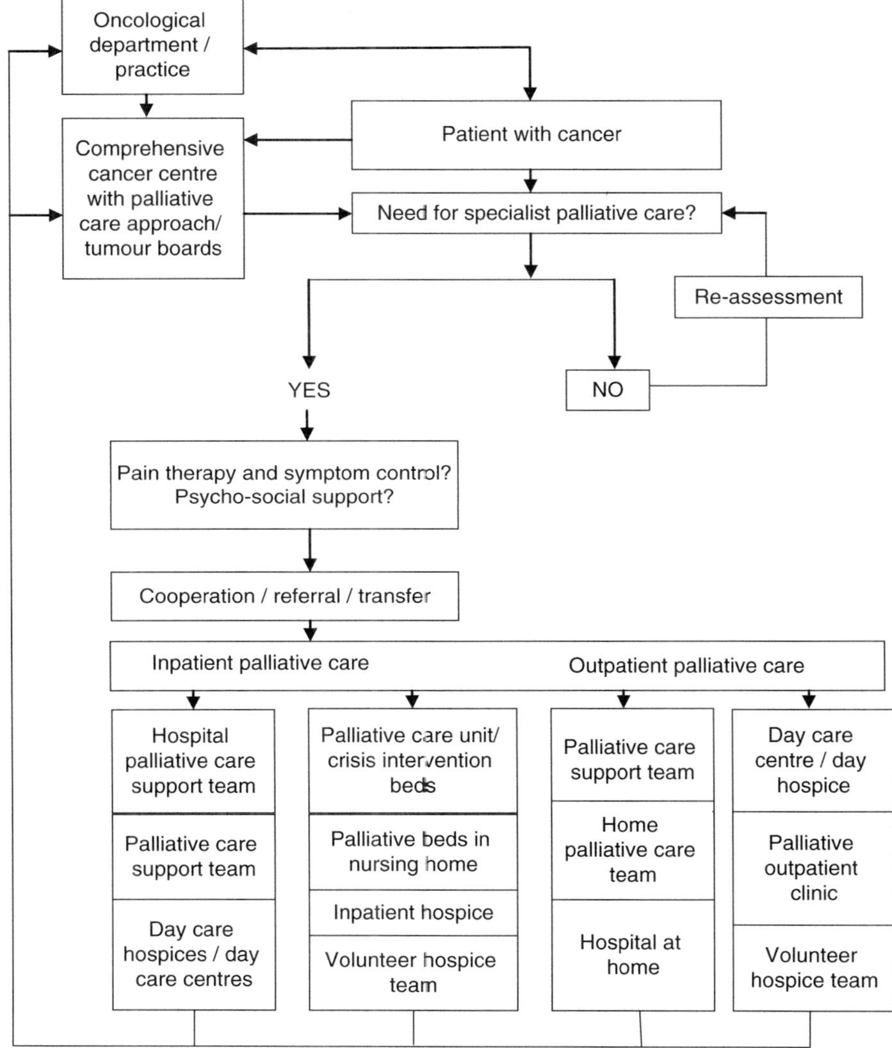

Fig. 12.1 Algorithm for the integration of palliative care across the trajectory of cancer for optimal symptom control

Psychosocial Support

Oncology practice	Home palliative care team, volunteer hospice team, day hospices or day-care centres
Oncology department in hospital	Hospital palliative care support teams, palliative care unit, volunteer hospice team

On the basis that the patient should not (for an interim phase or no longer at all) be the main responsibility of the treating oncologist or team of oncologists, the inclusion of specialist palliative care services, depending on national/regional resources and availability of services, may be useful as follows:

Symptom Control and Psychosocial Support

Oncology practice	Palliative care unit, inpatient hospice, hospice at home, home palliative care team
Oncology department in hospital	Palliative care unit, inpatient hospice, hospice at home, home palliative care team

Place of Care In case treating oncologists need to discuss, initiate or prepare a change of place of care, they may also approach one of the above-mentioned specialist palliative services for advice on and/or organising a patient transfer. Depending on the structure and legal regulations of national or regional healthcare systems, there may be a specific pathway of responsibilities for referral to another place of care, e.g. the general practitioner/family doctor or the organisation of a change of place of care may be the responsibility of the patient/family.

Directories of Palliative Care Services In some countries, there are national/regional directories of palliative care services that are updated on a regular basis. These directories provide contact details for available services and can be useful for healthcare professionals seeking a specific service in their vicinity for support with, for example, symptom control or referral or when trying to find a palliative care service in other regions or even a different country in case patients will no longer be staying at their current place of living. Directories are sometimes produced in form of books, but often (also) available on the Internet, e.g. UK and Ireland (http://www.helpthehospices.org.uk/media-centre/latest-news/hospice-and-palliative-care-directory-20122013/); Spain (http://www.secpal.com/directorio/), Germany (http://www.wegweiser-hospiz-palliativmedizin.de/), and other countries.

The inclusion of or referral to specialist palliative care services may also depend on the question if they are free of cost or affordable for the respective patient. An international project funded by the European Union has collected some data on this matter (see Table 12.1).

There may also be a need for oncologists to approach specialist palliative care services for support of physicians and/or treating teams themselves in matters of therapeutic decision-making, ethical reasoning or bereavement support.

In these cases, oncologists or oncology teams in hospitals may approach specialists from their hospital palliative care support team or the palliative care unit; if given, in some countries these services may come in from other hospitals too. Volunteer hospice teams located at the hospital or the religious/spiritual worker affiliated with the palliative hospital services may deliver bereavement support for professionals.

Oncologists in an oncology practice not attached to a hospital may seek bereavement support through volunteer hospice teams in the ambulatory sector; home

Table 12.1 Funding/financing of palliative care in seven European countries (reference year 2009/10) according to current legislation in the respective countries, mod (Jaspers 2010)

	France	Germany	The Netherlands	Poland	Spain	UK
Palliative care unit (in hospital)	C,E	A,D	A,D	A	A,D	A,D	A,E,G,I
Crisis intervention beds in hospital	Ø	A,D	A,D	A	Ø	A,D	E
Palliative outpatient clinic	Ø	A,D	A,D	A,D	A,D	A,D,H	D
Hospital palliative care support team	A,D	A,D	A,E,I	E,A	A,E,G	A,D,H	D
Palliative care support team	Ø	A,D	A,E,J	Ø	Ø	Ø	E,G
Inpatient hospice	Ø	Ø	B,E,I,J	B,E,I,J	A,D	A,D,G	E,G
Volunteer hospice team	Ø	Ø	A,E,G	Ø	A,D	A,D,G	E,G
Home palliative care team	A,E,G	A,D	A,D	B,E	A,D	A,D,G,H,I	E,G
Palliative beds in nursing homes	C,E	Ø	Ø	A,D	Ø	Ø	E,I
Day hospice/ day-care centre	E,G	A,D	Ø	A,D	A,E,G	A,D,I	E,G
Bereavement support	Ø	A,D,I	A,E,G,J	B	A,F	A,D,G	E,G

A free of cost for the patient, *B* partly financed by the patient, *C* minimal contribution of the patient, *D* fully financed by health system, *E* partly financed by health system, *F* fully financed by charity, *G* partly financed by charity, *H* fully financed by patient (out of pocket), *I* partly financed by social services, *J* partly not financed, *Ø* does not apply to this country

palliative care teams, for example, in Germany delivered by SAPV teams (special-ised ambulatory palliative care), may support oncologists in matters of ethical decision-making.

12.5   Summary

For the integration of palliative care into oncology care, oncologists need to have knowledge about the organisation of palliative care in their respective country, legal and financial regulations of collaboration, access and availability of palliative care services and potential benefits from such collaboration for their patients and/or the oncology team. From a structural point of view, integration and collaboration would benefit from national and international efforts to harmonise the terminology referring to palliative care (services) with consideration of such harmonising initiatives among the palliative care community.

References

Ahmedzai S, Gómez-Batiste X, Engels Y, Hasselar J, Jaspers B, Leppert W, Menten J, Mollard JM, Vissers K (eds) (2010) Assessing organisations to improve palliative care in Europe. Vantilt Publishers, Nijmegen, pp 265–274

Alt-Epping B, Nauck F (2010) Implications of modern anticancer therapies for palliative care concepts. Schmerz 24(6):633–641 [Article in German]

Alt-Epping B, Stäritz AE, Simon ST, Altfelder N, Hotz T, Lindena G, Nauck F, Hospice And Palliative Care Evaluation Hope Working Group (2012) What is special about patients with lung cancer and pulmonary metastases in palliative care? Results from a nationwide survey. J Palliat Med 15(9):971–977

Bakitas M, Lyons KD, Hegel MT, Balan S, Brokaw FC, Seville J, Hull JG, Li Z, Tosteson TD, Byock IR, Ahles TA (2009) Effects of a palliative care intervention on clinical outcomes in patients with advanced cancer: the Project ENABLE II randomized controlled trial. JAMA 302:741–749

Bakitas M, Lyons KD, Hegel MT, Ahles T (2013) Oncologists' perspectives on concurrent palliative care in a National Cancer Institute-designated comprehensive cancer center. Palliat Support Care 11:415–423

Bruera E, Hui D (2012) Conceptual models for integrating palliative care at cancer centers. J Palliat Med 15:1261–1269

Cancer Care Ontario (2013) Psycho-social and palliative care pathway. Version 2013.1. Available at: https://www.cancercare.on.ca (PsychosocialPalliativePathway.pdf)

Centeno C, Lynch T, Donea O, Rocafort J, Clark D, EAPC Atlas of Palliative Care in Europe 2013 – Full Edition (2013) EAPC (European Association for Palliative Care). Available at: http://dspace.unav.es/dspace/handle/10171/29291?locale=en. Last accessed 09 Apr 2014; cartographic edition available at: http://dspace.unav.es/dspace/handle/10171/29290?locale=en. Last accessed 09 Apr 2014

Cheng MJ, King LM, Alesi ER, Smith TJ (2013) Doing palliative care in the oncology office. J Oncol Pract 9:84–88

Gaertner J, Weingärtner V, Wolf J, Voltz R (2013) Early palliative care for patients with advanced cancer: how to make it happen? Curr Opin Oncol 25:342–352

Greer JA, Jackson VA, Meier DE, Temel JS (2013) Early integration of palliative care services with standard oncology care for patients with advanced cancer. CA Cancer J Clin 63:349–363

Howie L, Peppercorn J (2013) Early palliative care in cancer treatment: rationale, evidence and clinical implications. Ther Adv Med Oncol 5:318–323

http://www.eapcnet.eu/Themes/Organisation/EAPCStandardsNorms.aspx. Last accessed 9 Apr 2014

http://www.eapcnet.eu/Themes/Organisation/EAPCStandardsNorms/Translations.aspx. Last accessed 9 Apr 2014

Hui D, Mori M, Parsons HA, Kim SH, Li Z, Damani S, Bruera E (2012) The lack of standard definitions in the supportive and palliative oncology literature. J Pain Symptom Manage 43: 582–592

Jaspers B (2010) Tables. In: Ahmedzai S, Gómez-Batiste X, Engels Y, Hasselar J, Jaspers B, Leppert W, Menten J, Mollard JM, Vissers K (eds) Assessing organisations to improve palliative care in Europe. Vantilt Publishers, Nijmegen, pp 265–274

Kaasa S (2013) Integration of general oncology and palliative care. Lancet Oncol 14:571–572

Levy MH, Adolph MD, Back A, Block S, Codada SN, Dalal S, Deshields TL, Dexter E, Dy SM, Knight SJ, Misra S, Ritchie CS, Sauer TM, Smith T, Spiegel D, Sutton L, Taylor RM, Temel J, Thomas J, Tickoo R, Urba SG, Von Roenn JH, Weems JL, Weinstein SM, Freedman-Cass DA, Bergman MA (2012) Palliative care. J Natl Compr Cancer Netw 10:1284–1309. Available from www.nccn.org
Maciasz RM, Arnold RM, Chu E, Park SY, White DB, Vater LB, Schenker Y (2013) Does it matter what you call it? A randomized trial of language used to describe palliative care services. Support Care Cancer 21:3411–3419
Nauck F, Alt-Epping B (2008) Crises in palliative care–a comprehensive approach. Lancet Oncol 9(11):1086–1091
Ostgathe C, Gaertner J, Kotterba M, Klein S, Lindena G, Nauck F, Radbruch L, Voltz R, Hospice and Palliative Care Evaluation (HOPE) Working Group in Germany (2010) Differential palliative care issues in patients with primary and secondary brain tumours. Support Care Cancer 18(9):1157–1163
Pastrana T, De Lima L, Wenk R, Eisenchlas J, Monti C, Rocafort J, Centeno C (2012) Atlas of palliative care in Latin America ALCP, 1st edn. IAHPC Press, Houston. Available in English and Spanish at: http://cuidadospaliativos org/atlas-de-cp-de-latinoamerica/. Last accessed 9 Apr 2014
Quill TE, Abernethy AP (2013) Generalist plus specialist palliative care – creating a more sustainable model. N Engl J Med 368:1173–1175
Radbruch L, Payne S and the Board of Directors of the EAPC (2009) White paper on standards and norms for hospice and palliative care in Europe: part 1. Eur J Palliat Care 16:278–289
Radbruch L, Payne S and the Board of Directors of the EAPC (2010) White paper on standards and norms for hospice and palliative care in Europe: part 1. Eur J Palliat Care 17:22–33
Schenker Y, Park SY, Maciasz R, Arnold RM (2014) Do patients with advanced cancer and unmet palliative care needs have an interest in receiving palliative care services? J Palliat Med 17:667–672
Shin J, Temel J (2013) Integrating palliative care: when and how? Curr Opin Pulm Med 19:344–349
Smith TJ, Temin S, Alesi ER, Abernethy AP, Balboni TA, Basch EM, Ferrell BR, Loscalzo M, Meier DE, Paice JA, Peppercorn JM, Somerfield M, Stovall E, Von Roenn JH (2012) American Society of Clinical Oncology provisional clinical opinion: the integration of palliative care into standard oncology care. J Clin Oncol 30:880–887
Stavas M, Arneson K, Friedman J, Misra S (2014) From whole brain to hospice: patterns of care in radiation oncology. J Palliat Med 17:662–666
Van Beek K, Woitha K, Ahmed N, Menten J, Jaspers B, Engels Y, Ahmedzai SH, Vissers K, Hasselaar J (2013) Comparison of legislation, regulations and national health strategies for palliative care in seven European countries (Results from the Europall Research Group): a descriptive study. BMC Health Serv Res 13:275
Wedding U (2014) Palliative und supportive Betreuung onkologischer Patienten. Der Onkologe 20:66–71

Jan Gaertner, Jürgen Wolf, and Thomas J. Smith

Contents

J. Gaertner, MD (✉)
Palliative Care Center of Excellence for Baden-Württemberg (KOMPACT),
Baden-Württembers, Germany

Department of Palliative Medicine, Comprehensive Cancer Center Freiburg – CCCF,
University Medical Center Freiburg, Freiburg 79106, Germany
e-mail: jan.gaertner@uniklinik-freiburg.de

J. Wolf, MD, PhD
Department I of Internal Medicine, Centre for Integrated Oncology (CIO),
University of Cologne, Cologne 50937, Germany
e-mail: juergen.wolf@uk-koeln.de

T.J. Smith, MD
Department of Oncology, Johns Hopkins Sidney Kimmel Comprehensive Cancer Center,
600 N Wolfe St, Blalock 369, Baltimore, MD 21287, USA
e-mail: tsmit136@jhmi.edu

© Springer-Verlag Berlin Heidelberg 2015
B. Alt-Epping, F. Nauck (eds.), *Palliative Care in Oncology*,
DOI 10.1007/978-3-662-46202-7_13

13.1   Introduction

It takes a village to raise a child. (Earle 2012)

Health-care institutions and major stakeholders pointed out years ago that palliative care is a vital part of caring for patients with life-threatening diseases and applicable early in the course of the disease together with life-prolonging and disease-modifying therapies (WHO 2007). Yet, palliative care has been equated with end-of-life care by many physicians, including cancer specialists, the public, and policy makers (Parikh et al. 2013). Often, physicians have been rather reluctant to deliver basic palliative care interventions, such as the routine assessment and management of patients' psychosocial needs. Few have received specialist training for symptom control such as pain management (Breuer et al. 2011). Likewise, the routine integration of specialist palliative care services is still the exception and not the norm (Wentlandt et al. 2012).

In recent years, a number of studies have demonstrated the beneficial effects of early palliative care for patients and caregivers, whereupon medical associations such as the American Association of Clinical Oncology (ASCO) have stressed the importance of the topic. Recommendations for early palliative care have also been published (Smith et al. 2012). Meanwhile, the concept has emerged as one of the most intensely discussed topics in cancer care.

Despite widespread enthusiasm, there is also considerable skepticism among cancer specialists (Peppercorn et al. 2011; Mack and Smith 2012). Many cancer specialists feel uncomfortable with palliative care issues, and others hesitate to call upon specialist services because of their strong desire to care for their patients' palliative care needs on their own (Earle 2012). Both attitudes lead to a constant underutilization of early palliative care programs, even when they are readily available (Wentlandt et al. 2012). For instance, at two university hospitals in Philadelphia, only 8 % of cancer patients had a pain/palliative care consultation, usually for end-of-life care (Reville et al. 2010), and lack of a physician referral was the biggest barrier (Kumar et al. 2012). The authors of this chapter would like to share their experience of an early palliative care concept/model. This concept/model is based on collaborative (collegial) interdisciplinary patient care ("shared care") that supports the well-being of patients and relatives as well as cancer and palliative care specialists' satisfaction with their work. Once a cooperation between cancer and palliative care specialists has been established and each discipline has had the opportunity to share their views in the course of everyday collegial communication, we believe that such programs will be strongly endorsed by all disciplines involved. Based on interviews with oncologists who participated in a recently established early palliative care program, Bakitas et al. (2013) found that most cancer specialists report that early palliative care:

- "Completes my practice"
- "Shares the load"
- "Enhances patient care"

In the words of Earle (2012), we have learned,"It takes a village to raise a child," and it takes close collaboration of an interdisciplinary team to care for a patient. We will argue that such collaboration makes life easier for the patient, the family, and the treating oncologist.

> **Bottom Line**
> Early palliative care concepts/models are the cornerstone of state-of-the-art interdisciplinary (comprehensive) cancer care. Specialist palliative care services help oncologists and their teams to achieve their palliative care goals. This cooperation does not diminish the palliative care responsibilities of cancer specialists and does not lead to an over-delegation of palliative care assignments. This model does allow each specialty to use its strengths and to have different models when the oncologist wants to do more palliative care. This chapter provides insights into early palliative care along with practical suggestions for the clinical setting.

13.2   Situation Prior to Early Palliative Care

13.2.1   The Complexity of Cancer Care and Its Consequences for Patients and Physicians

When caring for patients with advanced cancer, medical oncologists (and other cancer specialists) are faced with numerous responsibilities. These physicians must correctly diagnose and stage the disease and also engage in time-consuming and difficult visits to inform patients about available treatment options. During visits with patients, cancer specialists must thoroughly discuss these treatment options with respect to the patients' individual priorities and fears. Subsequently, they must plan and apply disease-modifying interventions such as chemotherapy and coordinate the provision of therapies delivered by other specialists, such as radiotherapy and surgery. Moreover, oncologists are responsible for preventing and handling any complications. Patients must also be closely followed by oncologists to identify side effects and monitor the treatment effect. Often, additional visits and conferences with patients and their relatives are necessary to further discuss therapeutic goals and ensure the patient's autonomy based on participation and informed consent.

In addition to these regular responsibilities, it is also necessary to provide palliative care beginning in early stages of the disease. Therefore, oncologists (Smith et al. 2010) should:

  (i) Provide state-of-the-art symptom control
  (ii) Assure continuous care for family and friends (bereavement)
 (iii) Assess and identify the psychosocial and spiritual domains of suffering
 (iv) Provide competent care for all nonphysical domains of suffering
  (v) Actively initiate conversations about advanced care directives

(iv) Provide information and coordinate cross-sector care (e.g., home care)
(vi) Actively address end-of-life issues
(vii) Facilitate transition to hospice programs

Due to the multiple demands placed on cancer specialists and the work itself which involves repeated exposure to pain and suffering, optimal care for cancer patients and their families is a difficult and often burdensome challenge for physicians and their teams (Srivastava 2011; Walling et al. 2008).

A systematic review on burnout among cancer professionals revealed that the magnitude of personal resources (time, emotions, necessary expertise) needed to care for cancer patients results in a high incidence of burnout, depersonalization, and depression among oncology professionals (Trufelli et al. 2008). Unanimously, oncologists around the world indicate that especially the palliative care situation with all its challenges is a stressful and existential experience for patients and their carers (Ptacek et al. 2001; Baile et al. 2002). Patient-family discussions concerning the discontinuation of disease-modifying therapy are perceived as even more demanding and burdensome if cooperation with palliative care services has not occurred before discontinuation of chemotherapy (Morita et al. 2004). This is one of the main reasons patients often continue with chemotherapy until the end of life, when they have little or no chance of benefit and an overriding chance of harm (Braga 2011).

Interestingly, research has shown that the degree of emotional burden perceived by oncologists directly affects the extent of emotional distress experienced by the patient and their family (Morita et al. 2004). For the physician, emotional burden often results in a loss of professional self-confidence ("sense of failure") and can also lead to a pronounced loss of empathy and avoidance of emotionally demanding conversations (Pollak et al. 2007; Morse et al. 2008a, b).

In an ASCO survey, a majority of physicians dealing with patients suffering from incurable cancer expressed a need for support (Board I of MNCP 2001). Specifically, they reported that they often avoid conversations concerning end-of-life issues and require further training in this regard. Evading time-consuming communicative tasks can also negatively affect the personal and social situation of cancer patients and the welfare of their families (Zafar et al. 2013). Many oncologists reported that PC patients are "a traumatic experience" (Zafar et al. 2013) and indicated that they were inadequately prepared to provide competent symptom control. Another survey reassessed this self-reported competence in symptom control (Breuer et al. 2011) and confirmed early findings about deficits in symptom control (Portenoy 2011; Kearney et al. 2009). At least half of oncologists reported a mostly biomedical approach to cancer care, with little or no training in PC or end-of-life issues, a distant relationship with patients, a sense of failure upon the patient's death, and no ability to help patients cope (Jackson et al. 2008).

We have learned as much about the importance of good communication in the past 20 years as we have about genomic oncology. Modern-day oncology requires not only training in targeted therapy but in symptom management, communication about goals of care, and transition to hospice care. There is ample evidence

(Pham et al. 2014) that these skills can be learned at the resident and practicing oncologist level, either in person at communication skills training programs (Back et al. 2007) or with computerized distance learning (Tulsky et al. 2011). We expect oncologists to keep up with advances in targeted therapy, and good communication is just one example of truly personalized medicine (Peppercorn et al. 2011).

These shortcomings reported by oncologists are understood as a result of the heavy workload of cancer care professionals (Peppercorn et al. 2011). Although it first appears that deficits in symptom control and patient participation primarily affect quality of life and decision-making, they also have implications for the survival benefit of disease-modifying therapies (Maione et al. 2005). It is well known that a better quality of life in cancer patients increases the benefit of and response to chemotherapy (Sloan et al. 2012). Moreover, deficits in patient autonomy and participation during the decision-making process often increase the aggressiveness of care, which can itself reduce survival (Movsas et al. 2009; Pirl et al. 2008; Earle et al. 2008; Irwin et al. 2013). For instance, lung cancer patients in a recent randomized trial of standard oncology care versus usual care plus palliative care had a longer survival, which also strongly correlated with understanding their prognosis and goals of treatment better (Temel et al. 2011; Greer et al. 2012). Morever patients received less fourth and fifth line intravenous chemotherapy (Greer et al. 2012), which has no proven efficacy but some harm (Roeland et al. 2013).

> **Bottom Line**
> Providing both anticancer therapy and palliative care to patients with advanced cancer requires immense resources. According to the "solo-practice model," some physicians attempt to provide both anticancer therapy and palliative care completely on their own. In contrast, some physicians adhere to the "congress-practice model," in which they refer patients to multiple specialists (Bruera and Hui 2012). Unfortunately, neither of these practices allows for the best possible patient outcome and both result in significant burden for the cancer specialists. Therefore, we advocate the "integrated care model," in which oncologists and palliative care specialists actively work together.

13.3 The Difference Between General, Specialist, and Early Palliative Care

13.3.1 Clarifications

13.3.1.1 General Palliative Care

Palliative care is a broad *therapeutic approach* that aims to achieve the best quality of life of patients with life-threatening diseases and their families (WHO 2007). Details of this therapeutic approach have been outlined in detail earlier in this book.

All medical disciplines and professions should aim to possess the expertise to address the palliative care needs of their patients (Gaertner 2013). In fact, they have the obligation to do so and to actively engage in adequate training (Rangachari and Smith 2013; Sullivan et al. 2005). This is typically referred to as general or primary palliative care (Gaertner 2013; Rangachari and Smith 2013).

Hence, oncology teams should routinely provide core elements of general palliative care. Key tenets are:

- Routine symptom and (physical and psychosocial) distress assessment
- Routine spiritual assessment, with referral
- Symptom and (psychosocial and spiritual) distress management
- Routine screening for depression
- Sensitive communication, including advance care planning and end-of-life issues.

Practical recommendations for clinicians to comply with these key tenets are provided in one of the next sections of this chapter.

13.3.1.2 Specialist Palliative Care

In addition to general palliative care, specialist palliative care (syn. specialized palliative care) has emerged as a (medical) discipline.

Specialist palliative care is provided by multiprofessional teams on inpatient wards, in outpatient clinics, and in the form of palliative home care and consultation services (Gaertner et al. 2012a). According to the Center to Advance Palliative Care and the American Cancer Society Action Network definition, palliative care "is specialized medical care for people with serious illnesses. This type of care is focused on providing patients with relief from the symptoms, pain, and stress of a serious illness – whatever the diagnosis. The goal is to improve quality of life for both the patient and the family. Palliative care is provided by a team of doctors, nurses, and other specialists who work with a patient's other physicians to provide an extra layer of support. Palliative care is appropriate at any age and at any stage in a serious illness, and can be provided together with curative treatment."

Recently, specialist palliative care has become increasingly available. For example, the establishment of palliative care *consultation services* is developing rapidly, especially in large academic centers (Norton et al. 2011). For example, in the United States, the proportion of academic medical centers providing a palliative care consultation service increased fivefold (from 15 to 75 %) during the last decade (Gaertner et al. 2012a). By now, nine of ten US medical centers supported by the National Cancer Institute provide a palliative care consultation service (Norton et al. 2011).

In contrast, the institution of inpatient palliative care *wards* is not nearly as well-established in the United States, although there is a comparatively long tradition of such wards in Western Europe (Elsayem et al. 2011). While some institutions consider palliative care units to be a valuable component of specialized palliative care infrastructure, others report that the sole provision of state-of-the-art palliative care consulting services suffices to adequately care for the severely ill (Ellershaw et al. 2010). Reliable data to test either of these assumptions is scarce. However, according to the experiences of many palliative care teams, inpatients who are dying or suffering from severe or complex symptoms are best cared for on a specialist palliative care ward, even if the palliative care department provides a consultation service to help the teams of acute care wards with the care of such patients. Similar to intensive care unit staff that has special expertise in the recognition and management of severe heart failure, staff or PC units has special expertise in symptom assessment, management, and communication and is often able to deal with spiritual issues.

Despite the merits of inpatient palliative care, such specialist wards do not capture the full potential of palliative care (Gaertner et al. 2012b). For this, a cross-sector infrastructure including palliative *home care* is necessary (Gaertner et al. 2012b). Meta-analyses of studies assessing specialist palliative home care services support this assumption (Gomes et al. 2013). Patients are more likely to die at home and to receive adequate symptom control and psychosocial support if specialist palliative home care services are available. This is critically important, because most patients throughout the world prefer to die at home, (Higginson et al. 2013).

From an international perspective, it is noteworthy that there are substantial unsolved terminological issues when differentiating between hospice and palliative care services (von Gunten 2007; Hui et al. 2012). Therefore, it is necessary that readers acquire information about the hospice (and specialist palliative care) infrastructure in their region.

13.3.1.3 Early Palliative Care

Early palliative care has become a major issue in the field of cancer care since J. Temel's publication in the *New England Journal of Medicine* (Temel et al. 2010). Two years later, the study has already been cited by more than 130 PubMed listed publications. Temel and her team performed a randomized controlled trial in which they randomly assigned 151 patients with newly diagnosed metastatic non-small-cell lung cancer to receive either standard oncological care (control group) or additional care provided by a specialist multiprofessional (nurse/physician) palliative care team (intervention group). The palliative care team was to address the following components of cancer care in the initial visit: illness understanding, symptom management, decision-making, coping, planning, and referrals. Only patients with a moderate or good performance status were eligible (ECOG 0–2), and they had to enroll no later than 8 weeks after diagnosis. Despite the fact that 27 of the 151 randomized patients died after 12 weeks and only 107 (86 % of the remaining patients) completed assessments, the investigators were able to report statistically significant patient benefits for the intervention group. Patients who received the intervention had a better quality of life and a lower incidence of both anxiety and depression, despite understanding their prognosis and goals of treatment better. Furthermore, compared to the control group, early palliative care patients had a longer median survival despite receiving fewer aggressive end-of-life care treatments/therapies (aggressiveness defined as chemotherapy within 14 days before death, no hospice care, or admission to hospice 3 days or less before death). In detail, Kaplan-Meier estimates were as follows: 9.8 months (95 % CI, 7.9–11.7) in the entire sample (151 patients), 11.6 months (95 % CI, 6.4–16.9) in the group assigned to early palliative care (77 patients), and 8.9 months (95 % CI, 6.3–11.4) in the control group (74 patients) ($P=0.02$). After adjusting for age, sex, and baseline ECOG, the findings remained significant (hazard ratio for death in the control group, 1.70; 95 % CI, 1.14–2.54; $P=0.01$).

The findings have been actively discussed at different conferences and are still subject to debate. In addition to Temel's findings, other authors have reported similar results (Smith et al. 2012). Based on this evidence, the ASCO also published a provisional opinion on the matter (Smith et al. 2012).

> **Bottom Line**
> In fact, palliative care is *early* by definition, since it is a therapeutic approach that is applicable for all patients (cancer and noncancer) in early stages of life-threatening and life-limiting diseases (WHO 2007). Regardless of their discipline, physicians have the obligation to obtain the expertise to provide palliative care (Smith et al. 2012). This is most often referred to as *general* or *primary* palliative care. In addition to this, *specialist* palliative care has emerged as a (medical) discipline and is available for all patients with a life-threatening/serious illness. In the absence of a consensus definition, the authors of this chapter define early palliative care as:

> The provision of thoroughly delivered general palliative care in addition to close and early cooperation with specialist palliative care services.

13.4 General Palliative Care: The Oncologist's Assignment

13.4.1 Practical Recommendations

Oncology teams should routinely provide core elements of general PC (Rangachari and Smith 2013).

Therefore, basic expertise is mandatory for:

- Symptom assessment including psychosocial and spiritual issues
- Spiritual assessment, at least occasionally
- Sensitive communication, including advance care planning and end-of-life issues

13.4.2 Symptom Assessment

Patients with advanced cancer often suffer from burdensome symptoms that affect their quality of life and are a cause of suffering (Peppercorn et al. 2011). Therefore, actively inviting the patient to report the prevalence and intensity of possible symptoms and distress is an essential component of general PC early in the course of the disease and is necessary for identifying various aspects of the patient's suffering (Meldahl et al. 2012; Velikova et al. 2010).

For *symptom assessment* (e.g., pain, dyspnea, anxiety, insomnia, nausea), patient self-reported outcomes are the gold standard for ensuring patient-oriented care (Hughes et al. 2012). Such routine symptom assessment is advocated by all available guidelines, but adherence to this explicit recommendation is low and results in unnecessary suffering (Dudgeon et al. 2012). Consequently, recently established laws have made routine symptom assessment mandatory for all cancer patients in different regions across North America (Dudgeon et al. 2012).

Distress refers to psychosocial, existential, and spiritual aspects of suffering and may interfere severely with the ability to cope effectively with cancer (Carlson et al. 2012; NCCN 2012). Although distress often results from physical symptoms such as pain, it cannot reliably be detected with routine cancer symptom scales (i.e., ESAS and POS) (Carlson et al. 2012; NCCN 2012). Recent longitudinal studies have suggested that the routine implementation of distress screening may advance the identification and treatment of (existential) suffering in patients with advanced cancer (Carlson et al. 2012). As a result, different organizations have taken steps to recognize distress as "the 6th vital sign" in cancer care (Carlson et al. 2012). From a practical point of view, it must be acknowledged that the successful implementation of such initiatives depends on the *acceptability* and *sustainability* of routine distress screening. The utilized screening tools should be concise and easy to understand for cancer professionals and their patients. Currently, there are feasible single-item tools available that can help patients to provide a self-assessment of their distress (Holland et al. 2010; Goebel and Mehdorn 2011). For example, the *NCCN distress thermometer* is a brief screening tool that allows cancer patients to gauge their distress on a 10-point visual analogue scale NCCN 2012. To expand upon this tool, patients can be asked a single "help question" to identify specific unmet needs ("Do you want help for emotional or psychological concerns at this stage?") (Baker-Glenn et al. 2011).

It is essential to routinely assess the symptom and distress burden of patients with advanced cancer using self-reported and validated outcome measures (Hughes et al. 2012). For *symptom burden*, short and easy-to-use questionnaires should be implemented (Bausewein et al. 2011). A traditional choice is the well-established Edmonton Symptom Assessment System (ESAS) (Watanabe et al. 2012). ESAS has recently become available in a revised format and asks patients to rate the intensity of nine symptoms (e.g., pain, shortness of breath, nausea, anxiety) on an 11-point Likert scale (Watanabe et al. 2012). Another well-established, short, and validated questionnaire is the Palliative care Outcome Scale (POS) (Bausewein et al. 2011). One advantage of the POS is that it covers non-somatic PC issues, such as the patient's need for information and support.

13.4.3 Symptom Management

Physical symptoms are highly prevalent in advanced cancer and a major cause of significant emotional distress such as depression or anxiety (Dudgeon et al. 2012). Thus, basic skills in the treatment of cancer pain, dyspnea, nausea and vomiting, anxiety, gastrointestinal obstruction, delirium, and other frequent symptoms are paramount for cancer specialists. A number of organizations have developed concise treatment algorithms and general recommendations as part of evidence-based consensus guidelines (NCCN 2012; Bennett et al. 2012; Caraceni et al. 2012).

It is important to note that in advanced cancer, to "manage" the symptom must not be understood in the literal sense as "to control" or "to be in charge of" (www. hesaurus.com) each symptom. In advanced stages of the disease, many symptoms such as weakness or cachexia are part of the expected disease trajectory and cannot be reversed. We are simply unable to "control" them. A prominent example is the anorexia-cachexia syndrome (Fearon et al. 2011). In these cases, even novel pharmaceutical interventions are usually futile, and their use may cause patients to have unrealistic expectations. As a result of such interventions, patients may become more dissatisfied with care in the long run (Fearon et al. 2011). Sensitive and honest communication about the expected progress of the disease can lead to a greater patient satisfaction than ineffective treatments. During such conversations, it is important to understand how the symptom is affecting the patient and his/her family (Is the symptom causing anxiety worry? Who is worried?). Moreover, clinicians must reaffirm that they take the patients' concerns and worries seriously. When discussing (controversial and) emotional issues (e.g., withdrawal of nutritional support), it is crucial that the patient and his/her family receive the necessary emotional support (finding other ways of caring for the patient) as well as educational support (facts and information). In particular, the patient and his/her family should be informed about the following issues:

- Absence of hunger and thirst is normal among dying patients.
- Nutritional support may not be metabolized in patients with advanced cancer.
- Artificial nutrition and hydration may be associated with risks (e.g., fluid overload can result in burdening symptoms and hastened death).
- Symptoms like dry mouth are most often refractory/unresponsive to hydration.
- Withholding or withdrawing artificial nutrition and hydration may improve symptoms, is unlikely to hasten death, and is ethically permissible. The available randomized trial data show no benefit from applying 1 l of intravenous fluids daily for any symptom or for survival (Bruera et al. 2012).

Even with only a basic knowledge in palliative care, successful cancer pain management is feasible for the majority of patients, and comprehensive (pocket-size) recommendations are readily available (Table 13.1) (Portenoy 2011; Bennett et al. 2012; Schneider et al. 2012).

13.4.4 Must Knows

(i) Ensure the availability of comprehensive pain and symptom management guidelines in your clinical environment. Concise treatment recommendations fit in every pocket and may help physicians and their teams to adhere to basic rules (Table 13.1).

(ii) Foster close patient-physician communication by:
 – Providing information about the symptomatic treatment that is easy to understand
 – Writing a treatment plan

Table 13.1 Basic rules for the management of cancer pain (Portenoy 2011; Bennett et al. 2012; Schneider et al. 2012)

1. Rule out *noncancer-related causes* of pain! (e.g., gastritis, massive constipation, urinary tract infection, fractures, myocardial infarction)
2. *Opioid therapy:*
2.1. If pain is moderate to severe, initiate opioid therapy according to WHO Step III
2.2. Start with potent pure μ-agonist (e.g., morphine, hydromorphone, fentanyl, oxycodone)
2.3. Provide both a(n):
(i) Baseline ("regular" or "scheduled") opioid, e.g., sustained-release opioid (SRO)
(ii) On-demand ("rescue") opioid, e.g., immediate release (IR) morphine or nasal/buccal rapid-onset fentanyl (ROF)
Dosing of IRO: 1/6 or less than the daily dose of the SRO
Beware of strict dose "calculation" in case of high doses of SRO and opioid "patches"
Dosing of ROF: start with lowest available dose irrespective of SRO dose
2.4. Adjust SRO according to the *temporal pattern* of pain (e.g., if pain is stronger during the day, provide a double dose of SRO in the morning)
2.5. Identify *breakthrough pain* (pain episodes, pain attacks)
Identify triggers (e.g., physical activity)
Educate patient to take IR opioid in advance (e.g., 30 min *before* taking a walk)
If pain episodes need fast onset of analgesia use ROF
2.6. In the case of *dose escalation* (>240 mg oral morphine equivalent/day), consider opioid rotation (calculate carefully)
3. Identify concomitant *neuropathic* pain: initiate and titrate co-analgesic
4. Identify *other factors* that contribute to total pain
Other symptoms (e.g., dyspnea, anxiety, depression, etc.)
Psychosocial domain (e.g., loneliness, information deficits, feeling urged to "fight")
Spiritual burden (e.g., feeling of guilt, meaninglessness, perceived loss of dignity)
Existential suffering (e.g., hopelessness, wishing to hasten death)
5. *Non-opioids* should be provided on a regular basis (e.g., q 8 h), but risks and benefits of additional long-term therapy must be weighed critically
6. Consider analgesic indication for *radiotherapy*
7. Consider indication for *bisphosphonates* or *radionuclides* (if multiple bone metastases)
8. Consider indication for *glucocorticoids* in advanced disease
9. Ensure the availability and utilization of *specialist palliative care*

- Actively addressing frequent fears and prejudices concerning opioid therapy
- Considering new techniques to learn or relearn this information such as the Vital Talk app available at https://itunes.apple.com/us/app/vital-talk/id639969220?mt=8

(iii) Acknowledge the importance of psychosocial and spiritual issues (see below) that frequently relate to the patients' physical symptoms.

(iv) Some symptoms such as the anorexia-cachexia syndrome are part of the expected course of the disease. In these cases, sensitive and honest communication about the anticipated progress and prognosis of the disease is more important than pharmaceutical interventions.

13.4.5 Sensitive Communication, Including Advance Care Planning and End-of-Life Issues

Cancer care requires honest and sensitive disclosure and discussion of diagnosis, prognosis, and treatment options (NCCN 2012). Physicians often hesitate to break bad news, and most cancer patients do not actively communicate their most pressing questions (Mack and Smith 2012). However, once the oncologist actively suggests talking about worries and fears, patients are usually grateful to be offered the chance to discuss their distressing issues (Mack and Smith 2012). Despite the importance of such discussions for patient-oriented care and decision-making, doctors seldom document medical disclosure, advance care planning (ACP), and end-of-life issues (Mack and Smith 2012).

Current studies reveal that this often results in treatment decisions that are inconsistent with the patients' priorities, needs, and expectations (Del Rio et al. 2012). For example, the *Study to Understand Prognosis and Preferences for Outcomes and Risks of Treatments* (SUPPORT) reports that even in the last days of life, many patients were not treated according to their wish for "comfort care" (Mack and Smith 2012). The majority of patients with advanced cancer are offered systemic and often aggressive disease-modifying or intensive care treatment options even in very late stages of the disease. In contrast, palliative care options are not fully embraced (Mack and Smith 2012).

Notably, the majority of patients want to be involved in the disclosure of medical information and in the decision-making process regarding their treatments (alone or together with their families). It is crucial to specifically ask the patient during one of the first visits who should (and who should NOT) be involved in the information and decision-making process (identification of specific family members, friends, or others). These information preferences should be documented (Mack and Smith 2012; Del Rio et al. 2012). The timing of disclosures and discussion of end-of-life issues is crucial. Although this should be based on the individual needs of each patient, existing literature recommends minimum standards for clinical practice.

In this context, *hope* is an extremely crucial concept for physicians and patients (Mack and Smith 2012). In fact, health-care professionals frequently report that their "fear of destroying hope" is the central barrier to engaging in ACP and end-of-life discussions (Mack and Smith 2012). In accordance with Alfred Adler's notion that humans "cannot think, feel, will, or act without the perception of a goal," physicians have recognized that conveying hope is a key element of patient care (Mack and Smith 2012; Mack et al. 2007). All the available, albeit limited data, suggests that hope is strongly associated with honesty and truthful information, even if the news is bad or the prognosis is poor (Smith et al. 2010; Mack et al. 2007). Meanwhile, current guidelines for cancer care stipulate that the *provision of hope* is one aspect of palliative care (Gaertner 2013; NCCN 2012). It is important to note that for patients with advanced cancer (and other incurable and life-threatening diseases), physicians should not convey a one-dimensional concept of hope that is based on a cure or disease "control" (NCCN 2012). Instead, the provision of hope "relies on dignity, comfort, closure and growth at the end of life" (NCCN 2012). In a similar vein, a number of components that are relevant for the feeling of hope and existential suffering have been identified (Fallowfield and Jenkins 2004).

Central elements include:

1. Anxiety regarding death
2. Loss and change
3. Loss of control
4. Personal dignity
5. Fundamental loneliness
6. Quality of relationships
7. Search for meaning
8. Uncertainty regarding the unknowable

Due to their central role in cancer care, physicians can substantially add to their patients' sense of meaning, value, and purpose. Two core competences are required for physicians to practically approach this task:

1. *Empathy:* The willingness to perceive (identify and recognize) the existential dimension of our patients' suffering is essential for being able to provide hope (Fallowfield and Jenkins 2004). *Empathy* enables an adaptive response to the elements of suffering and promotes equanimity, peace, and fulfillment while also sustaining a commitment to life, creativity, and joy (Fallowfield and Jenkins 2004).
2. *Acceptance*: Core elements of existential suffering such as *the uncertainty of the unknowable* or loss and parting cannot be the subject of "treatment." Instead, physicians and their teams can help their patients to bear and accept the inevitable situation by affirming that they recognize their patients' suffering (Zafar et al. 2012; Kissane 2012).

13.4.6 Must Knows

Physicians should foster end-of-life conversations and can rely on available comprehensive (pocket-size) guidelines about physician-patient communication (Table 13.2) and basic frameworks for ACP (Table 13.3). In addition to communication directives, the two main core competences are *empathy* and *acceptance*. This means that the patients' uncertainty about the unknowable or loss and grief cannot

Table 13.2 Recommendations for conversations about end-of-life issues

(i) *Communication*
1. Use everyday language as much as possible
2. Be honest
3. Ask patients to restate information as a way to ensure they have understood it
4. Encourage patients to ask questions
5. Allow intervals of silence
6. Engage in active listening
7. Allow adequate time for discussion
8. Give at least some negative information along with the positive, to ensure understanding (Robinson et al. 2008)
9. Repeat and summarize
(ii) *Responses to strong emotions*
1. Recognition and legitimation: "It's only natural to feel that…."
2. Validation: "Yes, this is a very anxiety-provoking time for you."
3. Empathy: "This is making you both worried and sad, is that right?"
4. Tangible help: "I think I can help by…."
(iii) *Decision-making*
Patients should be fully informed about the realistic goals of different treatment options. So-called *decision aids* are helpful. These tools are designed to advance patient participation and information by ensuring the provision of a minimum amount of written information about the benefits and disadvantages of treatment interventions and the alternatives.
Adapted from Walling et al. (2008), Gaertner (2013), Rodin et al. (2009)

Table 13.3 Basic elements of advance care planning (ACP)

1. Making ACP a routine part of provider-patient communication
2. Identifying existing ACP documents or advance directives (AD)
3. Assessing decision-making capacity and the need for a surrogate decision-maker
4. Addressing anxiety and fear about dying
5. Encouraging the designation of a health-care proxy, medical power of attorney, or patient surrogate for health care
6. Considering patient diversity, including cultural differences
7. Documenting ACP discussions, including the patient's values and care preferences (may involve completion of an AD)
8. Including discussion of options for a range of potential patient-specific events, e.g., cardiopulmonary resuscitation and do-not-resuscitate orders, withholding/withdrawing nutrition or hydration and tube feeding, mechanical ventilation, admission to intensive care, blood transfusions, use of other life-saving or sustaining interventions, hospice, place of death, and organ donation
9. Recognizing medical uncertainty and inability to plan for all possible situations (limitations of advance directives and the value of ethics consultations)
10. Confirming the patient's understanding of the actual information
11. Ensuring cross-facility and cross-discipline communication on ACP
12. Conducting periodic review or revision of ACP, particularly when the patient's circumstances change
13. Referring to state and institutional guidelines for additional guidance

AD advance directives

be the subject of "treatment." Instead, physicians and their teams can help their patients to bear and accept the inevitable situation by affirming that they recognize their patient' suffering. The necessary skills, knowledge, and attitudes can be best acquired by participation in formal education courses. We suggest the use of smartphone "apps" for those who need support.

> **Bottom Line**
> Basic palliative care expertise is mandatory for all physicians, especially for cancer specialists and their teams. Routine symptom assessment and basic knowledge about symptom control and end-of-life communication are necessary components. Comprehensive (pocket-size) recommendations are available for most of these issues, and further training is recommended.

13.5 Integration of Specialist Palliative Care

13.5.1 Cooperation Is Key

This section refers to the second part of the definition for early palliative care as provided above: *early* PC is also characterized by the need for "early cooperation" between the primary treating cancer specialists and specialized PC teams.

Therefore, in addition to the general PC skills and attitudes of primary treating physicians, close cross-sector cooperation with primary care (such as family doctors and nursing services) and specialized PC services is warranted (Gaertner 2013; Smith et al. 2012).

For example, Temel et al. (2010) reported in the abovementioned study that patients with advanced non-small-cell lung cancer significantly benefit from the provision of an additional *specialized* PC team. Accordingly, close cooperation between medical oncology and specialized PC teams has been advocated by many international associations and institutions (WHO 2007; Smith et al. 2012; Project 2009; (NICE 2004).

In spite of the indisputable benefits of cooperation models involving oncology and PC specialists, there are also concerns. For example, Hoffman et al. (2012) pointed out that an over-delegation of general PC assignments, e.g., from medical oncology to specialized PC, could lead to a fragmented type of care. In line with other authors, they suggest that the field of medical oncology should pursue the development of instructional frameworks for hematology-oncology fellowship programs to address current deficiencies in PC and communication skills (Smith et al. 2012b).

Another concern is the role of primary care in these concepts. Notably, primary care (family medicine) is an important source of general PC provision (Gardiner et al. 2012). In everyday life, family doctors (general practitioners) and nursing services tend to most of the patients' and families' PC needs. The available data show that when the primary care physician remains involved in decision-making and support, patients suffer less distress (Aubin et al. 2011) and have a better quality of life.

Moreover, Quill and Abernethy (2013) have pointed out that the approach of Temel et al. (2010) would require enormous resources. In their model, each patient with advanced cancer is seen by a specialist palliative care team on a regular basis every 4 weeks beginning at the time the (e.g., stage IIIb lung) cancer is diagnosed.

We agree that close communication between the different PC providers is necessary to avoid:

(i) Burdening patients and their families with contradictory opinions about the reasonable means and realistic goals of therapy
(ii) Ambiguity about which doctor holds the main responsibility for the patient and should be contacted in the case of medical problems and questions
(iii) Uncoordinated (poly)pharmacy
(iv) Unnecessary appointments and futile resource utilization

13.5.2 A Practical Framework

As a reaction to concerns described above, our working groups (e.g., Rangachari and Smith (2013) and Gaertner et al. (2013)) are dedicated to the development and implementation of concepts that provide coordinated interdisciplinary palliative care in close cooperation with cancer and palliative care specialists. These concepts are described here:

From our perspective, the key to timely and routine specialist palliative care integration is an "introductory/exploratory visit." To ensure this, the identification and routine assessment of "green flags" is helpful (Table 13.4). Such an "initiation visit" does not necessarily generate the need for further routine specialist palliative care appointments (as, e.g., in the work of Temel et al. (2010)). Yet, it reduces the patients', caregivers', and oncologists' barriers to access specialist palliative care once it becomes necessary.

Oncologists have repeatedly expressed their difficulty to explain the need for specialist palliative care involvement to their patients (Breuer et al. 2011; Wentlandt et al. 2012). Therefore, we recommend that physicians communicate what palliative care is and why specialist palliative care is necessary as proposed in Box 13.1.

It is important that specialist palliative care visits are not viewed as an ambiguous "black box." Rather, specialist palliative care assignments and proceedings should be as transparent as possible to other colleagues. To achieve this, many teams

Table 13.4 ("Green flags") for first specialist palliative care team visit

(a) Time of first progression
(b) Once the patient begins receiving opioids (suggested by Craig C Earle, MD)
(c) Presence of modest to severe distress (measured by the NCCN distress thermometer)
(d) Presence of modest to severe symptoms (e.g., dyspnea, pain, depression)
(e) Patient expresses the wish to die (desire to hasten death)
(f) Patient expresses feeling of hopelessness
(g) Presence of unmet palliative care needs is suspected by oncology team members or family caregivers

find it helpful to consent and create an outline ("timetable," "schedule," or "algorithm") for these visits. Such an outline is presented in Table 13.5. Key tenets are No. 1.3 ("responsibility split" or "dividing responsibility") and No. 5 ("back coupling"). These ensure the coordinated and collegial provision of palliative care by cancer and palliative care specialists.

> **Box 13.1 Possible explanation why the specialist palliative care visit is initiated**
> Doctor: *We want to fight your cancer and make you live as long as possible. But it is also important to fight for you and how you feel. We call this "quality of life".*
>   *We can manage most of your quality of life needs, but medicine has become a complex business. The palliative care team members are our specialists for quality of life, so it might be very helpful for you to get to know them and better understand where you and your family can get additional help in case this is necessary*

Table 13.5   Potential outline for a first (specialist) palliative care ((S)PC) visit (Gaertner 2013)

1.	**Informing the patient and family** – "mission statement"	
	Description	**Possible statements**
1.1	**Scope** *What is PC all about?*	PC is focused on maintaining quality of life (Qol)
		PC helps patients (pt) and families (fam) to:
		– Live with cancer
		– Treat symptoms (e.g., pain)
		– Find things they can do to care for themselves
		– Find out what is important to them
		– Organize help if it is necessary
		– Live a life as normal as possible
1.2	**Reason** *Why does additional SPC makes sense?*	Treatment of severe illness is difficult
		It helps all involved to have a team dedicated to treating symptoms and helping the patient cope with the illness
		Cooperation of specialists helps to provide the best treatment (i) **against** cancer and (ii) **for** Qol
1.3	**Dividing responsibility** *Who is primarily in charge?*	The oncologist (in close cooperation with the family doctor) is the main contact person
		SPC provides *additional* advice in close communication with the oncologist/family doctor (congruency of concepts, see No. 5 below)
1.4	**Availability** *When will I see the SPC team?*	SPC is provided "*on demand*" and "*as needed*"
		If pt, fam, or other doctors feel that additional support or advice could be helpful, neither one should hesitate to contact the SPC team (flyer or card should be provided to pt and fam)

(continued)

Table 13.5 (continued)

2	**Identification of suffering and information needs** – "listen and assess"	
2.1	**Open questions** *Opportunity for pt and fam to find out and/or express what they need*	Possible questions:
		How are you?
		Is there anything you would like to know?
		What bothers you most?
		What are you thinking about right now?
		What is important to you right now?
		What are you hoping for?
2.2	**Structured PC assessment**	Edmonton Symptom Assessment Scale (ESAS)
		Palliative Care Outcome Scale (POS)
		NCCN Distress Thermometer, etc.
3	**Clinical and biographic assessment** – "the whole picture"	
3.1	**Patient history**: including medical, psychosocial, and spiritual domains	
3.2	**Patient autonomy:**	
	Identify state of pt (and fam) information (What does the pt know about the prognosis?)	
	Identify preferred mode of pt information	
	(i) What information does the pt *want* to receive in the future?	
	(ii) Does the pt want fam members be involved in this process?	
	Advance Directives (AD):	
	(i) Document current AD	
	(ii) Inform pt and fam that AD are advisable in the case of severe illness	
	(iii) Offer help and counseling for formulating an AD	
3.3	**Physical examination**: (i) if applicable (ii) symptom oriented	
3.4	**Review of records**: *I*dentify causes for symptoms and understand prognosis of disease	
4	**Provision of PC suggestion** – "advice"	
4.0	**Preview of records**: Ensure congruity of care through close interdisciplinary communication (see No. 5)	
4.1	**Medication** (if applicable):	
	Provide and explain medication plan	
	Actively address possible opioid myths	
	Assure pt and fam that they can call back in case of questions/concerns	
	Assure appropriate follow-up (e.g., visit or phone call)	
4.2	**Non-pharmacologic interventions** (if applicable):	
	For example, fan, wound dressing, aromatherapy, and mouth care	
	Consider helpfulness of further counseling (e.g., psycho-oncology, chaplaincy, social work)	
4.3	**Patient and family information needs** (if applicable)	
4.4	**Diagnostic procedures** (if applicable)	
5	**Short personal interdisciplinary communication with cancer specialist** – "back coupling"	
	Agree and ensure:	
	(i) Common understanding of therapeutic goals	
	(ii) Common information basis about pt and fam information needs	
	(ii) Congruity of care	
	(iii) Availability of PC suggestions	
	(iv) That the oncologist and family doctor remain the primary contacts	

In later follow-up visits, component No. 1 ("*mission statement*") may be omitted

Bottom Line

In summary, the Latin prefix "Co" (together, jointly) is the basis of the main pillars of an early palliative care "*Co*-ncept":

1. *Co-operation:*
   Patients' and families' palliative care needs are best addressed by close triangular cooperation between (i) cancer specialists, (ii) primary care (family medicine, nursing services, etc.), and (iii) specialist palliative teams.
2. *Co-mmunication and Co-ngruity of care*
   This triangular approach requires close communication about the relevant aspects of care for each patient to (i) avoid contradictory communication of treatment goals and (ii) futile or hazardous medication and to (iii) assure the utilization of synergies of the different disciplines involved.
3. *Co-ordination*
   At all times, patients and their families should know who is primarily responsible for their care and who they should contact in case of questions, concerns, or medical problems.
4. *Co-llegiality* (and *Co-ntracts*)
   Cooperation, communication, coordination, and congruity of cancer care can be facilitated through formal agreements (contracts). This may also foster a collegial understanding of interdisciplinary care and reduce barriers toward the integration of specialized palliative care services. Specifications and agreements can be helpful for organizing the *timing* and responsibilities of specialized palliative care. For example, agreeing about "green flags" helps to ensure the timely integration of specialist palliative care (Table 13.4). The "dividing *responsibility*" should be a formal agreement between oncology, primary care, and specialized palliative care specialists aimed at enhancing the congruity of care and supporting a teamwork understanding of interdisciplinary care.

   For example, it may be helpful to formally agree that (i) patients and their families must not be confronted with contradictory recommendations and suggestions and that (ii) oncology (or radiotherapy, radio-oncology and other cancer specialists) remains fully in charge of treatment decisions regarding disease-modifying therapy. According to this concept, specialized palliative care is provided as a *consultation* (to provide advice) to the oncology or primary care team and patients. As such, the primary responsibility for patient care remains with the other disciplines unless specialized palliative home care or admission to a specialized inpatient ward becomes necessary. Ideally, specialist palliative care consultation should take place in the out- and inpatient units of the other disciplines. This procedure can help avoid unnecessary appointments and convey the team approach to patients and caregivers.

Box 13.2 Personal Experience: The Medical Oncologist (J.W.)

When we thought about integrating our colleagues from the palliative care team in terms of establishing an *early integration of palliative care* model, we were just starting to build up a new central interdisciplinary outpatient unit in our comprehensive cancer center. There was a lot of enthusiasm among the colleagues in my team with all these new ideas and structures: patient navigators, interdisciplinary consultation hours, new programs in molecular diagnostics, and personalized early phase clinical trials. I was responsible for this program and thus absolutely shared this enthusiasm. However, personally, I also felt some discomfort realizing the imbalance between our great new ideas on the one hand and the still unchanged disastrous prognosis of most of our solid cancer patients with advanced disease.

To give an example, a patient with stage IV lung cancer and without any favorable mutation in his tumor has a chance of about 20–40 % for response to first-line chemotherapy and a median overall survival expectation of only one year. Especially in the science-driven setting of a comprehensive cancer center with innovative clinical trials, the interaction of the medical oncologist and the patients first of all is focused on the cancer-specific treatment and the hope for tumor control (which is absolutely justified). However, a substantial proportion of these patients will not benefit from this therapy at all (and the ratio is still worse in the relapsed setting), and these patients (and not much later also the patients who respond initially to therapy) will be faced with all the problems and questions arising during the final stage of their disease: how to control symptoms like pain and fatigue, how to cope with the fear of death, how to interact with family members, and how to select the right place for dying? My feeling was increasingly that raising hope in our patients with new drugs and new treatment strategies would be only justified if, in parallel, these existential needs would also be addressed.

Thus, the early integration of palliative care – for all noncurative patients from the beginning of their treatment in our institution – was the ideal answer to my concerns and I strongly supported the implementation of these programs. And despite concerns of colleagues related to the generation of competing treatment strategies and unnecessary frightening of patients and families the program immediately became a great success in our cancer center. It is well accepted by doctors, patients, and family members. Not only did symptom control become better in general – what might be at least of equal importance: the patients and their families, besides hoping for the effects of new treatment strategies, have the chance to talk unhurriedly about all the fundamental questions arising in the context of an approaching death and thus are better prepared for the final period of their life.

Box 13.3 Personal Experience: The Palliative Care Specialist (J.G.)

Years ago, after approaching the team of our comprehensive cancer center to initiate an early palliative care program, I was not too sure whether this had been a good idea. The palliative care team did not show much enthusiasm for this project. The objections were in part related to the fear of being a stopgap for situations that would otherwise run out of control. Literally, one member of the team said that "you may become the psychosocial fig leaf and symptom controller for the oncology team."

My personal reluctance had different causes. I thought, "What can I really DO with this fit (ECOG 1), young NSCLC stage IV EGFR pos patient?" and "What will the patients and families think during the 1st visit?" The latter is indeed an interesting question. What really helped was the fact that we were introduced as "experts for quality of life." Patients valued knowing how to get additional support to maintain quality of life if this became necessary.

Meanwhile, I have learned to appreciate the value of this approach. Patients that I have not seen for months or even years after the initiation visit repeatedly say that "it was so valuable to have your card with us." The card (or leaflet) is often perceived as the assurance of a close network or a "Plan B." This seems to calm patients and their families.

But also for my colleagues and me, the close interdisciplinary concept was a real treasure. The experience of working together closely with nephrologists, cardiologists, neurologists, oncologists, radiotherapists, urologists, and surgeons (and many more) leads to incredible growth of clinical knowledge. This is an opinion that all of us share. As experienced seniors within our own discipline, such a concept allows for an ongoing growth of clinical competence – a wonderful experience.

Collegiality and teamwork are key tenets. The concept only works when we appreciate each other's core competences. For example, a specialist palliative care team should not provide a second opinion on the already initiated chemotherapy. Offering a second opinion when it is not necessary not only damages relationships between colleagues but also confuses and bothers the patients. Of course I sometimes have different opinions about the indication for this or that treatment. But, it is best to discuss these matters in the colleague's office. Interdisciplinary care is key. This leads to the last point I want to make. As a palliative care specialist, I have often perceived that in many centers and private practices, patients are not receiving the specialist palliative care support they need. On the other hand, however, I must be honest in saying that some palliative care departments (wards, home care services, outpatient clinics) also (paradoxically) underutilize oncological expertise because not all palliative care colleagues are dedicated to such interdisciplinary care – even though this is a mainstay of our specialty.

References

Aubin M, Vézina L, Verreault R, Fillion L, Hudon E, Lehmann F et al (2011) Family physician involvement in cancer care and lung cancer patient emotional distress and quality of life. Support Care Cancer 19(11):1719–1727

Back AL, Arnold RM, Baile WF, Fryer-Edwards KA, Alexander SC, Barley GE et al (2007) Efficacy of communication skills training for giving bad news and discussing transitions to palliative care. Arch Intern Med 167(5):453–460

Baile WF, Lenzi R, Parker PA, Buckman R, Cohen L (2002) Oncologists' attitudes toward and practices in giving bad news: an exploratory study. J Clin Oncol 20:2189–2196

Baker-Glenn EA, Park B, Granger L, Symonds P, Mitchell AJ (2011) Desire for psychological support in cancer patients with depression or distress: validation of a simple help question. Psychooncology 20:525–531

Bakitas M, Lyons KD, Hegel MT, Ahles T (2013) Oncologists' perspectives on concurrent palliative care in a National Cancer Institute-designated comprehensive cancer center. Palliat Support Care 11(5):415–423

Bausewein C, Le Grice C, Simon S, Higginson I (2011) The use of two common palliative outcome measures in clinical care and research: a systematic review of POS and STAS. Palliat Med 25:304–313

Bennett MI, Graham J, Schmidt-Hansen M, Prettyjohns M, Arnold S (2012) Prescribing strong opioids for pain in adult palliative care: summary of NICE guidance. BMJ 344:e2806

Board I of MNCP (2001) In: Foley K, Gelband H (eds) AACN advanced critical care. National Academies Press, Washington, DC

Braga S (2011) Why do our patients get chemotherapy until the end of life? Ann Oncol 22(11):2345–2348

Breuer B, Fleishman SB, Cruciani RA, Portenoy RK (2011) Medical oncologists' attitudes and practice in cancer pain management: a national survey. J Clin Oncol Off J Am Soc Clin Oncol 29(36):4769–4775

Bruera E, Hui D (2012) Conceptual models for integrating palliative care at cancer centers. J Palliat Med 15(11):1261–1269

Bruera E, Hui D, Dalal S, Torres-Vigil I, Trumble J, Roosth J et al (2012) Parenteral hydration in patients with advanced cancer: a multicenter, double-blind, placebo-controlled randomized trial. J Clin Oncol [Internet]. Available from: http://www.ncbi.nlm.nih.gov/pubmed/23169523

Caraceni A, Hanks G, Kaasa S, Bennett MI, Brunelli C, Cherny N et al (2012) Use of opioid analgesics in the treatment of cancer pain: evidence-based recommendations from the EAPC. Lancet Oncol 13:e58–e68

Carlson LE, Groff SL, Maciejewski O, Bultz BD (2010) Screening for distress in lung and breast cancer outpatients: a randomized controlled trial. J Clin Oncol 28(33):4884–4891

Carlson LE, Waller A, Groff SL, Zhong L, Bultz BD (2012) Online screening for distress, the 6th vital sign, in newly diagnosed oncology outpatients: randomised controlled trial of computerised vs personalised triage. Br J Cancer 107:617–625

Del Rio MI, Shand B, Bonati P, Palma A, Maldonado A, Taboada P et al (2012) Hydration and nutrition at the end of life: a systematic review of emotional impact, perceptions, and decision-making among patients, family, and health care staff. Psychooncology 21:913–921

Dudgeon D, King S, Howell D, Green E, Gilbert J, Hughes E et al (2012) Cancer Care Ontario's experience with implementation of routine physical and psychological symptom distress screening. Psychooncology 21:357–364

Earle CC (2012) It takes a village. J Clin Oncol 30:353–354

Earle CC, Landrum MB, Souza JM, Neville BA, Weeks JC, Ayanian JZ (2008) Aggressiveness of cancer care near the end of life: is it a quality-of-care issue? J Clin Oncol 26:3860–3866

Ellershaw J, Dewar S, Murphy D (2010) Achieving a good death for all. BMJ 341:c4861

Elsayem A, Calderon BB, Camarines EM, Lopez G, Bruera E, Fadul NA (2011) A month in an acute palliative care unit: clinical interventions and financial outcomes. Am J Hosp Palliat Care 28:550–555

Fallowfield L, Jenkins V (2004) Communicating sad, bad, and difficult news in medicine. Lancet 363:312–319

Fearon K, Strasser F, Anker SD, Bosaeus I, Bruera E, Fainsinger RL et al (2011) Definition and classification of cancer cachexia: an international consensus. Lancet Oncol 12:489–495

Gaertner JWV (2013) Early Palliative care for patients with advanced cancer: how to make it work. Curr Opin Oncol 25:342–352

Gaertner J, Frechen S, Sladek M, Ostgathe C, Voltz R (2012a) Palliative care consultation service and palliative care unit: why do we need both? Oncologist 17(3):428–435

Gaertner J, Drabik A, Marschall U, Schlesiger G, Voltz R, Stock S (2012b) Inpatient palliative care: a nationwide analysis. Health Policy [Internet]. Available from: http://www.ncbi.nlm.nih.gov/pubmed/22889468

Gardiner C, Gott M, Ingleton C (2012) Factors supporting good partnership working between generalist and specialist palliative care services: a systematic review. Br J Gen Pract 62:e353–e362

Goebel S, Mehdorn HM (2011) Measurement of psychological distress in patients with intracranial tumours: the NCCN distress thermometer. J Neurooncol 104:357–364

Gomes B, Calanzani N, Curiale V, McCrone P, Higginson IJ (2013) Effectiveness and cost-effectiveness of home palliative care services for adults with advanced illness and their caregivers. Cochrane Database Syst Rev (Online) (6):CD007760

Greer JA, Pirl WF, Jackson VA, Muzikansky A, Lennes IT, Heist RS et al (2012) Effect of early palliative care on chemotherapy use and end-of-life care in patients with metastatic non-small-cell lung cancer. J Clin Oncol 30(4):394–400

Higginson IJ, Sarmento VP, Calanzani N, Benalia H, Gomes B (2013) Dying at home – is it better: a narrative appraisal of the state of the science. Palliat Med 27(10):918–924

Hoffman MA, Raftopoulos H, Roy R (2012) Oncologists as primary palliative care providers. J Clin Oncol 30(22):2801–2802; author reply 2802

Holland JC, Andersen B, Breitbart WS, Compas B, Dudley MM, Fleishman S et al (2010) Distress management. J Natl Compr Cancer Netw 3:448–485

Hughes EF, Wu AW, Carducci MA, Snyder CF (2012) What can I do? Recommendations for responding to issues identified by patient-reported outcomes assessments used in clinical practice. J Support Oncol 10:143–148

Hui D, Mori M, Parsons HA, Kim SH, Li Z, Damani S et al (2012) The lack of standard definitions in the supportive and palliative oncology literature. J Pain Symptom Manage 43:582–592

Irwin KE, Greer JA, Khatib J, Temel JS, Pirl WF (2013) Early palliative care and metastatic non-small cell lung cancer: potential mechanisms of prolonged survival. Chron Respir Dis 10(1):35–47

Jackson VA, Mack J, Matsuyama R, Lakoma MD, Sullivan AM, Arnold RM et al (2008) A qualitative study of oncologists' approaches to end-of-life care. J Palliat Med 11(6):893–906

Kearney MK, Weininger RB, Vachon MLS, Harrison RL, Mount BM (2009) Self-care of physicians caring for patients at the end of life: "Being connected… a key to my survival.". JAMA 301(11):1155–1164, E1

Kissane DW (2012) The Relief of Existential Suffering. Arch Intern Med 3:1–5

Kumar P, Casarett D, Corcoran A, Desai K, Li Q, Chen J et al (2012) Utilization of supportive and palliative care services among oncology outpatients at one academic cancer center: determinants of use and barriers to access. J Palliat Med 15:923–930

Mack JW, Smith TJ (2012) Reasons why physicians do not have discussions about poor prognosis, why it matters, and what can be improved. J Clin Oncol 30:2715–2717

Mack JW, Wolfe J, Cook EF, Grier HE, Cleary PD, Weeks JC (2007) Hope and prognostic disclosure. J Clin Oncol 25:5636–5642

Maione P, Perrone F, Gallo C, Manzione L, Piantedosi F, Barbera S et al (2005) Pretreatment quality of life and functional status assessment significantly predict survival of elderly patients with advanced non-small-cell lung cancer receiving chemotherapy: a prognostic analysis of the multicenter Italian lung cancer in the elderly study. J Clin Oncol 23(28):6865–6872

Meldahl ML, Acaster S, Hayes RP (2012) Exploration of oncologists' attitudes toward and perceived value of patient-reported outcomes. Qual Life Res [Internet]. Available from: http://www.ncbi.nlm.nih.gov/pubmed/22684493

Morita T, Akechi T, Ikenaga M, Kizawa Y, Kohara H, Mukaiyama T et al (2004) Communication about the ending of anticancer treatment and transition to palliative care. Ann Oncol 15:1551–1557

Morse DS, McDaniel SH, Candib LM, Beach MC (2008a) "Enough about me, let's get back to you": physician self-disclosure during primary care encounters. Ann Intern Med 149(11):835–837

Morse DS, Edwardsen EA, Gordon HS (2008b) Missed opportunities for interval empathy in lung cancer communication. Arch Intern Med 168:1853–1858

Movsas B, Moughan J, Sarna L, Langer C, Werner-Wasik M, Nicolaou N et al (2009) Quality of life supersedes the classic prognosticators for long-term survival in locally advanced non-small-cell lung cancer: an analysis of RTOG 9801. J Clin Oncol 27:5816–5822

NCCN (2012) NCCN clinical practice guidelines in oncology: palliative care [Internet]. Available from: www.nccn.org

(NICE) NI for CE (2004) Improving supportive and palliative care for adults with cancer [Internet]. London. Available from: www.nice.org

Norton SA, Powers BA, Schmitt MH, Metzger M, Fairbanks E, Deluca J et al (2011) Navigating tensions: integrating palliative care consultation services into an academic medical center setting. J Pain Symptom Manage 42(5):680–690

Parikh RB, Kirch RA, Smith TJ, Temel JS (2013) Early specialty palliative care – translating data in oncology into practice. N Engl J Med 369(24):2347–2351

Peppercorn JM, Smith TJ, Helft PR, Debono DJ, Berry SR, Wollins DS et al (2011) American society of clinical oncology statement: toward individualized care for patients with advanced cancer. J Clin Oncol 29(6):755–760

Pham AK, Bauer MT, Balan S (2014) Closing the patient-oncologist communication gap: a review of historic and current efforts. J Cancer Educ Off J Am Assoc Cancer Educ 29:106–113

Pirl WF, Temel JS, Billings A, Dahlin C, Jackson V, Prigerson HG et al (2008) Depression after diagnosis of advanced non-small cell lung cancer and survival: a pilot study. Psychosomatics 49:218–224

Pollak KI, Arnold RM, Jeffreys AS, Alexander SC, Olsen MK, Abernethy AP et al (2007) Oncologist communication about emotion during visits with patients with advanced cancer. J Clin Oncol 25:5748–5752

Portenoy RK (2011) Treatment of cancer pain. Lancet 377:2236–2247

Project NC (2009) National Consensus Project for Quality Palliative Care [Internet]. Clinical practice guidelines for quality palliative care, 2nd edn. Available from: http://www.nationalconsensusproject.org

Ptacek JT, Ptacek JJ, Ellison NM (2001) "I'm sorry to tell you …" physicians' reports of breaking bad news. J Behav Med 24:205–217

Quill TE, Abernethy AP (2013) Generalist plus specialist palliative care–creating a more sustainable model. N Engl J Med 368:1173–1175

Rangachari D, Smith TJ (2013) Integrating palliative care in oncology: the oncologist as a primary palliative care provider. Cancer J Sudbury Mass 19(5):373–378

Reville B, Miller MN, Toner RW, Reifsnyder J (2010) End-of-life care for hospitalized patients with lung cancer: utilization of a palliative care service. J Palliat Med 13(10):1261–1266

Robinson TM, Alexander SC, Hays M, Jeffreys AS, Olsen MK, Rodriguez KL et al (2008) Patient-oncologist communication in advanced cancer: predictors of patient perception of prognosis. Support Care Cancer 16(9):1049–1057

Rodin G, Mackay JA, Zimmermann C, Mayer C, Howell D, Katz M et al (2009) Clinician-patient communication: a systematic review. Support Care Cancer 17:627–644

Roeland E, Loprinzi C, Moynihan TJ, Smith TJ, Temel J (2013) In chemotherapy for lung cancer, sometimes less is more. J Natl Compr Cancer Netw 11(3):232–235

Schneider G, Voltz R, Gaertner J (2012) Cancer pain management and bone metastases: an update for the clinician. Breast Care (Basel) 7:113–120

Sloan JA, Zhao X, Novotny PJ, Wampfler J, Garces Y, Clark MM et al (2012) Relationship between deficits in overall quality of life and non-small-cell lung cancer survival. J Clin Oncol 30(13):1498–1504

Smith TJ, Dow LA, Virago E, Khatcheressian J, Lyckholm LJ, Matsuyama R (2010) Giving honest information to patients with advanced cancer maintains hope. Oncology (Williston Park) 24:521–525

Smith TJ, Temin S, Alesi ER, Abernethy AP, Balboni TA, Basch EM et al (2012a) American Society of Clinical Oncology provisional clinical opinion: the integration of palliative care into standard oncology care. J Clin Oncol 30(8):880–887

Smith TJ, Coyne PJ, Cassel JB (2012b) Practical guidelines for developing new palliative care services: resource management. Ann Oncol 23(Suppl 3):70–75

Srivastava R (2011) Critical conversations: navigating between hope and truth. Lancet 378(9798):1213–1214

Sullivan AM, Lakoma MD, Billings JA, Peters AS, Block SD, PCEP Core Faculty (2005) Teaching and learning end-of-life care: evaluation of a faculty development program in palliative care. Acad Med J Assoc Am Med Coll 80(7):657–668

Temel JS, Greer JA, Muzikansky A, Gallagher ER, Admane S, Jackson VA et al (2010) Early palliative care for patients with metastatic non-small-cell lung cancer. N Engl J Med 363(8):733–742

Temel JS, Greer JA, Admane S, Gallagher ER, Jackson VA, Lynch TJ et al (2011) Longitudinal perceptions of prognosis and goals of therapy in patients with metastatic non-small-cell lung cancer: results of a randomized study of early palliative care. J Clin Oncol 29(17):2319–2326

Trufelli DC, Bensi CG, Garcia JB, Narahara JL, Abrao MN, Diniz RW et al (2008) Burnout in cancer professionals: a systematic review and meta-analysis. Eur J Cancer Care (Engl) 17:524–531

Tulsky JA, Arnold RM, Alexander SC, Olsen MK, Jeffreys AS, Rodriguez KL et al (2011) Enhancing communication between oncologists and patients with a computer-based training program: a randomized trial. Ann Intern Med 155(9):593–601

Velikova G, Keding A, Harley C, Cocks K, Booth L, Smith AB et al (2010) Patients report improvements in continuity of care when quality of life assessments are used routinely in oncology practice: secondary outcomes of a randomised controlled trial. Eur J Cancer 46:2381–2388

Von Gunten CF (2007) Humpty-Dumpty Syndrome. Palliat Med 21:461–462

Walling A, Lorenz KA, Dy SM, Naeim A, Sanati H, Asch SM et al (2008) Evidence-based recommendations for information and care planning in cancer care. J Clin Oncol 26(23):3896–3902

Watanabe SM, Nekolaichuk CL, Beaumont C (2012) Palliative care providers' opinions of the Edmonton Symptom Assessment System Revised (ESAS-r) in clinical practice. J Pain Symptom Manag [Internet]. Available from: http://www.ncbi.nlm.nih.gov/pubmed/23017606

Wentlandt K, Krzyzanowska MK, Swami N, Rodin GM, Le LW, Zimmermann C (2012) Referral practices of oncologists to specialized palliative care. J Clin Oncol 30(35):4380–4386

World Health Organisation (WHO 2007) Palliative care. Geneva, p 62

Zafar SY, Malin JL, Grambow SC, Abbott DH, Kolimaga JT, Zullig LL et al (2012) Chemotherapy use and patient treatment preferences in advanced colorectal cancer: a prospective cohort study. Cancer [Internet]. Available from: http://www.ncbi.nlm.nih.gov/pubmed/22972673

Zafar SY, Peppercorn JM, Schrag D, Taylor DH, Goetzinger AM, Zhong X et al (2013) The financial toxicity of cancer treatment: a pilot study assessing out-of-pocket expenses and the insured cancer patient's experience. Oncologist 18(4):381–390

Psycho-oncology and Palliative Care: Two Concepts That Fit into Comprehensive Cancer Care

14

Daniela Weber, Matthias Gründel, and Anja Mehnert

We must somehow give everything we can to these people that says "you matter because you are you," everything to enable the patient to live up until he dies, and the family to go on living afterwards. Cicely Saunders "A death in the family: a professional view". British Medical Journal, 1973, pp 30–31.

Contents

D. Weber, MSc (✉)
Department of Palliative Medicine, University Medical Center,
Göttingen, Germany
e-mail: daniela.weber@med.uni-goettingen.de

M. Gründel, PhD
Department of Haematology/Oncology, University Medical Center,
Göttingen, Germany
e-mail: mgruend1@gwdg.de

A. Mehnert, PhD
Department of Medical Psychology and Medical Sociology,
University Medical Center, Leipzig, Germany
e-mail: Anja.Mehnert@medizin.uni-leipzig.de

© Springer-Verlag Berlin Heidelberg 2015
B. Alt-Epping, F. Nauck (eds.), *Palliative Care in Oncology*,
DOI 10.1007/978-3-662-46202-7_14

14.1 Introduction

For a variety of different tumor entities, early diagnosis and multimodal cancer treatments have markedly improved survival rates during the last years, resulting in the fact that cancer is increasingly regarded as a chronic disease (Globocan 2012). Nevertheless, for many patients, the diagnosis of cancer is associated with significant limitations on their quality of life and a shortened lifetime. Research has shown that early integration of palliative care leads to significant improvements in quality of life and even enhances survival rates among patients with advanced cancer (Temel et al. 2010). These developments have been addressed in models of comprehensive cancer care where palliative care begins at diagnosis or at an early disease stage and is integrated throughout the course of cancer care (Irwin and von Gunten 2010). It is recommended that clinicians increase their focus on the patient's experience of illness to improve congruence of treatment with patient goals and preferences (Hartenstein 2002). Palliative care should be integrated as a component of assessment of goals of treatment and treatment planning. Thus, according to a patient's disease status, his or her goals and priorities should determine which treatment approaches and care plans might be the most valuable and should be negotiated within an interdisciplinary health-care team. Along the palliative care continuum including acute illness, chronic illness, end-of-life and hospice care, as well as bereavement care, within this approach, abrupt transitions are avoided. Early palliative care models adequately reflect the course of psychosocial distress in patients and their families and indicate patients' and families' psychosocial supportive care needs.

14.1.1 Physical Symptom Burden and Emotional Distress in Patients with Advanced Cancer

Cancer and multimodal treatments are associated with a variety of biological and physical stressors for the patient including physical symptom distress such as pain, fatigue, physical and cognitive impairments, as well as neurobiological changes that are likely to influence psychological and behavioral stress responses (Li et al 2010). Medical conditions and medication associated with psychological distress, anxiety, or depression include metabolic, cardiovascular, and pulmonary conditions as well as neurological conditions such as pain or central nervous system neoplasms, endocrine factors, and medication including corticosteroids or interferon (Breitbart et al. 1995; Pessin et al. 2008; Levin and Alici 2010).

Patients with advanced cancer and their families are often confronted with difficult treatment decisions, lack of information and discontinuity or abrupt transitions of care, and changing health-care professionals, resulting in difficulties to build and maintain a trustworthy doctor-patient relationship. Psychosocial consequences of cancer progression include multiple stressors and challenges for both the patient and the family. These include loss of function, increasing dependency, and changes in appearance that can represent a threat to the sense of control as well as the identity and the sense of dignity of a patient (Chochinov et al. 2009). Patients and family caregivers also face uncertainty as well as changes in relationships, attachment security, and social roles (Tan et al. 2005; Rodin et al. 2007). Depending on their individual situation in life, their personality, and cultural background, patients experience significant levels of psychosocial distress but also exhibit a variety of coping strategies in facing advanced cancer and death. The emotional suffering might be greater than their physical pain or discomfort.

Research on the understanding of the psychological adaptation to a cancer diagnosis has convincingly shown high levels of mental or emotional distress among various cancer populations (Zabora et al. 2001; Teunissen et al. 2007; Delgado-Guay et al. 2009; Kolva et al 2011; Lam et al. 2013). Physical symptom distress, the impact of treatments, and psychological distress are often closely interrelated in patients with advanced disease. The continuum of psychological and behavioral stress responses consists of a wide range of emotional states. These include worry, anxiety, fear of death, feelings of helplessness and regret, shame, fears of abandonment and insecurity, guilt or anger, sadness, demoralization, loss of meaning and hope, and (anticipatory) grief (Li et al 2010; Vehling et al. 2013). The demoralization syndrome has been described as a clinically relevant syndrome of existential distress and despair with particular relevance for patients with severe and advanced physical illness (de Figueiredo 1993; de Figueiredo and Frank 1982; Kissane et al. 2001; Clarke and Kissane 2002). Some patients experience a loss of sense of dignity, suicidal thoughts, and desire for hastened death particularly during the end-of-life phase (Oechsle et al. 2014; Robinson et al. 2014; Rosenfeld et al. 2014).

In a significant proportion of patients, the level of distress meets the strict diagnostic criteria for a mental disorder. Epidemiological studies show that the 4-week prevalence for any mental disorder in cancer patients across major tumor entities is 32 % including anxiety disorders (11.5 %), adjustment disorders (11 %), and affective disorders such as depression (6.5 %) as the most prevalent mental disorders (Mehnert et al. 2014). In the palliative care setting, Mitchell and colleagues (2011) found prevalence rates of 16.5 % for depression, 15 % for adjustment disorders, and 10 % for anxiety disorders.

Adjustment disorders are characterized as clinically relevant emotional or behavioral symptoms arising from a specific stressful event such as the diagnosis or recurrence of a life-threatening illness and are one of the most common psychiatric differential diagnoses on oncology (Li et al 2010; Mitchell et al. 2011; Mehnert et al. 2014). Frequent subtypes comprise adjustment disorder with depressed mood, anxiety, or mixed anxiety and depressed mood.

Anxiety disorders are characterized by cognitive, affective, physiological, and behavioral symptoms including excessive anxiety and worry, difficulties of controlling the worry, difficulty concentrating or irritability, and shortness of breath. Generalized anxiety disorder, panic disorder, and post-traumatic stress disorder were found with an incidence of 6–14 % in patients with advanced disease using clinical psychiatric interviews (Miovic and Block 2007; Mitchell et al. 2011; Vehling et al. 2012).

Affective disorders such as depression are characterized by a persistent depressed mood or loss of pleasure. Other symptoms are related to psychomotor changes, such as cognitive and somatic complaints. Depression is a common disorder for patients with advanced disease, with consistently high rates of clinically significant levels of depressive symptomatology between 14 and 37 %(Massie 2004; Miovic and Block 2007; Mitchell et al. 2011; Mellor et al. 2013). In patients with advanced cancer, depressive symptomatology and sadness are common and appropriate human grief responses when confronted with a terminal illness and the approaching of the end of life (Pessin et al. 2008). However, clinical depression is an adverse condition that causes additional physical and psychosocial burden for these patients and needs to be adequately diagnosed and treated.

Suicidal thoughts and desire for hastened death: Depression, severe pain and high unrelieved physical symptom burden, feelings of help- and hopelessness, delirium, low family support, and feelings of being a burden to others are major factors in the occurrence of suicidal thoughts and the desire for hastened death (Hudson et al. 2006; Rodin et al. 2009; Breitbart et al. 2010; Rosenstein 2011). Occasional thoughts of suicide in patients with advanced or terminal disease often represent an attempt to regain a sense of control in a situation experienced primarily as uncontrollable. Suicide thoughts occur on average in 15 % of advanced cancer patients (Henderson and Ord 1997; Druss and Pincus 2000; Akechi et al. 2001, 2002, 2010; Rasic et al. 2008). However, few patients experience persistent suicidal thoughts and express the desire for hastened death. The reasons for patients' desire for hastened death are often multiple and complex. Factors associated with the desire for hastened death are the expression of feelings and current reactions to the circumstances such as the loss of autonomy and the sense of dignity, communicating distress and suffering or exploring options for relieving distress, seeking information about suicide or euthanasia, and seeking health professional assistance with hastened death or acknowledging a suicidal intent (Hudson et al. 2006).

The assessment of suicide risk and early administration of appropriate interventions are critical. It is recommended to evaluate the patient's understanding of his/her symptoms and assess the mental status, vulnerability, pain control, the support system, recent losses, as well as prior psychiatric history, including alcohol and substance abuse as well as prior suicide attempts and threats. This should also assess the need for patient observation and formulate a short- and long-term treatment plan (Pessin et al. 2008).

14.1.2 Psychosocial Distress in Family Caregivers

Emotional distress does not only affect patients but also family, friends, and other caregivers. Especially in palliative care, many studies have shown high levels of emotional distress and anticipatory grief in caregivers, which is triggered by signs of clinical instability, sudden health changes, depression, cognitive impairments, and end-stage disease. Previous research has shown levels of distress, sadness, anxiety, and depression of about 40–70 % in caregivers of patients with advanced cancer, particularly in the late palliative phase (Costa-Requena et al. 2012; Friethriksdottir et al. 2011; Grov et al. 2005, 2006; Rosenberger et al. 2012). A recent study reported that 55 % of male caregivers and 36 % of female caregivers of patients with advanced and terminal disease had moderate or severe anxiety and 36 % of male caregivers compared to 14 % of female caregivers had moderate or severe depression (Oechsle et al. 2013a). In addition, significant rates of unmet needs and a significant decrease in quality of life in caregivers compared to normal population cohorts have been reported (Friethriksdottir et al. 2011; Grov et al. 2005).

Factors influencing anxiety and depression in caregivers of palliative care patients are heterogeneous. Some studies discuss differences between male or female relatives, the family caregivers' or the patients' age, the patients' symptom profile, as well as the relatives' self-esteem, unmet needs, or quality of life (Costa-Requena et al. 2012; Friethriksdottir et al. 2011; Grov et al. 2005, 2006; Rosenberger et al. 2012). Furthermore, difficult treatment decisions encountered by caregivers in the process of care for a patient with a terminal disease are stressful situations (Huang et al. 2012) and can lead to conflicts between the patient, caregivers, and health-care providers. During bereavement time, support offers for caregivers include supportive counseling, psychodynamic and interpersonal psychotherapies, cognitive behavioral therapy, and family therapy (Lichtenthal et al. 2010).

14.1.3 Assessment of Psychological Distress and Mental Disorders

Psychological distress often represents a response to the life-threatening disease, the deterioration of the patients' health, and the multimodal medical treatments (Kelly et al. 2006). However, only few patients with psychosocial distress and mental disorders that are identified early by the primary care team are referred to receive psychosocial services (Passik et al. 1998; Fallowfield et al. 2001; Kelly et al. 2006). Thus, recommendations have been developed to provide guidance in how best to assess patients with advanced disease and help to ensure adequate care.

The assessment of psychological distress and the diagnosis of mental disorders in patients with severe physical diseases are crucial yet comprise a range of challenges for the clinician. A comprehensive psychological or psychiatric assessment in palliative care should be balanced against the many possible causes that can be identified easily using minimally invasive procedures and effectively be treated to avoid additional distress for the patient and the caregiver by additional diagnostic procedures.

Given the complex medical issues and treatment interactions, the etiology of physical and psychological symptoms often remains unclear. The interpretation of somatic symptoms is particularly challenging. It often remains unclear whether a particular symptom such as difficulty concentrating or weight loss is a treatment consequence or a symptom of a mental disorder such as depression (Pessin et al. 2005). It has been recommended (e.g., in the DSM) to focus on the cognitive and psychological symptoms such as hopelessness or guilt rather than on somatic symptoms (Passik et al. 2000; Pessin et al. 2005). Other diagnostic approaches include all symptoms regardless of their etiology, probably leading to an overidentification of mental disorders (Cassem 1990). Endicott (1984) suggested a substitutive approach and replaced somatic symptoms by somatic diseases in the assessment of depression in patients. However, it also can be difficult to distinguish whether psychological symptoms are symptoms of elevated distress or a normal adaptive emotional response to the end-of-life, e.g., if hopelessness is present in patients with a poor prognosis.

A range of brief and ultra-brief screening tools for the assessment of psychological distress has been developed and evaluated. The US National Comprehensive Cancer Network (NCCN) (2003) has established the distress thermometer, a single-item measure to assess distress and to identify and measure various sources of distress. Chochinov and colleagues (1997) suggested a single screening item approach for depression. Kelly and colleagues (2006) provide an overview about further screening tools and the measurement of psychological distress in palliative care.

14.2 Discussing Palliative and End-of-Life Care, Dying, and Death

Negotiating the goals of care often represents a challenge for the cancer patient with advanced cancer, the family caregivers, and the health-care team. This is of particular relevance since palliative care physicians tend to underestimate their patients' symptom burden, while family caregivers tend to overestimate the patient's symptom distress (Oechsle et al. 2013b). Advanced cancer patients may thus have difficulties in dealing with different or conflicting needs of family members, their own preferences, and evidence-based medicine care guidelines. Therefore, adequate symptom treatment and psychosocial care can only be successful in a close dialogue between patients, their caregivers, and a multidisciplinary team. Effective communication with patients and family members is a therapeutic basis for both medical and psychological interventions. The prerequisite is a trusting relationship with the therapist or mental health professional who himself helps creating this trust through empathic and honest behavior.

What are primary goals in discussing end-of-life care, dying, and death? Advance care planning is a collaborative process among patients, family members, and health-care professionals. It aims to educate patients and their families about the treatment and palliative care options at the end-of-life such as termination of treatment decisions and advance directives and to encourage patients and family members to think about end-of-life preferences. Further goals include supporting patients and their families in end-of-life discussions, communicating evidence-based information that is relevant to end-of-life decisions, and advocating patients' end-of-life preferences.

There might be several trigger situations that invite the patient, family members or caregivers, and the health-care provider to reflect upon and discuss goals of care

(Irwin and von Gunten 2010). These situations include the advance care planning at the time of diagnosis as well as subsequent episodes of progression or relapse and when end-of-life care or hospice care is initiated or recommended.

Evidence shows that patients are open to such discussion, but there might also be conflicting communication when individual preferences about the goals of care differ between patients and family caregivers and/or between the patient, family caregivers, and the health-care team. These conversations are not simple to execute. The challenges are related to the processes in the health-care system itself, including deficient communication strategies, psychological barriers, and the actual advanced care approach.

What are the goals of effective communication in palliative care? In negotiating transitions and goals of care, Irwin and von Gunten (2010) emphasize a stepwise approach of six steps to setting goals: (1) establishing an appropriate setting for the discussion, (2) asking the patient and the family caregiver(s) about their understanding of the patient's health situation, (3) exploring the patient's and the family caregivers' expectations about the future and about what they want to know, (4) discussing overall goals and treatment options, (5) responding to the patient's and the family caregiver's emotions, and (6) establishing and implementing an (early) palliative care plan (Irwin and von Gunten 2010). The SPIKES protocol (Baile et al. 2000) is one of the most prominent models for breaking bad news (Table 14.1).

However, there might be emotional and psychological barriers that impede the quality of early as well as advance care planning conversations. Emotional states such as overwhelming fears and anxiety, depression, or anger are likely to influence the quality of communication in palliative care. Often, the doctor or another member of the health-care team faces the difficult task to discuss a patient's treatment situation, sad news, or palliative care options honestly, while he or she is also asked

Table 14.1   Spikes – a six step protocol (Baile et al. 2000)

STEP 1:	S –	*SETTING UP* the Interview (the talk should take place in a quiet and private setting. The physician should be seated facing the patient)
STEP 2:	P –	ASSESSING THE PATIENT'S *PERCEPTION* (through questioning, the clinician tries to ascertain how the patient perceives his situation and what information he already has)
STEP 3:	I –	OBTAINING THE PATIENT'S *INVITATION* (it is important to find out how much information the patient would like to receive because he may not always want to know all the details)
STEP 4:	K –	GIVING *KNOWLEDGE* AND INFORMATION TO THE PATIENT (it is important to give the information in clear and comprehensible language)
STEP 5:	E –	ADDRESSING THE PATIENT'S *EMOTIONS* WITH EMPATHIC RESPONSES (this step allows for sufficient time and space for the patient's emotional response)
STEP 6:	S –	*STRATEGY* AND *SUMMARY* (in this last step the physician discusses the treatment strategy with the patient, and the contents of the discussion are summarized by either the physician or the patient)

to deal with patients' and families' emotions and at the same time to promote hope and future perspectives.

The aim of discussing palliative and end-of-life care is to guide the patient and family to understand the goals of care relevant to the palliative approach, focusing on maintaining quality of life (Clayton and Kissane 2011). A typical sequence of steps involved in communicating about the transition of palliative care include (1) recognizing the patient's emergent clinical reality; (2) establishing understanding of disease progression, treatment efficacy, and prognosis; (3) discussing patient's values and priorities, negotiating new goals of care based on patient's values and priorities as well as the burden versus benefit ratio of available treatments; (4) responding empathically to emotions; (5) negotiating the shift to discuss the process of dying; (6) promoting understanding of change and illness transitions; (7) addressing caregivers and family concerns; (8) effecting referral to palliative care services whenever appropriate; and (9) closing the consultation (Clayton and Kissane 2011).

According to Coyle and colleagues (2012), it is often difficult when patients or families become emotionally upset, and there may not appear to be any verbal consolation one can give to issues such as fear of dying, overwhelmed caregivers, or finding meaning through the course of the illness. During such times, the ability to open up conversations focusing on these issues may be the sole intervention available. For example, honest discussion and validation of emotion without false reassurance or premature advice can be effective in providing comfort and diffusing an emotionally charged discussion (Coyle et al. 2012).

14.3 Psycho-oncological Interventions

Psycho-oncological interventions and clinical work in palliative care comprise a wide spectrum of objectives aiming at reducing psychosocial distress and maintaining the quality of life in patients and their caregivers. Psychosocial care for patients with progressing disease comprises different interventions and techniques committed to a multidisciplinary supportive approach. Those interventions and techniques include, among others, cognitive behavioral therapy, cognitive analytic therapy, narrative interventions, relaxation and guided imagery, mindfulness-based interventions, meaning-focused interventions, art therapy, and dignity therapy. The use of psychopharmacological medication in combination with psychotherapeutic interventions can be indicated in patients with severe distress and should be further clarified with the medical care team.

14.3.1 Psychotherapeutic Goals and Approaches

Psychotherapeutic interventions in palliative care include multimodal and supportive approaches addressing the supportive care needs of patients and caregivers. Supportive psychotherapy is defined as a therapeutic intervention that aims to help patients and caregivers deal with distressing emotions and to promote existing resources, strengths, and adaptive coping with the disease (Lederberg and Holland 2011). Patients and family caregivers often want to make sure that everything has been done by the palliative care team to help the patient. In relation to these issues, the objectives of psychotherapeutic interventions include the enhancement of adaptive coping efforts, reducing psychological symptom burden (e.g., anxiety and depression), mobilizing individual and family resources, maintaining hope and life goals, clarification of misunderstandings and (mis-) expectations, clarification and/ or strengthening of interpersonal relationships, strengthening of self-esteem, acknowledgement of strengths and achievements in life, reduce feelings of isolation and loneliness, maintaining a sense of dignity, finding meaning in life and a sense of peace, as well as acknowledgement of feelings of grief and sadness about loss and saying good-bye (MacLeod 2008).

Relaxation and image-based interventions comprise techniques such as guided imagery, visualization, and progressive muscle relaxation. Those techniques are easy to learn and help patients to regain a sense of control and mastery, to develop coping skills for side effects such as fatigue or nausea, and to maintain or regain psychological well-being (Lewis and Sharp 2011). In patients with severe health conditions, however, it should be considered that an intervention such as visualization of the body or body parts can also increase anxiety or even induce panic. Therefore, whether an intervention is appropriate or helpful for a patient should be carefully considered (Lewis and Sharp 2011).

Cognitive behavioral therapy (CBT) has been shown to be very effective in treating emotional distress and particularly depression in patients with chronic health conditions (Horne and Watson 2011). In palliative care settings, CBT has not been used as much as in patients with nonlife-threatening conditions. However, cognitive techniques such as cognitive restructuring/reframing and behavioral techniques such as activity scheduling and distraction can help to relieve specific symptom distress such as anxiety, depression, fatigue, and pain. Contraindications include organic mental syndromes, schizoaffective disorders, and delirium (Horne and Watson 2011).

Mindfulness interventions such as mindfulness-based stress reduction (MBSR) have been found useful in patients with life-threatening and advanced diseases (Payne 2011). They usually address two areas: (a) self-regulating attention of immediate experience, allowing for greater awareness of mental events in the present moment, and (b) adopting a curiosity, openness, and acceptance toward one's experiences in the present moment (Payne 2011). MBSR has been found effective to reduce a variety of unpleasant psychological states such as anxiety and depression, fatigue, and insomnia. MBSR further promotes hope and quality of life.

Meaning-centered psychotherapy comprises specific approaches that promote a sense of meaning and purpose in the life of patients. During recent years growing efforts have been made to develop meaning-based interventions for patients with life-threatening diseases. Meaning-based interventions are often realized as group therapy approaches to reduce emotional and spiritual distress and to promote hope, courage, and control, to mobilize internal resources, and to discuss future goals despite a noticeable limited life expectancy. However, also individual interventions have been realized (Nissim et al. 2012; Breitbart et al. 2012). Further aims include strengthening a patient's self-esteem and sense of dignity to appreciate strengths and past achievements, to reduce feelings of isolation, to strengthen the relation with the partner and family members, and to improve the communication with the professional health-care team (LeMay and Wilson 2008).

Dignity-centered psychotherapy: Dignity and respect for the patient and his or her care needs represent an essential attitude in the palliative treatment. A sense of dignity for patients comprises feelings of respect and being worthy despite increasing physical and psychological symptoms and is often mediated by both intrinsic and extrinsic factors and particularly social interactions (Chochinov and McKeen 2011). Dignity-centered therapy is particularly designed for patients at the end of life. Based on the empirical dignity model by Chochinov et al. (2002), dignity therapy aims to reduce suffering and promote emotional and spiritual well-being, quality of life, and a sense of meaning and purpose by encouraging patients to reflect on their memorable life events (Chochinov and McKeen 2011). The intervention includes a dignity therapy interview and one or two therapy sessions. The interview sessions are transcribed, edited, and read to the patient again, and (after corrections) the patient is given the document to share it with family members, friends, or others (Chochinov and McKeen 2011). Dignity therapy was found to be effective to increase sense of dignity and improve quality of life, spiritual well-being, and appreciation through the family based on self-report end-of-life experiences (Chochinov et al. 2011).

Grief counseling: In palliative care, grief counseling is an integral part of psychosocial interventions. Grief is a reaction to (anticipated) loss, disappointment, and departure. Grieving is an individual process and can be expressed by different behaviors and different emotional reactions. Family members and friends receive support in dealing with their loss and help in coping with their grief. The ultimate goal is to alter the condition of the bereaved person. In grief counseling it is most important to listen closely and to empathize with the person grieving who often initially cannot be consoled. As a result, no effort should be made to relativize his loss. It is necessary to give the bereaved enough time for the grieving process and simply accompany him in his deep sorrow. However, one must be careful that the feeling of helplessness does not lead to more complicated grieving and social isolation (Jerneizig 2006). The goals and results of grief work are that the relationship to the deceased is appropriately reestablished (a dead person is not necessarily an absent one), the relationship to the outside world and to the social environment can be redefined, one's own changes in personality can be encountered with interest and acceptance, the desire and the reasons to live can be revived, a place of belonging is found for the deceased; integration into the life of the bereaved takes place (Melching 2012).

14.3.2 Psychotherapeutic Requirements

During recent years, a variety of effective psychological and psychosocial interventions has been developed, implemented, and evaluated that specifically address psychosocial distress and supportive care needs in patients suffering from advanced and life-threatening diseases and in their caregivers (Watson and Kissane 2011). The psychotherapeutic work and goals in palliative care settings differ in several respects from psychological interventions for patients with early or curative diseases or physically healthy individuals.

The time frame for psychosocial and psychotherapeutic interventions is limited. Usually, patients can be seen only a few times, depending on the physical condition, the course of the disease, and the inpatient or outpatient setting. Having limited time has several implications for the development of a trusting and sustainable therapeutic relationship and the psychotherapeutic treatment planning. The latter often depends on the course of the disease and sometimes quickly changing supportive care needs of patients and/or their caregivers. Clinical psycho-oncological work in palliative care requires medical and therapeutic knowledge including information about common treatments and treatment side effects such as cognitive impairments or treatment-induced psychological distress and close contact and collaboration with the palliative care team. The often unpredictable course of the disease and changes in the supportive care needs further place high demands with regard to flexibility, empathy, and understanding of the patients' situation.

Communication with the patient and the caregiver can be hampered not only by severe health conditions such as delirium or organic mental syndromes, but also by unclear or divergent perceptions about the goals of treatment and the curability of the disease. Temel and colleagues showed that despite having terminal cancer, about one-third of patients newly diagnosed with metastatic non-small cell lung cancer reported that their cancer was curable at baseline, and a majority endorsed getting rid of all of the cancer as a goal of therapy (Temel et al. 2011). In addition, patients experience hope and hopelessness often as closely linked constructs (Sachs et al. 2012). Rodin and Zimmermann used the term "double awareness" to describe the situation of patients with advanced – yet not terminal – disease and their challenges to deal with issues of death and dying and at the same time remaining engaged in life (e.g., dealing with complex treatment decisions, managing changing relationships; Rodin and Zimmermann 2008).

The psycho-oncologist is often faced with the difficult task of encouraging patients and caregivers to cope adaptively with the palliative care situation, helping to maintain hope and quality of life and reduce psychological stress, and simultaneously promote acceptance and enable patients and caregivers to face "realistic" treatment goals and treatment decisions also affecting the psychosocial well-being of the patient and the family in the course of the disease. Emotional responses of the patient and the caregiver can include frustration and anger, disappointment, despair (anticipatory) grief, and high levels of distress that may lead to difficult therapeutic interactions. Finally, psycho-oncologists working in palliative care settings are often confronted with the threat of death and dying, their own helplessness and existential or spiritual questions about the meaning of life and death.

14.3.3 Caring for the Professional Team

Psychologists are not only mere members of a multi-professional palliative care team. They may also adopt mediating functions in cases of communicative problems within the team, e.g., when perspectives on therapeutic decisions diverge between different disciplines. Working with gravely ill and dying people is a constant challenge with varying stress factors for the entire team. This makes it also the task of the psychologist to support the team members both emotionally and professionally. To accomplish this, the psychologist should be accessible, recognize the stress and strains that each team member is experiencing, respond to individual needs, and listen carefully. Also, the collaborative preparation of structures, processes, and solutions can contribute to improving the dealings with colleagues and with patients (Gaspar 2012).

Formal interventions are scheduled meetings that take place on a weekly, monthly, or on a regular basis. Informal talks are a form of counseling that is important to understand and process actions and situations that may have just occurred; this may be particularly important in palliative care. In addition, supervision and intervision are well-defined options to reflect team-related or clinical situations and should be offered on a regular basis. Supervision comprises five main steps (Scobel 2002):

1. Reflecting upon and analyzing professional experience and actions in external perception, in terms of clients, colleagues, institution, and hierarchy, in internal perception, and in the form of self-reflection.
2. Introspection, self-awareness, and self-analysis.
3. Processing inner conflicts caused by one's own professional duties.
4. Processing interpersonal conflicts, for example, within the team.
5. Analyzing the institution, reflecting upon the institutional system (e.g., hospital and palliative ward) and its implications for the teams, groups, and individuals.

As a rule, supervision should be conducted by an external, qualified supervisor. Intervision is carried out by the team members themselves and addresses individual needs within the team. Here the team members draw on and develop the resources at their disposal to provide themselves and others with the support they need.

14.3.4 Caring for Oneself

From a psychological point of view, working with palliative care patients means stress for the team members but also offers unique opportunities. The awareness of one's own finiteness is constantly present and forces carers to deal with their primal fear of death. The confidence that one will live a normal life of growing old into the distant future and then die after a full life can be challenged through daily dealings with people who have to die before their time. On the other hand, many team members see great meaning in accompanying people through the last phase of their life.

Close and meaningful contact to patients, often over an extended period of time, enables these team members to experience a sense of connectedness. This inner fulfillment may often be more rewarding than the satisfaction gained in other professions. The balance between opportunity and stress means that the risk of "burn out" or excessive job fluctuation is not higher than in other areas of medicine (Müller and Pfister 2012). Everybody working in this area is advised to find and promote his own balance. While the following guidelines have proven to be helpful, they need to be adapted to one's individual needs:

- Establishing a work-life balance through professional and leisure activities that allow distance to be gained from clinical work.
- Promoting good teamwork so that team members can process together what they are experiencing and support each other.
- Creating a framework for work, whether it be spiritual, social, philosophical, or simply your view of the world, which allows you to extract meaning from what you experience in your work.

People working in palliative care should not assume that close and continual work with severely ill people is not stressful, nor should they expect that they will not suffer from this stress. That would be denial. But if they follow the above advice, adjusting them when necessary, they can more than compensate for the stress. From a psychological perspective, the chances are good to have meaningful work that contributes significantly to satisfaction in their life as a whole (Yalom 1980).

14.4 Summary

It can be safely assumed that psychological expertise is helpful in palliative care to create a sustainable and livable context for both caregivers and patients. On the one hand, psychologists can support the professions in their contact with patients and help them cope with the stress that they experience. On the other hand, the main part of their work comprises therapeutic interventions with patient and family members. Here psychologists make use of methods from, and elements of, all major psychotherapeutic approaches (depth, humanistic, systemic, and cognitive behavioral). They aid patients and families in coping with conflicts and fears in end-of-life situations. Another aspect of psycho-oncology is to focus on fundamental questions of human existence, of life and death, and of finding meaning to life. This plays a disproportionately larger role in psycho-oncology (especially in the palliative care setting) than in other psychotherapeutic approaches. In this regard, existential psychotherapy (Yalom 1980) has proven to be helpful. By including philosophy, in particular existentialism, as well as spiritual aspects and elements from the American Human Potential Movement, psychologists widen their perspectives. A new sounding board emerges that allows both patients and caregivers to explore existential questions and problems. Experiencing the meaning in life despite the suffering can be the reward.

References

Akechi T, Okamura H, Yamawaki S et al (2001) Why do some cancer patients with depression desire an early death and others do not? Psychosomatics 42(2):141–145

Akechi T, Okamura H, Nishiwaki Y et al (2002) Predictive factors for suicidal ideation in patients with unresectable lung carcinoma. Cancer 95(5):1085–1093

Akechi T, Okamura H, Nakano T et al (2010) Gender differences in factors associated with suicidal ideation in major depression among cancer patients. Psychooncology 19(4):384–389

Baile WF, Buckmann R, Lenzi R et al (2000) Spikes – a six-step protocol for delivering bad news: application to the patient with cancer. Oncologist 5:302–311

Breitbart W, Bruera E, Chochinov H et al (1995) Neuropsychiatric syndromes and psychological symptoms in patients with advanced cancer. J Pain Symptom Manage 10(2):131–141

Breitbart W, Rosenfeld B, Gibson C (2010) Impact of treatment for depression on desire for hastened death in patients with advanced AIDS. Psychosomatics 51(2):98–105

Breitbart W, Poppito S, Rosenfeld B, Vickers AJH (2012) Pilot randomized controlled trial of individual meaning-centered psychotherapy for patients with advanced cancer. J Clin Oncol 30(12):1304–1309

Cassem EH (1990) Depression and anxiety secondary to medical illness. Psychiatr Clin North Am 13(4):597–612

Chochinov HM, McKeen NA (2011) Dignity therapy. In: Watson M, Kissane DW (eds) Handbook of psychotherapy in cancer care. Wiley, West Sussex, pp 79–88

Chochinov HM, Wilson KG, Enns M et al (1997) 'Are you depressed?' Screening for depression in the terminally ill. Am J Psychiatry 154(5):674–676

Chochinov HM, Hack TF, McClement S, Kristjanson LJ (2002) Dignity in the terminally ill: a developing empirical model. Soc Sci Med 54:433–443

Chochinov HM, Hassard T, McClement S (2009) The landscape of distress in the terminally ill. J Pain Symptom Manage 38(5):641–649

Chochinov HM, Kristjanson LJ, Breitbart W, McClement S (2011) Effect of dignity therapy on distress and end-of-life experience in terminally ill patients: a randomised controlled trial. Lancet Oncol 12(8):753–762

Clarke DM, Kissane DW (2002) Demoralization: its phenomenology and importance. Aust N Z J Psychiatry 36(6):733–742

Clayton JM, Kissane DW (2011) Communication about transitioning patients to palliative care. In: Kissane DW, Bultz BD, Butow PM et al (eds) Handbook of communication in oncology and palliative care. Oxford University Press, Oxford, pp 203–214

Costa-Requena G, Cristófol R, Cañete J (2012) Caregivers' morbidity in palliative care unit: predicting by gender, age, burden and self-esteem. Support Care Cancer 20:1465–1470

Coyle N, Krueger CA, Banerjee SC (2012) Discussing death, dying and end-of-life goals of care: COMSKIL nurse training. Memorial Sloan-Kettering Cancer Center, New York

de Figueiredo JM (1993) Depression and demoralization: phenomenologic differences and research perspectives. Compr Psychiatry 34(5):308–311

de Figueiredo JM, Frank JD (1982) Subjective incompetence, the clinical hallmark of demoralization. Compr Psychiatry 23(4):353–363

Delgado-Guay M, Parsons HA, Li Z, Palmer JL et al (2009) Symptom distress in advanced cancer patients with anxiety and depression in the palliative care setting. Support Care Cancer 17(5):573–579

Druss B, Pincus H (2000) Suicidal ideation and suicide attempts in general medical illnesses. Arch Intern Med 160(10):1522–1526

Endicott J (1984) Measurement of depression in patients with cancer. Cancer 53(10):2243–2249

Fallowfield L, Ratcliffe D, Jenkins V et al (2001) Psychiatric morbidity and its recognition by doctors in patients with cancer. Br J Cancer 84(8):1011–1015

Friethriksdottir N, Saevarsdottir T, Halfdanardottir SI et al (2011) Family members of cancer patients: needs, quality of life and symptoms of anxiety and depression. Acta Oncol 50:252–258

Gaspar M (2012) Die Rolle des Psychologen im multiprofessionellen Team. In: Fegg M, Gramm J, Pestinger M (eds) Psychologie und Palliative Care. Aufgaben, Konzepte und Interventionen in der Begleitung von Patienten und Angehörigen, 1st edn. Kohlhammer, Stuttgart, pp 48–55

Globocan (IARC) (2012) Section of cancer information. http://globocan.iarc.fr/Pages/fact_sheets_cancer.aspx. Accessed 22 Sept 2014

Grov EK, Dahl AA, Moum T et al (2005) Anxiety, depression, and quality of life in caregivers of patients with cancer in late palliative phase. Ann Oncol 16:1185–1191

Grov EK, Fosså SD, Sørebø O et al (2006) Primary caregivers of cancer patients in the palliative phase: a path analysis of variables influencing their burden. Soc Sci Med 63:2429–2439

Hartenstein R (2002) Stellenwert der Palliativmedizin in der Onkologie. Onkologie 25(1):60–64

Henderson JM, Ord RA (1997) Suicide in head and neck cancer patients. J Oral Maxillofac Surg 55(11):1217–1221

Horne D, Watson M (2011) Cognitive-behavioral therapies in cancer care. In: Watson M, Kissane DW (eds) Handbook of psychotherapy in cancer care. Wiley, West Sussex, pp 15–26

Huang HL, Chiu TY, Lee LT et al (2012) Family experience with difficult decisions in end-of-life care. Psychooncology 21(7):785–791

Hudson PL, Kristjanson LJ, Ashby M et al (2006) Desire for hastened death in patients with advanced disease and the evidence base of clinical guidelines: a systematic review. Palliat Med 20(7):693–701

Irwin S, von Gunten C (2010) The role of palliative care in cancer care transitions. In: Holland J, Breitbart W, Jacobsen P et al (eds) Psycho-oncol, 2nd edn. Oxford University Press, New York, pp 277–283

Jerneizig R (2006) Psychologie der Trauer und Trauerverarbeitung – Beratung und Therapie. In: Koch U, Lang K, Mehnert A (eds) Die Begleitung schwer kranker und sterbender Menschen. Grundlagen und Anwendungshilfen für Berufsgruppen in der Palliativversorgung, 1st edn. Schattauer, Stuttgart, pp 213–220

Kelly B, McClement S, Chochinov HM (2006) Measurement of psychological distress in palliative care. Palliat Med 20(8):779–789

Kissane DW, Clarke DM, Street AF (2001) Demoralization syndrome–a relevant psychiatric diagnosis for palliative care. J Palliat Care 17(1):12–21

Kolva E, Rosenfeld B, Pessin H et al (2011) Anxiety in terminally ill cancer patients. J Pain Symptom Manage 42(5):691–701

Lam WWT, Soong I, Yau TK et al (2013) The evolution of psychological distress trajectories in women diagnosed with advanced breast cancer: a longitudinal study. Psychooncology 22:2831–2839

Lederberg M, Holland J (2011) Supportive psychotherapy in cancer care: an essential ingredient of all therapy. In: Watson M, Kissane DW (eds) Handbook of psychotherapy in cancer care. Wiley, West Sussex, pp 3–14

LeMay K, Wilson KG (2008) Treatment of existential distress in life threatening illness: a review of manualized interventions. Clin Psychol Rev 28(3):472–493

Levin T, Alici Y (2010) Anxiety disorders. In: Holland J, Breitbart W, Jacobsen P et al (eds) Psycho-oncology, 2nd edn. Oxford University Press, New York, pp 324–331

Lewis EJ, Sharp DM (2011) Relaxation and image based therapy. In: Watson M, Kissane DW (eds) Handbook of psychotherapy in cancer care. Wiley, West Sussex, pp 49–58

Li M, Hales S, Rodin G (2010) Adjustment disorders. In: Holland J, Breitbart W, Jacobsen P et al (eds) Psycho-oncology, 2nd edn. Oxford University Press, New York, pp 303–310

Lichtenthal W, Prigerson H, Kissane DW (2010) Bereavement: a special issue in oncology. In: Holland J, Breitbart W, Jacobsen P (eds) Psycho-oncology, 2nd edn. Oxford University Press, New York, pp 537–543

MacLeod R (2008) Setting the context: what do we mean by psychosocial care in palliative care? In: Lloyd-Williams M (ed) Psychosocial issues in palliative care. Oxford University Press, New York, pp 1–20

Massie MJ (2004) Prevalence of depression in patients with cancer. J Natl Cancer Inst Monogr 32:57–71

Mehnert A, Brähler E, Faller H et al (2014) Four-week prevalence of mental disorders in cancer patients across major tumor entities. J Clin Oncol 32:3540–3546

Melching H (2012) Trauer. In: Fegg M, Gramm J, Pestinger M (eds) Psychologie und Palliative Care. Aufgaben, Konzepte und Interventionen in der Begleitung von Patienten und Angehörigen, 1st edn. Kohlhammer, Stuttgart, pp 84–92

Mellor D, McCabe MP, Davison TE et al (2013) Barriers to the detection and management of depression by palliative care professional carers among their patients: perspectives from professional carers and patients' family members. Am J Hosp Palliat Care 30(1):12–20

Miovic M, Block S (2007) Psychiatric disorders in advanced cancer. Cancer 110(8):1665–1676

Mitchell AJ, Chan M, Bhatti H (2011) Prevalence of depression, anxiety, and adjustment disorder in oncological, haematological, and palliative-care settings: a meta-analysis of 94 interview-based studies. Lancet Oncol 12(2):160–174

Müller M, Pfister D (2012) Wie viel Tod verträgt das Team. Vandenhoeck & Ruprecht, Göttingen

National Comprehensive Cancer Network (NCCN) (2003) Distress management. Clinical practice guidelines. J Natl Compr Canc Netw 1(3):344–374

Nissim R, Freeman E, Lo C (2012) Managing Cancer and Living Meaningfully (CALM): a qualitative study of a brief individual psychotherapy for individuals with advanced cancer. Palliat Med 26(5):713–721

Oechsle K, Goerth K, Bokemeyer C, Mehnert A (2013a) Anxiety and depression in caregivers of terminally ill cancer patients: impact on their perspective of the patients' symptom burden. J Palliat Med 16(9):1095–1101

Oechsle K, Goerth K, Bokemeyer C, Mehnert A (2013b) Symptom burden in palliative care patients: perspectives of patients, their family caregivers, and their attending physicians. Support Care Cancer 21(7):1955–1962

Oechsle K, Wais MC, Vehling S (2014) Relationship between symptom burden, distress, and sense of dignity in terminally ill cancer patients. J Pain Symptom Manage 48(3):313–321

Passik SD, Dugan W, McDonald MV et al (1998) Oncologists' recognition of depression in their patients with cancer. J Clin Oncol 16(4):1594–1600

Passik SD, Lundberg JC, Rosenfeld B (2000) Factor analysis of the Zung Self-Rating Depression Scale in a large ambulatory oncology sample. Psychosomatics 41(2):121–127

Payne D (2011) Mindfulness interventions for cancer patients. In: Watson M, Kissane DW (eds) Handbook of psychotherapy in cancer care. Wiley, West Sussex, pp 39–47

Pessin H, Olden M, Jacobson C (2005) Clinical assessment of depression in terminally ill cancer patients: a practical guide. Palliat Support Care 3(4):319–324

Pessin H, Evcimen YAA, Breitbart W (2008) Diagnosis, assessment, and treatment of depression in palliative care. In: Lloyd-Williams M (ed) Psychosocial issues in palliative care. Oxford University Press, New York

Rasic DT, Belik SL, Bolton JM (2008) Cancer, mental disorders, suicidal ideation and attempts in a large community sample. Psychooncology 17(7):660–667

Robinson S, Kissane DW, Brooker J et al (2014) A systematic review of the demoralization syndrome in individuals with progressive disease and cancer: a decade of research. J Pain Symptom Manage pii:S0885-3924(14)00407-2

Rodin G, Zimmermann C (2008) Psychoanalytic reflections on mortality: a reconsideration. J Am Acad Psychoanal Dyn Psychiatry 36(1):181–196

Rodin G, Walsh A, Zimmermann C et al (2007) The contribution of attachment security and social support to depressive symptoms in patients with metastatic cancer. Psychooncology 16(12):1080–1091

Rodin G, Lo C, Mikulincer M et al (2009) Pathways to distress: the multiple determinants of depression, hopelessness, and the desire for hastened death in metastatic cancer patients. Soc Sci Med 68(3):562–569

Rosenberger C, Hocker A, Cartus M et al (2012) Outpatient psycho-oncological care for family members and patients: access, psychological distress and supportive care needs. Psychother Psychosom Med Psychol 62:185–194

Rosenfeld B, Pessin H, Marziliano A et al (2014) Does desire for hastened death change in terminally ill cancer patients? Soc Sci Med 111:35–40

Rosenstein DL (2011) Depression and end-of-life care for patients with cancer. Dialogues Clin Neurosci 13(1):101–108

Sachs E, Kolva E, Pessin H et al (2012) On sinking and swimming: the dialectic of hope, hopelessness, and acceptance in terminal cancer. Am J Hosp Palliat Care 30(2):121–127

Scobel W (2002) Supervision im Krankenhaus. Kommunikation ist das Rezept, 1st edn. Hans Huber, Bern

Tan A, Zimmermann C, Rodin G (2005) Interpersonal processes in palliative care: an attachment perspective on the patient-clinician relationship. Palliat Med 19(2):143–150

Temel JS, Greer JA, Muzikansky A et al (2010) Early palliative care for patients with metastatic non–small-cell lung cancer. N Engl J Med 363(8):733–742

Temel JS, Greer JA, Admane S (2011) Longitudinal perceptions of prognosis and goals of therapy in patients with metastatic non-small-cell lung cancer: results of a randomized study of early palliative care. J Clin Oncol 29(17):2319–2326

Teunissen SCCM, de Graeff A, Voest EE et al (2007) Are anxiety and depressed mood related to physical symptom burden? A study in hospitalized advanced cancer patients. Palliat Med 21(4):341–346

Vehling S, Koch U, Ladehoff N et al (2012) Prevalence of affective and anxiety disorders in cancer: systematic literature review and meta-analysis. Psychother Psychosom Med Psychol 62(7):249–258

Vehling S, Oechsle K, Koch U et al (2013) Receiving palliative treatment moderates the effect of age and gender on demoralization in patients with cancer. PLoS One 8(3):e59417

Watson M, Kissane DW (eds) (2011) Handbook of psychotherapy in cancer care. Wiley, West Sussex

Yalom I (1980) Existential psychotherapy. New York, Basic Books

Zabora J, Brintzenhofeszoc K, Curbow B (2001) The prevalence of psychological distress by cancer site. Psychooncology 10:19–28

Cancer Therapy in Developing Countries: The Role of Palliative Care

Richard A. Powell, Charmaine L. Blanchard, Liliana de Lima, Stephen R. Connor, and M.R. Rajagopal

Contents

R.A. Powell, MD (✉)
Global Health Researcher, PO Box 459-00621, Village Market, Nairobi, Kenya
e-mail: richard2powell@yahoo.co.uk

C.L. Blanchard, MPhil Pall Med
Wits Centre for Palliative Care, University of the Witwatersrand, Gauteng Centre
of Excellence for Palliative Care, Chris Hani Baragwanath Academic Hospital,
PO Bertsham, 2013 Johannesburg, South Africa
e-mail: Charmaine.blanchard@wits.ac.za; vervet@iafrica.com

L. de Lima
International Association for Hospice and Palliative Care,
5535 Memorial Dr. Suite F – PMB 509, Houston, Texas 77007, USA
e-mail: ldelima@iahpc.com

S.R. Connor, PhD
Worldwide Palliative Care Alliance, 10990 Rice Field Pl, Fairfax Station,
Virginia 22039, USA
e-mail: sconnor@icloud.com

© Springer-Verlag Berlin Heidelberg 2015
B. Alt-Epping, F. Nauck (eds.), *Palliative Care in Oncology*,
DOI 10.1007/978-3-662-46202-7_15

M.R. Rajagopal, MD
Pallium India, Trivandrum, Kerala, India

Trivandrum Institute of Palliative Sciences Trivandrum, Trivandrum, Kerala, India
e-mail: mrraj47@gmail.com

15.1   Introduction

Non-communicable diseases (NCDs) are globally the principal cause of mortality, accounting for 66 % of 54.6 million (m) deaths in 2011, primarily cardiovascular diseases, diabetes, chronic respiratory diseases, and cancer (World Health Organization 2013). In developing countries they are forecasted to supersede communicable diseases and nutrition-related disorders as the primary causes of mortality by 2030 (Wagner and Brath 2012).

In 2012 there were an estimated 14.1 m new cases and 8.2 m deaths from cancer worldwide – the latter projected to rise by 2030 to 13.2 m, attributable to an increasing and ageing population and adoption of risk-factor lifestyles (Bray et al. 2012). Most cancers occur in developing countries (Jemal et al. 2011), a variously defined and accepted term that refers to nations with a lower living standard, underdeveloped industrial base, and low Human Development Index compared with that of other nations. Sixty per cent of cancer incidences and 70 % of cancer deaths occur in Africa, Asia, and Central and South America, where the disease increasingly is a public health concern given these regions' populous nature and often deficient preventive and curative oncological approaches and treatment access (Gulland 2014). Moreover, despite recent improvements (Lynch et al. 2013), palliative care service provision and patient coverage in developing regions is variable at best and is generally not integrated into mainstream health-care services.

By addressing oncology and palliative care in developing country settings, this chapter discusses the illustrative countries and regions outlined in Table 15.1, drawing upon the World Bank's four income group classification of countries (World Bank nd).

These countries are not intended to be representative of these regions' stage of development of palliative care and oncology services or of these nations' phase of economic development. Instead, they are countries with an established palliative care and oncological service, so the relative role of these countries in addressing cancer needs can be discussed. India was selected as the sole country from South Asia because of its substantial population (more than 1.2 billion) and growing palliative care services profile. Three of these countries – Brazil, India, and South Africa – are BRICS countries (others comprising the acronym are Russia and China), considered to be at a similar stage of newly advanced economic development. This chapter includes these countries as a means of

Table 15.1 Countries reviewed by the World Bank 2012, gross national income estimations

Category[a]	Region	Country[b]	GNI per capita
Low-income economies	Africa	Kenya	US$1,035 or less
		Malawi	
		Uganda	
Lower middle-income economies	–	India	US$1,036–$4,085
	Eastern Europe	Georgia	
		Ukraine	
Upper middle-income economies	Africa	South Africa	US$4,086–$12,615
	Eastern Europe	Albania	
		Serbia	
	Latin America[c]	Argentina	
		Brazil	
		Colombia	
		Peru	

Source: Adapted from World Health Organization (2011)
Notes:
[a]Low- and middle-income countries are sometimes referred to as developing economies. However, this aggregating term is not intended to suggest that all economies in the group are experiencing similar development or that other economies have reached a preferred or final stage of development (World Bank nd).
[b]The World Bank list of economies, July 2012 (Anon nd).
[c]Latin America refers to the 19 countries with Spanish or Portuguese as official languages.

contrasting palliative care and oncology services in the countries where oncology services are negligible with the previously developing nations where more substantial oncology services exist.

15.2 Disease Burden

The comparative mortality contribution of communicable (especially HIV/AIDS) and NCD diagnoses varies in the reviewed countries. As Table 15.2 shows, NCDs currently account for a considerably lower percentage of the total number of deaths in the African nations (ranging from 25 to 29 %) than in the nations of Eastern Europe (86–95 %), India (53 %), and Latin America (60–80 %). However, with the exception of South Africa, the data from Africa are subject to a high level of uncertainty, resulting in a problematic reliance on estimates (Pisani 2011). In general terms, age-standardised death rates per 100,000 varied in Africa from 83.5 (male)/105.5 (female) in Malawi to 207.2 (m)/123.9 (f) in South Africa; in Eastern Europe from 116.3 (m)/77.8 (f) in Georgia to 211.2 (m)/129.1 (f) in Serbia; in India, 78.8 (m)/71.8 (f); and in Latin America from 109.5 (m)/118.9 (f) in Peru to 167.7 (m)/107.0 (f) in Argentina.

Table 15.2 NCD and cancer deaths (total and age standardised) in selected review countries

| Region/country | 2010 population (millions) | Total NCD deaths (000s)[a] | | Age-standardised death rate per 100,000 | | | | NCD % of all deaths |
| | | | | All NCDs | | Cancers | | |
		m	f	m	f	m	f	
Africa								
Kenya	40.5	56.5	46.6	779.6	575.0	118.8	113.0	28 %
Malawi	14.9	39.7	28.1	1208.2	811.5	83.5	105.5	28 %
South Africa	50.1	92.4	98.1	733.7	555.2	207.2	123.9	29 %
Uganda	33.4	64.1	42.3	1094.7	684.9	126.5	140.3	25 %
Eastern Europe								
Albania	3.2	11.2	13.7	755.0	623.2	171.6	126.3	89 %
Georgia	4.4	23.0	22.0	858.4	490.8	116.3	77.8	91 %
Serbia	9.9	59.1	58.6	804.2	577.7	211.2	129.1	95 %
Ukraine	45.4	310.9	338.0	1121.9	582.5	159.3	79.2	86 %
India	1,224.6	2,967.6	2,273.8	781.7	571.0	78.8	71.8	53 %
Latin America								
Argentina	40.4	128.7	130.0	612.7	365.5	167.7	107.0	80 %
Brazil	194.9	474.0	419.9	614.0	428.1	136.3	94.7	74 %
Colombia	46.3	66.3	68.2	437.6	351.3	112.9	92.1	66 %
Peru	29.1	41.4	41.2	407.6	338.8	109.5	118.9	60 %

Source: Adapted from World Health Organization (2011)
Note:
[a]2008 estimates

Based upon this infectious and NCD disease burden, it is estimated that globally, the number of patients in need of end-of-life palliative care[1] for adults and children is 20.4 m, 19.2 m of whom are adults, with approximately one-third (34 %) of these adults suffering from cancer and 78 % located in low- and middle-income countries (Connor and Bermedo 2014). Among these global cancer cases, an estimated 6.6 m patients are in need of end-of-life palliative care, 6.5 m of whom are adults. Regionally, the total in Africa was 1.8 m, 346,203 of whom had cancer; in the European region 4.2 m adults needed end-of-life care, 1.6 m of whom had cancer; in South East Asia (India is subsumed in the regional data) the total number was 4.1 m, 1 m of whom had cancer; and in the region of the Americas (with Latin America subsumed in the regional data) the total number was 2.6 m, 1 m of whom had cancer (Connor and Bermedo 2014).

15.2.1 Africa

Africa stands out because of its significant burden of communicable and non-communicable diseases, especially sub-Saharan Africa. The relative distribution is predicted to shift by 2030 (Mathers and Loncar 2006). By 2011, 23.5 m people in the subregion suffered from HIV/AIDS, 69 % of the global disease burden, with 1.8 m new cases (Joint United Nations Programme on HIV/AIDS 2012), and the prevalence rate among adults (aged 15–49) in the review countries ranged from 1.6 % (Kenya) to 17.9 % (South Africa) (UNAIDS 2014).

Regionally, cancer is an emerging public health problem (Jemal et al. 2012). In 2008 there were 715,000 new cases and 542,000 cancer-related deaths in Africa; this number is predicted to nearly double (1.28 m new cases and 970,000 deaths) by 2030 because of population growth and ageing (Ferlay et al. 2010). Of the cancers, 36 % are infection related, which is twice the global average (Parkin 2006). Sankaranarayanan et al. (2010) reported that late presentation to services meant that for cancers where prognosis depends upon the stage at diagnosis, survival rates did not exceed 22 % for any cancer site in Gambia and no more than 13 % for any cancer (except for breast cancer) in Uganda. Poor health outcomes for patients are aggravated by limited access to appropriate analgesics, especially for moderate-to-severe pain, because they are surrounded to a high degree by legal and regulatory restrictions, inadequate training of health-care providers, procurement difficulties, and inefficient health systems (O'Brien et al. 2013; Cleary et al. 2013b).

Consequently, the most common diseases referred for palliative care on the continent are HIV/AIDS and cancer. For example, in South Africa and Uganda, a recent

---

[1] Calculated as the number of total deaths from disease requiring palliative care at the end of life multiplied by the percentage pain prevalence – with pain used as a proxy indicator of palliative care need – by disease at the end of life. However, these estimates do not capture the need for palliative care in its entirety, which would include the need from the point of diagnosis, as well as one or two involved caregivers, orphans, vulnerable children, and the bereaved (Connor and Bermedo 2014).

study reported that 80.7 % of palliative care patients were diagnosed with HIV, 17.9 % with cancer, and 1.4 % other conditions (Selman et al. 2011). In Malawi a retrospective review of patient case notes found that 54 % of patients seen by the hospital team were HIV positive, while 42 % had HIV-related diagnoses – including AIDS-defining malignancies – and 48 % had non-AIDS-related cancers (Tapsfield and Bates 2011). However, in a continent characterised by socio-economic heterogeneity and genetic diversity, variation exists within and between nations in the incidence of different cancer types. In 2008, the most common cancers in men and women varied between Northern Africa (i.e. lung, urinary bladder, and non-Hodgkin lymphoma for men and breast, cervix uteri, and colorectal for women) and sub-Saharan Africa (i.e. prostrate, liver, and lung for men and breast, cervix uteri, and liver for women) (American Cancer Society 2011a).

15.2.2 Eastern Europe

The prevalence of HIV in the region is very low compared with rates in Africa, with adult (aged 15–49) prevalence rates in the review countries ranging from <0.1 % (Serbia) to 0.9 % (Ukraine) (UNAIDS 2014).

In the 40 countries of the four United Nations-defined areas of Europe and the 27 countries of the European Union (EU), there were an estimated 3.45 m new cancer cases in 2012 – excluding non-melanoma skin cancer – and 1.75 m cancer deaths (Ferlay et al. 2013). The most common causes of death were cancers of the lung (353,000), colorectal (215,000), breast (131,000), and stomach (107,000) (Ferlay et al. 2013). Indeed, in 2008 cancer was the second most common cause of death in the EU, 29 % of deaths among men and 23 % among women (Eurostat 2008), while in 2008 there were an estimated 985,200 new cases of cancer in Central and Eastern Europe (American Cancer Society 2011b).

However, the survival rates vary across European states. In a retrospective observational study of 107 cancer registries for more than 10 m patients with cancer diagnosed up to 2007 and followed for 1 year across 29 European countries, De Angelis et al. and the EUROCARE group found that while 5-year relative survival generally increased steadily over time for all European regions, survival in eastern Europe was generally low and below the European mean (De Angelis et al. 2013). Similarly, examining survival trends between 2000 and 2004 for 20 common cancers, Gondos et al. (2008) found that among the 12 participating cancer sites, major geographical differences in patient prognosis persisted, with a lower survival observed in Eastern European countries.

15.2.3 India

While HIV adult prevalence in the country is low (0.3 %), the size of the Indian population means that a considerable number of people are living with the illness (2.1 m) (UNAIDS 2014).

Cancer prevalence is estimated to be 2.5 m (Directorate General of Health Services, India 2014), with in excess of half a million dying from cancer annually (Dikshit et al. 2012). It has been reported that annually, more than 9.8 m die in India, with the number requiring palliative care estimated to be approximately 6 m, assuming that 60 % of all who die would benefit from palliative care (Kumar 2013). However, fewer than 2 % of the needy have access to palliative care in the country (Kumar 2013). Of at least 1 m people with cancer in moderate-to-severe pain at any point of time, pain relief is only provided to between <0.4 % and <4 % (Rajagopal and Joranson 2007; Human Rights Watch 2010), with multiple formulary restrictions on opioid availability and use (Cleary et al. 2013c).

15.2.4 Latin America

HIV prevalence in Latin America is also low, with adult (aged 15–49) prevalence rates in the review countries ranging from 0.4 % (Argentina, Brazil, and Peru) to 0.5 % (Colombia) (UNAIDS 2014).

Cancer is becoming an increasing problem regionally. In 2008 there were an estimated 176,600 new cases of cancer in Central America and 650,000 in South America (American Cancer Society 2011b). Cancer is a leading cause of death in Latin America, with cancer rates among the 10 % of the population who are indigenous found to be higher than for nonindigenous peoples for cervical cancer in parts of Brazil, Ecuador, and Guyana and for stomach cancer in regions of Chile and for gallbladder in Chile and Bolivia, while breast cancer rates were lower in Ecuador, Brazil, and Chile (Moore et al. 2013).

15.3 Palliative Care and Cancer Treatment

This section discusses the status of palliative care services in each country and region before exploring the role of the discipline in addressing the needs of patients with non-cancer and cancer diagnoses.

15.3.1 Africa

15.3.1.1 Status of Palliative Care Services

During the 30 years after the formation of the first services were initiated in Zimbabwe (Wright and Clark 2006), palliative care development across the continent was minimal for many years (Mwangi-Powell et al. 2010). Based upon the World Health Organization's (WHO 2002) definition of palliative care, these services aspired to the organisation's public health approach, founded upon appropriate government policies, the adequate availability of medicines, the education of health professionals, and integration of palliative care at all levels in national healthcare systems (Sternsward et al. 2007).

In 2004–2005 a global study of hospice and palliative care services was conducted using a four-part typology to depict levels of service development by country:

- Group 1: No known hospice/palliative care activity
- Group 2: Capacity-building activity
- Group 3: Localised hospice/palliative care provision
- Group 4: Countries where hospice/palliative care services were reaching a measure of integration with the mainstream health-care system (Clark et al. 2007)

The study not only reported that 21 of 47 African countries surveyed had no identified hospice or palliative care activity, but also that just 4 of the 47 (8.5 %) could be classified as having services approaching some measure of integration with mainstream health services. While the 26 countries with palliative care activity constituted approximately 136 hospice and palliative care organisations operating in 15 countries and a capacity-building presence in the other 11 (Wright and Clark 2006), the majority were based in South Africa.

Five years later, research noted a number of significant advances against these baseline data (Lynch et al. 2013). Nine countries progressed from no known activity/capacity building (groups 1/2) to isolated provision (group 3a), while four countries moved from group 3 to group 4a (preliminary integration into mainstream service provision). In the review countries, the service development levels were Kenya (4a), Malawi (4a), Uganda (4b – advanced integration into mainstream services), and South Africa (4a). Despite the pressing clinical and public health challenge (Harding et al. 2013a), paediatric palliative care provision on the continent is less developed than adult services, with a recent mapping study finding that among 53 African countries, 43 were ranked at level 1 (no known activities) and only 1 at level 4 (provision reaching mainstream) (Knapp et al. 2011).

Despite this progress in advancing service provision in Africa (Mwangi-Powell et al. 2013), palliative care coverage on the continent remains deficient (Grant et al. 2011; Powell et al. 2011), as does the research needed to underpin it (Harding et al. 2013b; Powell et al. 2014a). Where it is available, palliative care is primarily provided by non-governmental organisations (NGO) with limited geographic and patient coverage rather than integrated fully within national health systems, using a home-based care (HBC) model of service provision based on trained health professionals, community-based volunteers, and family carers (Powell and Hunt 2013).

15.3.1.2 Addressing the Needs of Non-cancer and Cancer Patients

For many years, NCDs have been "left in the shadows" by disease-specific HIV programmes (Lemoine et al. 2012). There is now, however, a growing recognition of not only NCDs and cancer specifically as a public health priority (Kingham et al. 2013), with no discrimination based upon diagnosis, but also a growing recognition of palliative care (Powell et al. 2014b). However, while globally many organisations are contributing to the fight against cancer, in Africa these efforts are generally yet to be structured into coherent plans for effective cancer control (Stefan et al. 2013).

Table 15.3 Country capacity to address and respond to cancer and other NCDs in the selected review countries

Region/country	Has body responsible for NCDs[a]	National health reporting system for cause-specific mortality	Has national, population-based cancer registry	Has operational cancer plan[b]
Africa				
Kenya	Yes	Yes	No	No
Malawi	Yes	No	No	No
South Africa	Yes	Yes	Yes	Yes
Uganda	Yes	Yes	No	No
Eastern Europe				
Albania	No	Yes	No	No
Georgia	Yes	Yes	No	No
Serbia	Yes	Yes	Yes	No
Ukraine	Yes	Yes	No	Yes
India	Yes	Yes	No	Yes
Latin America				
Argentina	Yes	Yes	No	Yes
Brazil	Yes	Yes	Yes	Yes
Colombia[c]	ND	ND	ND	ND
Peru	Yes	Yes	No	No

Source: Adapted from World Health Organization (2011)

Note:

[a]"Body" could be a unit, branch, or department in the Ministry of Health

[b]"Plan" could be an integrated or topic-specific policy, programme, or action plan

[c]Country did not respond to country capacity survey

In 2010 only 17 countries reported policies, strategies, or action plans for cancer care, but only 17 % of the NCD programmes are funded (Stefan et al. 2013).

The current capacity of the review countries, in and outside Africa, to address and respond to cancer and other NCDs is outlined in Table 15.3. While many have a recognised body responsible for NCDs and cause-specific mortality-reporting systems, a considerable number lack national, population-based cancer registries to monitor the disease prevalence and operational plans to implement corrective programmes, as well as the infrastructure capacity (e.g. pathology and radiotherapy services) needed for the treatment and care of cancer patients (Sylla and Wild 2012; Abdel-Wahab et al. 2013).

Palliative care needs of patients across Africa differ from those in more developed nations because of the levels of impoverishment and differing sociocultural attitudes to illness, life, and death (Powell et al. 2014c). Often these needs do not require specialist palliative care interventions. In addition to pain and symptom control and psychological counselling, these needs can include financial support for food, shelter, funeral costs, school fees, income generation schemes, and orphan care (Harding and Higginson 2004). In these instances, the palliative care approach to address these needs can be employed by a combination of non-palliative care specialist doctors, nurses, and volunteers, supported by appropriate protocols and built on a community-based model of care provision. However, in some countries specialist palliative care centres offer interventions for referred patients presenting with complex cases (Grant et al. 2012).

The importance of palliative care in patient management on the continent is heightened by their late presentation to health services, when curative options are often unattainable. However, limited oncological treatment opportunities also contribute to the critical role of palliative care. In addition to the lack of national cancer policies, there is a generalised deficit of material resources and skilled personnel in Africa to treat cancer effectively. Radiation therapy is generally indicated in more than 50 % of cancers, with its availability sometimes indicating cancer treatment capability (Abdel-Wahab et al. 2013). However, according to Abdel-Wahab et al. (2013), of 52 African countries only 23 offered external beam radiotherapy, with 60 % of the 277 instruments on the continent located in Egypt (76) and South Africa (92), and approximately 198 m people, roughly one-fifth of the continent's population, having no access to teletherapy. Indeed, among the seven African countries with the highest levels of palliative care integration into mainstream health systems (Kenya, Malawi, South Africa, Tanzania, Zambia, Zimbabwe, and Uganda), one has no radiotherapy service (Lynch et al. 2013; Abdel-Wahab et al. 2013), while 20 of the 21 countries with no reported palliative care activity reportedly have no radiotherapy services.

15.3.2 Eastern Europe

15.3.2.1 Status of Palliative Care Services

Subsequent to the political upheavals of the 1990s, and following years of minimal significant developments during the years of communist rule, there has been a steady development of palliative care services among countries in Central and Eastern Europe. Using data from a recent regional atlas of palliative care, the status of services in the reviewed countries is outlined in Table 15.4. Georgia reports the most adult palliative care services, while Ukraine is alone in having no official palliative care strategy, with poor levels of palliative care education in medical schools across all four nations, and Serbia having significantly more strong opioid consumption levels.

In 2006, barriers to the progressive development of services were (1) financial and material resources, (2) problems relating to opioid availability, (3) lack of public awareness and government recognition of palliative care as a field of specialisation, and (4) lack of palliative care education and training programmes (Lynch et al. 2009). The problem of restrictive formulary deficiencies and excessive regulatory barriers that interfere with appropriate patient care remains a problem in many European countries (Cherny et al. 2010). Indeed, the development of palliative care in many countries remains uneven and uncoordinated, with poor integration across wider health-care systems.

The specialty of palliative care is only beginning to be recognised across Eastern Europe. While countries such as Poland and Romania have been at the forefront of service development, gaining wider acceptance for the discipline (Mosoiu et al. 2000), in most nations there is a tendency among medical bodies to discourage the acceptance of new specialisations. However, many countries are seeking approval

Table 15.4 Status of palliative care services and activity in the selected Eastern European review countries

| Country | Service type | | | | | Total/ million inhabitants | Natl PC Association (date of formation) | Official national strategy | Legislation on PC | Level of development | PC in medical schools[a] | Strong opioid consumption 2010 (ME MG/capita/year (Europe average = 80.55) |
	Total # of adult services	Inpatient service	Home care team	Hospital service	Mixed team							
Albania	3	0	2	0	1	0.93	Yes (2002)	Yes	No	3b	No PC subject (100 %)	1.8
Georgia	16	1	13	2	0	3.72	Yes (2009)	Yes	Yes	3b	Mandatory subject (10 %)	2.17
Serbia	2	0	1	1	0	0.20	In development	Yes	No	4a	No PC subject (100 %)	24.2
Ukraine	3	0	3	0	0	0.07	Yes (2007 & 2010)	No	No	3a	0[b]	1.31[c]

Source: Adapted from Centeno et al. (2013)

Note:

Children care services, reported in three countries, are:

Albania: 1 home care paediatric team, 2 mixed paediatric care support teams, and 8 mixed paediatric beds available for day-care services only

Georgia: 4 paediatric home palliative care support teams

Ukraine: Fewer than 100 paediatric hospital palliative care teams throughout Ukraine (4,000 beds) and 1 paediatric home palliative care support team

[a]Palliative care educational activity – of various types – as a percentage of all country medical schools

[b]This may represent the absence of any medical schools in the country

[c]In May 2013, the country's Cabinet of Ministers lifted Decree #333, which for decades had placed burdensome procedural impediments that severely limited access to opioids for pain relief (Tymoshevska and Shapoval-Deinega 2013)

for specialisation as an important milestone in the development of palliative care: currently, Poland has full specialisation, while Romania, Slovakia, the Czech Republic, and Georgia have subspecialisation status.

As in many countries, recognition of nurses and social workers lags behind that of the medical profession. Indeed, professional nursing is relatively new to the region, where in Soviet times nurses were poorly trained and served to assist physicians without a broad scope of practice. However, although university degree programmes for nurses are recent developments in the region, a number of countries have introduced basic palliative care education for undergraduate and postgraduate nurses. Similarly, social work as a profession is new, with many university programmes only formed in the past 5–10 years.

15.3.2.2 Addressing the Needs of Non-cancer and Cancer Patients

As occurred worldwide, palliative care in Eastern Europe began with a major focus on cancer (Traue and Ross 2005; Boland and Johnson 2013). This was attributable to the high symptom burden, lower prevalence of infectious diseases (like HIV), more readily determined prognosis, associated stigma and significant need for family support, and the acknowledgement that addressing the needs of all persons with life-threatening illnesses in such a resource-limited setting is beyond the capacity of emerging service providers (Sloan and Gelband 2007). However, in some countries there remain deficiencies in health-care provision, for example, in Romania where screening to detect and subsequently address psychological problems arising from a cancer diagnosis is suboptimal (Dégi 2013).

Regionally, non-cancer patients are usually ineligible to receive strong opioid medication, even though there is a high level of moderate-to-severe pain among this group. In many countries, only oncologists are legally permitted to prescribe morphine, with some formulary regulations limiting opioids to cancer patients (Cleary 2010). However, many palliative care providers in the region have attempted to embrace non-cancer patients.

In this setting, while no palliative care specialist explicitly promotes the discipline as an alternative for, or substitute to, modern anticancer treatment interventions, health-care systems in the former Soviet Union and socialist republics of Eastern Europe are in a period of transition, with evident disparities in access to oncological treatment. Indeed, the emergence of market economies has resulted in the development of two-tiered health-care systems: the overburdened state-run system and private facilities providing superior levels of care for those with the financial resources to receive it.

In this context, patient access to prevailing anticancer treatments is determined by available personal economic resources. For patients with limited finances forced to access the state-run health system, however, there are multiple problems securing cancer therapies: for instance, there are limited numbers of radiation therapy equipment, specific chemotherapy medicines are often unavailable, and a patient needs to wait months before accessing the correct type of chemotherapy.

15.3.3 India

15.3.3.1 Status of Palliative Care Services

In 1985 palliative care originated in India in the Shanti Avedna Sadan, an inpatient hospice dedicated to patients with cancer based in Mumbai, in the state of Maharashtra (Khosla et al. 2012). During the next 8 years, two more such care centres were created by the hospice's founder in Goa and Delhi. Further foundational work was initiated to form Cancer Relief India (Burn 2001), while Dr Jan Stjernsward, then Chief of Cancer and Palliative Care at the World Health Organization (WHO), and Dr Robert Twycross, as head of the WHO Collaborating Centre for Palliative Care based in Oxford, England, promoted teachings that sensitised the next generation of the country's palliative care pioneers.

Major breakthroughs occurred in the early 1990s when, based on a government medical college in Calicut, Kerala, a new NGO named the Pain and Palliative Care Society (PPCS) initiated an outpatient palliative care service. The PPCS' work brought pain management and the concept of palliative care to the public's attention, emphasising quality of life (Seamark et al. 2000), with volunteers involved in the management of the organisation as well as patient care, providing it with a unique service feature. The PPCS attracted considerable public attention, initiating regular home visit programmes for the needy that actively involved the community, and was declared a WHO demonstration project in 1995. During the following years, interested volunteers established palliative care programmes in villages and towns in Kerala that were supported by part-time doctors and nurses who received training from PPCS.

From the outset, the service was provided to people with non-cancer and cancer diagnoses, with the extent of disease-related suffering and not diagnosis being the criteria for care provision. In this way, PPCS embraced a systematic evaluation and management of patients' problems as far as possible based in the patient's home. Inpatient facilities addressing the needs of patients who experienced problematic symptoms and required end-of-life care when the patient or family found their life situation intolerable domestically – with the service promoting the use of opioids and thereby establishing its safety (Rajagopal et al. 2001) – were appended later. Moreover, the PPCS services were not restricted to symptom control. Trained professionals and volunteers provided emotional and social support (Sureshkumar and Rajagopal 1996), while the organisation also initiated educational programmes for professionals and volunteers across the country (Rajagopal and Sureshkumar 1999).

Another major development in that decade was the formation of the Indian Association of Palliative Care in 1994, with the involvement of the Government's Ministry of Health, which created an avenue for palliative care pioneers across the nation to meet, network, share experience, and plan service development together. In the following years, many palliative care units emerged across the country, primarily in major cities. However, many were housed in cancer hospitals or founded by cancer survivors and consequently catered only to people with a cancer diagnosis, while other organisations – many inspired by the experience of the PPCS – provided care to patients irrespective of their disease.

The network of Kerala-based palliative care centres, catalysed by the PPCS, expanded to approximately 30 in the first 7 years, while later the community network was strengthened by the development of the Neighbourhood Network in Palliative Care (NNPC) (Kumar and Numpeli 2005; Smith 2012). In 2007 it was reported that the network had more than 60 units covering a population of in excess of 12 m (Kumar 2007).

In 2003, and acknowledging that a palliative care development in the country was significantly centred in Kerala – with the exception of a few major metropolitan cities – the voluntary organisation Pallium India was formed to promote development of palliative care nationally (www.palliumindia.org). The organisation identifies potential individuals and institutions to collaborate with to develop new palliative care facilities and upgrade promising ones to training centres (Rajagopal and Twycross 2009). During the following decade, Pallium India successfully established or catalysed the development of 3 palliative care training centres across the country, as well as the development of 11 palliative care centres, 9 of which were in separate states that previously had no palliative care service. However, currently, while India's available palliative care services are rated at level 3b (isolated palliative care provision) (Lynch et al. 2013), they are very unevenly distributed across the nation, with the state of Kerala, with 3 % of the country's population, having more than 90 % of the country's palliative care services (Kumar 2013).

15.3.3.2 Addressing the Needs of Non-cancer and Cancer Patients

While India's 28 Regional Cancer Centres (RCCs) and more than 140 medical colleges provide radiotherapy services, these are inadequate to reach all in need, particularly in rural areas where more than 80 % of India's population live. In some states, basic cancer treatment is free or subsidised for those falling below the poverty line, whereas in most parts of the country, treatment costs are out-of-pocket, borne by individual patients. Consequently, a significant proportion of the population do not have access to cancer treatment.

On this basis, access to palliative care as a substitute to cancer treatment might be perceived as undesirable but inevitable. However, in reality patient access to palliative care is much scarcer than it is for cancer treatment. Approximately half of all RCCs and most of the medical colleges that offer cancer treatment do not have palliative care facilities. Moreover, in the way health-care services in the country are planned and developed, it is unlikely that in the near future, access to palliative care will exceed access to cancer treatment.

15.3.4 Latin America

15.3.4.1 Status of Palliative Care Services

Palliative care in the region originated in the early 1980s with the formation of the Pain and Palliative Care Clinic in Medellin, Colombia, and the provision of home-based care in San Nicolas, Argentina (Pastrana et al. 2012). With additional services emerging in the following decade, 84 % of countries in the region had a palliative care presence of some description by the start of the twenty-first century.

The development of the discipline has, however, been very heterogeneous. By 2011, 3 countries were classified as being in Group 2 (capacity building), 12 in Group 3a (isolated provision), 1 in Group 3b (generalised provision), and 3 in Group 4a (preliminary integration, the latter comprising Chile, Costa Rica, and Uruguay (Lynch et al. 2013)).

By 2012, there were an estimated 922 palliative care services across the region, 1.63 services/units/teams per 1 m inhabitants (mi), ranging from 16.06 (/mi) in Costa Rica to 0.24 (/mi) services in Honduras, with 46 % of existing services (in Argentina and Chile) serving 10 % of the regional population (Pastrana et al. 2012). The most prevalent service type are home-based care teams (0.4/mi), followed by hospital support services/teams (0.34/mi) and multilevel teams (0.33/mi).

Four countries have palliative care officially accredited as a medical speciality/ subspeciality, and in six countries it is a course or diploma. It is estimated that approximately 600 palliative care doctors are accredited in the region, with 70 % based in Argentina, Chile, and Mexico. Argentina has the highest number of educational programmes and services and has served as an aspirational model for other countries in the region since palliative care started locally in 1989. Chile and Costa Rica initiated national programmes in 1990 and have made important advances, as has Venezuela, which began in 2001 and is progressing well. Panama designed a palliative care programme for the entire country, which is currently being implemented (Pastrana et al. 2012).

Eleven countries have at least one palliative care association, and active research groups are evident in Chile (10), Argentina (5), Mexico (5), Cuba (4), Colombia (4), Peru (3), Panama (2), Brazil (1), and the Dominican Republic (1). In terms of health policy, three countries have a national palliative care law, with national palliative care plans/programmes reported in seven countries, five of which are integrated with cancer or pain work. Two-fifths (42 %) of countries have active research groups, but these are not prodigious (Wenk et al. 2008). Of only 106 original articles emanating from Latin America and the Caribbean, more than half of their authors originated in Brazil. The status of palliative care in the reviewed countries is presented in Table 15.5.

15.3.4.2 Addressing the Needs of Non-cancer and Cancer Patients

Treatment regimens for patients with advanced cancer are primarily directed to curative rather than palliative care approaches, with patients usually confronted by two choices: if it is assumed that no restorative interventions will succeed, they are abandoned by the health-care system, with the responsibility of care transferred in its entirety to the family or primary caregiver; secondly, they are admitted to a hospital where they usually face futile treatment regimens and isolation from family and loved ones (Pan American Health Organization 1997).

Given the nature of the disease burden, most palliative care models focus on cancer patients; while some groups are providing palliative care for patients with non-cancer conditions, it is not widespread. In a recent survey by the Latin American

Table 15.5 Status of palliative care services and activity in the selected Latin American review countries

| Country | Service type | | | | | | | | Accreditation | Medical school with PC (%) | National association | Standards, norms of guidelines | National law | National programme/ plan | Level of development[c] |
	Full services (per million inhab.)	Hospice inpatient (per million inhab.)	Home care (per million inhab.)	Community Centre (per million inhab.)	Services/ units in 2nd level hospitals (per million inhab.)	Services/ units in 3rd level hospitals (per million inhab.)	Multilevel services/ teams (per million inhab.)	Hospital services/ Support teams (per million inhab.)							
Argentina	151 (3.76)	11 (0.27)	21 (0.52)	0 (0.00)	2 (0.05)	21 (0.52)	16 (0.40)	80 (1.99)	Yes	6 (22.2)	1	Yes	No[a]	No	3b
Brazil	93 (0.48)	6 (0.03)	24 (0.12)	0 (0.00)	0 (0.00)	16 (0.08)	26 (0.14)	21 (0.11)	Yes	3 (1.7)	2	Yes	No	Yes[b]	3a
Colombia	23 (0.50)	4 (0.09)	2 (0.04)	0 (0.00)	1 (0.02)	13 (0.28)	3 (0.07)	0 (0.00)	Yes	3 (5.3)	1	No	Yes[b]	No	3a
Peru	12 (0.42)	0 (0.00)	0 (0.00)	0 (0.00)	1 (0.03)	7 (0.24)	4 (0.14)	0 (0.00)	No	0 (0.0)	1	No	No	Yes[b]	3a

Source: Adapted from Pastrana et al. (2012)

Note:

[a]Federal, state, or municipal laws exist

[b]Linked to cancer or pain programmes

[c]Lynch et al. (2013)

Association for Palliative Care, 86 % of respondents reported that their countries have national HIV/AIDS programmes in their Ministries of Health (Selwyn and De Lima 2008). The vast majority of these programmes included prevention and active treatment (92 and 98 %, respectively), while palliative care was included in only seven programmes. The limited availability of palliative care programmes for HIV/AIDS in the region may also be attributed to political negligence or to the lacking recognition of palliative care as a crucial care component. Indeed, a publication by the Pan American Health Organization (PAHO) that outlines a regional plan for HIV/AIDS omits palliative care (Organización Panamericana de la Salud 2005).

In terms of cancer care and treatment, 16 countries in the region have a national cancer control programme, 13 of which include palliative care (Pastrana et al. 2012). This care is predominantly provided by oncologists, with a survey of 777 physicians and nurses from Argentina, Brazil, Cuba, Mexico, and Peru showing that over half (55 %) of patients receiving advanced cancer care do so in a hospital setting, while 34 % received care at home, and only 10 % received professional end-of-life care at home or in a hospice (Torres-Vigil et al. 2008). The study participants also identified multiple barriers to the progress of palliative care in cancer, including lack of appropriate health legislation regarding end-of-life care, socio-economic disparities, poverty levels, ethnic and cultural diversities, low educational levels, lack of information on diagnosis and prognosis given to patients and families, fear of diversion of opioids to illegal markets, oncologists' concern that palliative care eliminates hope, inadequate palliative care policies in the countries of the region, and limited availability of potent analgesics, a finding reported elsewhere (Cleary et al. 2013a).

15.4   The Future of Cancer Treatment and Palliative Care

In many developing nations, patients with advanced-stage, incurable cancers present late to health services, partly as a consequence of the absence of early detection programmes and the ignorance of, and stigma surrounding, the illness. Oncological treatment in developing countries has made substantial progress during the recent decades, even if it is often overreliant on basic chemotherapy – where this exists.

However, palliative care has often been forced to occupy the service gap left by inadequate oncology treatment options. Faced with this reality, while it could be argued that palliative care has evolved in many developing nations into a substitute for modern anticancer treatment, this is more a case by omission rather than commission, a product of de facto infrastructure and human resource limitations rather than by conscious design. As shown above, for example, many African nations face a considerable burden of infectious and NCDs that consume a significant proportion of limited national health budgets. Against this backdrop, innovative, cutting-edge treatment modalities are not only resource intensive, but they may exert a limited impact in addressing the care gap between palliation and cure, and that between developed and developing countries, only benefiting a small minority at a significant financial cost.

By definition, palliative care alone will not cure the disease, but attempt to alleviate any associated troubling pain and other symptoms to improve patients' quality of life. Indeed, given that state-of-the-art oncological treatment is currently unrealistic in many such countries – given the exorbitant costs – there is an argument that contends that patients with incurable diagnoses should at least have access to palliative care to optimise their comfort, function, and social support, and that of their family, when the illness is no longer remediable (Schrijvers 2007). Consequently, and this argument is evident across many developing nations, a suggested significant investment in cancer treatment services may be more optimally spent on primary preventative measures for those unaffected by cancer – eliminating or reducing exposure to recognised risk factors in vulnerable populations – and enhanced palliative care services with much greater patient coverage for those with a cancer diagnosis, thereby potentially impacting upon a greater percentage of a population.

While ethically this might sound an unjustifiable argument – potentially depriving cancer interventions for people with curable illnesses for the prolongation of a life of reasonable quality – it is a valid question for health-care system planners with ultimately morally problematic choices in the light of heavily constrained finances at their disposal.

Looking to the future, it is interesting to speculate as to the extent to which palliative care will continue to be a de facto substitute for modern anticancer treatment for the vast majority of peoples in developing nations. Similarly, it will be interesting to follow whether the gap that exists between developing and developed countries regarding cancer care provision will be widened further by the advent of a combination of targeted oncological therapies unaffordable in low-resource settings and the emergence of specialised palliative care in developed nations.

In BRICS countries, of course, the possibility of a more holistic, integrated approach to illness and well-being is enhanced given the greater financial resources. In India, there is a planned expansion of cancer treatment facilities within a hierarchical system of cancer centres that entails:

(a) Three national cancer centres – one each in North, South, and East of India
(b) 20 state cancer centres, to function as centres of excellence
(c) 100 tertiary cancer centres in regional cancer centres, medical colleges, or other institutions
(d) Cancer services in all of the 640 districts in the country, each of which will have a palliative care component

Importantly, each of the district services will include a palliative care component, with the latter seen as a component part of the cancer care continuum – that includes prevention, early detection, and treatment – and not as a substitute for effective oncological care (Ministry of Health & Family Welfare, Government of India 2012). But in non-BRICS countries, provision of such holistic care along the cancer care continuum is less realistic.

Conclusions

There is widespread recognition that among NCDs, cancer is a "global and growing, but not uniform, problem", with an increased proportion of its burden borne by low- and middle-income developing countries (Vineis and Wild 2014). It has been argued that, using a warfare metaphor, a new "military battlespace vision" – a strategic approach taking an integrative, rounded view of war that incorporates detailed information on the pathogenic enemy, its strengths, weaknesses, and related warzone intelligence – is required that supplements, if not supersedes, the hundreds of new anticancer drugs, including the so-called advance therapy magic bullets, that have had variable success (Hanahan 2014).

A global agenda that constitutes this "battlespace vision" and embraces cancer in developing country settings – where the cost of new medications and modern oncological technologies are generally prohibitive or logistically impractical to deliver to sufficient numbers of patients – is certainly welcome. Currently, however, and in the absence of additional funding, many health planners and governments have to operate under the premise that, assuming one cannot do everything in health-care provision, one has to consider deliberative models (e.g. cost-benefit analysis) upon which rational, informed health system planning decisions can be formed.

In developing countries, an argument can be postulated that what is required is a combination of the societally rather than individual-focused – in the form of regulatory controls among industries linked with unhealthy commodities (e.g. tobacco, alcohol, foods high in sugar, fat, and salt) (Vineis and Wild 2014) – approach to the primary prevention of cancer cases. This should be complemented by secondary prevention and treatment options as part of an overall cancer control strategy and a mainstreamed, enhanced palliative care service addressing all patients with a life-threatening, progressive illness. Without governmental action in developing nations to develop and implement effective cancer prevention policies in the absence of funding for cancer care continuum interventions, however, the notion that palliative care is a poor man's alternative to good oncological care will persist.

There are a number of recent policy initiatives that suggest that an integrated approach to cancer care provision is increasingly possible within the confines of restricted national budgets. From the focus on NCDs following the high-level UN General Assembly meeting in September 2011 (Wild 2012) to the imminent adoption by the WHO of the integration of palliative care services into existing health systems (Burki 2014), and, for example, the 2013 consensus statement on palliative care adopted by 34 African health ministries (Gwyther 2014), there is potential to see a reduction in the occurrence of cancers and a meaningful improvement – through effective pain and symptom management – in their treatment. This is more likely, however, to exert a meaningful impact if we avoid a replication of the HIV/AIDS vertical funding model so that systems as a whole are strengthened, placing the individual rather than their diagnosis at the centre of health systems (Knaul et al. 2011).

References

Abdel-Wahab M, Bourque J-M, Pynda Y et al (2013) Status of radiotherapy resources in Africa: an international atomic energy agency analysis. Lancet Oncol 14:e168–e175

American Cancer Society (2011a) Cancer in Africa. American Cancer Society, Atlanta

American Cancer Society (2011b) Global cancer facts and figures, 2nd edn. American Cancer Society, Atlanta

Anon (nd) The World Bank list of economies, July 2012. Source: http://librarians.acm.org/sites/default/files/world%20bank%20List%20of%20Economies%20(as%20of%20July%202012).pdf. Accessed 31 Jan 2014

Boland J, Johnson MJ (2013) End-of-life care for non-cancer patients. BMJ Support Palliat Care 3:2–3

Bray F, Jemal A, Grey N et al (2012) Global cancer transitions according to the Human Development Index (2008-2030): a population-based study. Lancet Oncol 13:790–801

Burki TK (2014) WHO resolution on access to palliative care. Lancet Oncol http://dx.doi.org/10.1016/S1470-2045(14)70034-8

Burn G (2001) A personal initiative to improve palliative care in India: 10 years on. Palliat Med 15:159–162

Centeno C, Pons JJ, Lynch T, Donea O, Rocafort J, Clark D (2013) APC atlas of palliative care in Europe 2013 – Cartographic edition. EAPC Press, Milan

Cherny NI, Baselga J, de Conno F et al (2010) Formulary availability and regulatory barriers to accessibility of opioids for cancer pain in Europe: a report from the ESMO/EAPC Opioid Policy Initiative. Ann Oncol 21:615–626

Clark D, Wright M, Hunt J et al (2007) Hospice and palliative care development in Africa: a multi-method review of services and experiences. J Pain Symptom Manage 33:698–710

Cleary J (2010) Access to therapeutic opioid medications in Europe by 2011? Fifty years on from the single convention on narcotic drugs. Palliat Med 24:109–110

Cleary J, De Lima L, Eisenchlas J et al (2013a) Formulary availability and regulatory barriers to accessibility of opioids for cancer pain in Latin America and the Caribbean: a report from the Global Opioid Policy Initiative (GOPI). Ann Oncol 24(Suppl 11):xi41–xi50

Cleary J, Powell RA, Munene G, Mwangi-Powell FN, Luyirika E, Kiyange F, Merriman A, Scholten W, Radbruch L, Torode J, Cherny NI (2013b) Formulary availability and regulatory barriers to accessibility of opioids for cancer pain in Africa: a report from the Global Opioid Policy Initiative (GOPI). Ann Oncol 24(Suppl 11):xi14–xi23

Cleary J, Simha N, Panieri A, Scholten W, Radbruch L, Torode J, Cherny NI (2013c) Formulary availability and regulatory barriers to accessibility of opioids for cancer pain in India: a report from the Global Opioid Policy Initiative (GOPI). Ann Oncol 24(Suppl 11):xi33–xi40

Connor SR, Bermedo MCS (2014) Global atlas of palliative care at the end of life. World Health Organization/Worldwide Palliative Care Alliance, Geneva/London

De Angelis R, Sant M, Coleman MP et al (2013) Cancer survival in Europe 1999 – 2007 by country and age: results of EUROCARE-5 – a population-based study. Lancet Oncol. doi:10.1016/S1470-2045(13)70546-1

Dégi CL (2013) In search of the sixth vital sign: cancer care in Romania. Support Care Cancer 21:1273–1280

Dikshit R, Gupta PC, Ramasundarahettige C et al (2012) Cancer mortality in India: a nationally representative survey. Lancet 379:1807–1816

Directorate General of Health Services, Ministry of Health & Family Welfare, Government of India (nd) National programme for prevention and control of cancer, diabetes, cardiovascular diseases and stroke: operational guidelines. Directorate General of Health Services, Ministry of Health & Family Welfare, Government of India. Available at: http://health.bih.nic.in/Docs/Guidelines/Guidelines-NPCDCS.pdf. Accessed 3 Mar 2014

Eurostat (2012). Eurostat Regional yearbook, 2012: Health. Available at: http://ec.europa.eu/eurostat/documents/3217494/5734884/KS-HA-12-001-03-EN.PDF/1cd9cc21-562a-4c74-92cb-77c0430b961d?version=1.0. Accessed 13 Nov 2013

Ferlay J, Shin H-R, Bray F et al (2010) Estimates of worldwide burden of cancer in 2008: GLOBOCAN 2008. Int J Cancer 127:2893–2917

Ferlay J, Steliarova-Foucher E, Lortet-Tieulent J et al (2013) Cancer incidence and mortality patterns in Europe: estimates for 40 countries in 2012. Eur J Cancer 49:1374–1403

Gondos A, Bray F, Brewster DH et al (2008) Recent trends in cancer survival across Europe between 2000 and 2004: a model-based period analysis from 12 cancer registries. Eur J Cancer 44:1463–1475

Grant L, Brown J, Leng M et al (2011) Palliative care making a difference in rural Uganda, Kenya and Malawi: three rapid evaluation field studies. BMC Palliat Care 10:8

Grant L, Downing J, Leng M, Namukwaya L (2012) Models of delivering palliative care in Sub-Saharan Africa: advocacy summary. The Diana, Princess of Wales Memorial Fund, London. Available at: www.dianaprincessofwalesmemorialfund.org/information-and-resources/publications. Accessed 31 Oct 2013

Gulland A (2014) Global cancer prevalence is growing at 'alarming pace', says WHO. BMJ 348:g1338

Gwyther L (2014) Palliative care in chronic disease. S Afr Med J 104:114–115

Hanahan D (2014) Rethinking the war on cancer. Lancet 383:558–563

Harding R, Higginson IJ (2004) Palliative care in sub-saharan Africa: an appraisal 2004. The Diana, Princess of Wales Memorial Fund. King's College London, London. Available at: www.dianaprincessofwalesmemorialfund.org/information-and-resources/publications. Accessed 31 Oct 2013

Harding R, Albertyn R, Sherr L, Gwyther L (2013a) Paediatric palliative care in Sub-Saharan Africa: a systematic review of the evidence for care models, interventions, and outcomes. J Pain Symptom Manage. doi:10.1016/j.jpainsymman.2013.04.010

Harding R, Selman L, Powell RA et al (2013b) Research into palliative care in sub-Saharan Africa. Lancet Oncol 14:e183–e188

Human Rights Watch (2010) Unbearable pain: India's obligation to ensure palliative care. Human Rights Watch, New York

Jemal A, Bray F, Center MM et al (2011) Global cancer statistics. CA Cancer J Clin 61:69–90

Jemal A, Bray F, Forman D et al (2012) Cancer burden in Africa and opportunities for prevention. Cancer 118:4372–4384

Joint United Nations Programme on HIV/AIDS (2012) UNAIDS report of the global AIDS epidemic. UNAIDS, Geneva

Khosla D, Patel FD, Sharma SC (2012) Palliative care in India: current progress and future needs. Indian J Palliat Care 18:149–154

Kingham TP, Alatise OI, Vanderpuye V et al (2013) Treatment of cancer in sub-Saharan Africa. Lancet Oncol 14:e158–e167

Knapp C, Woodworth L, Wright M et al (2011) Paediatric palliative care provision around the world: a systematic review. Pediatr Blood Cancer 57:361–368

Knaul FM, Frenk J, Shulman L, for the Global Task Force on Expanded Access to Cancer Care and Control in Developing Countries (2011) Closing the cancer divide: a blueprint to expand access in low and middle income countries. Harvard Global Equity Initiative, Boston

Kumar SK (2007) Kerala, India: a regional community-based palliative care model. J Pain Symptom Manage 33:623–627

Kumar S (2013) Models of delivering palliative and end-of-life care in India. Curr Opin Support Palliat Care 7:216–222

Kumar S, Numpeli M (2005) Neighbourhood network in palliative care. Indian J Palliat Care 11:6–9

Lemoine M, Girard PM, Thursz M et al (2012) In the shadow of HIV/AIDS: forgotten diseases in sub-Saharan Africa: global health issues and funding agency responsibilities. J Public Health Policy 33:430–438

Lynch T, Clark D, Centeno C et al (2009) Barriers to the development of palliative care in the countries of Central and Eastern Europe and the Commonwealth of Independent States. J Pain Symptom Manage 37:305–315

Lynch T, Connor S, Clark D (2013) Mapping levels of palliative care development: a global update. J Pain Symptom Manage 45:1094–1106

Mathers CD, Loncar D (2006) Projections of global mortality and burden of disease from 2002 to 2030. PLoS Med 3:e442

Ministry of Health & Family Welfare, Government of India (2012) Proposal of strategies for palliative care in India. Available at: http://palliumindia.org/cms/wp-content/uploads/2014/01/National-Palliative-Care-Strategy-Nov_2012.pdf. Accessed 25 Jan 2014

Moore SP, Forman D, Piñeros M et al (2013) Cancer in indigenous people in Latin America and the Caribbean: a review. Cancer Med. doi:10.1002/cam4.134

Mosoiu D, Andrews C, Perolls G (2000) Global perspectives: palliative care in Romania. Palliat Med 14:65–67

Mwangi-Powell FN, Downing J, Ddungu H et al (2010) Palliative care in Africa. In: Ferrell BR, Coyle N (eds) Textbook of palliative nursing, 3rd edn. Oxford University Press, New York, pp 1319–1329

Mwangi-Powell FN, Powell RA, Harding R (2013) Models of delivering palliative and end-of-life care in sub-Saharan Africa. Curr Opin Support Palliat Care 7:223–228

O'Brien M, Mwangi-Powell F, Adewole IF et al (2013) Improving access to analgesic drugs for patients with cancer in sub-Saharan Africa. Lancet Oncol 14:e176–182

Organización Panamericana de la Salud (2005) Plan Regional de VIH/ITS para el Sector Salud 2006-2015. Organización Panamericana de la Salud, Washington, DC

Pan American Health Organization (1997) Framework for a regional project on cancer palliative care in Latin America and the Caribbean. Pan American Health Organization, Washington, DC. Source: www.paho.org/english/Hcp/HCN/doc214.pdf. Accessed 27 Feb 2014

Parkin DM (2006) The global health burden of infection-associated cancers in the year 2002. Int J Cancer 118:3030–3044

Pastrana T, De Lima L, Wenk R et al (2012) Atlas of palliative care in Latin America. IAHPC Press, Houston

Pisani P (2011) The cancer burden and cancer control in developing countries. Environ Health 10(Supp 1):S2

Powell RA, Hunt J (2013) Family care giving in the context of HIV/AIDS in Africa. Prog Palliat Care 21:13–21

Powell RA, Harding R, Namisango E et al (2014a) Palliative care research in Africa: consensus building for a prioritized agenda. J Pain Symptom Manage 47:315–324

Powell RA, Mwangi-Powell FN, Kiyange F et al (2011) Palliative care development in Africa: how we can provide enough quality care? BMJ Support Palliat Care 1:113–114

Powell RA, Radbruch L, Mwangi-Powell FN, Cleary J, Cherny NI (2014b) Failing to numb the pain: the untreated epidemic. S Afr Med J 104:117–118

Powell RA, Selman L, Galimaka-Kabalega D (2014c) Perspectives on end-of-life care in global context. In: Lazenby M, McCorkle R, Sulmasy D (eds) Safe passage: a global spiritual sourcebook for religion at the end of life care in Africa. Oxford University Press, Oxford, pp 20–35

Rajagopal MR, Joranson DE (2007) India: opioid availability – an update. J Pain Symptom Manage 33:615–622

Rajagopal MR, Sureshkumar K (1999) A model for delivery of palliative care in India – the Calicut experience. J Palliat Care 15:44–49

Rajagopal MR, Twycross RG (2009) Providing palliative care in resource-poor countries. In: Hanks G, Cherny NA, Fallon M et al (eds) Oxford textbook of palliative medicine, 4th edn. Oxford University Press, Oxford

Rajagopal MR, Joranson DE, Gilson AM (2001) Medical use, misuse and diversion of opioids in India. Lancet 358:139–143

Sankaranarayanan R, Swaminathan R, Brenner H et al (2010) Cancer survival in Africa, Asia, and Central America: a population-based study. Lancet Oncol 11(2):165–173

Schrijvers D (2007) Should palliative care replace palliative treatment for cancer in resource-poor countries? Lancet Oncol 8:86–87

Seamark D, Ajithakumari K, Burn G (2000) Palliative care in India. J R Soc Med 93:292–295

Selman LE, Higginson IJ, Agupio G et al (2011) Quality of life among patients receiving palliative care in South Africa and Uganda: a multi-centred study. Health Qual Life Outcomes 9:21

Selwyn P, De Lima L (2008) Los Cuidados Paliativos en VIH/SIDA en Latinoamérica: Propuesta para un enfoque integral en la atención de la salud. Actualizaciones en SIDA 16:59–62

Sloan FA, Gelband H (eds) (2007) Institute of Medicine (US) Committee on cancer control in low and middle-income countries. National Academies Press, Washington, DC

Smith R (2012) A way to provide palliative care globally. Available at: http://blogs.bmj.com/bmj/2012/06/25/richard-smith-a-way-to-provide-care-globally/. Accessed 25 Jan 2014

Stefan DC, Ahmed M, Elzawawy AM et al (2013) Developing cancer control plans in Africa: examples from five countries. Lancet Oncol 14:e189–e195

Sternsward J, Foley K, Ferris F (2007) The public health strategy for palliative care. J Pain Symptom Manage 33:486–493

Sureshkumar K, Rajagopal MR (1996) Palliative care in Kerala: problems at presentation in 440 patients with advanced cancer in a South Indian State. Palliat Med 10:293–298

Sylla BS, Wild CP (2012) A million Africans a year dying from cancer by 2030: what can cancer research and control offer to the continent? Int J Cancer 130:245–250

Tapsfield JB, Bates MJ (2011) Hospital based palliative care in sub-Saharan Africa; a six month review from Malawi. BMC Palliat Care 10:12

Torres-Vigil I, Aday LA, Reyes-Gibby C et al (2008) Health care providers' assessments of the quality of advanced-cancer care in Latin American medical institutions: a comparison of predictors in five countries – Argentina, Brazil, Cuba, Mexico and Peru. J Pain Palliat Care Pharmacother 22:7–20

Traue DC, Ross JR (2005) Palliative care in non-malignant disease. J R Soc Med 98:503–506

Tymoshevska V, Shapoval-Deinega K (2013) A win for palliative care in Ukraine. Available at: www.opensocietyfoundations.org/voices/win-palliative-care-ukraine. Accessed 16 Feb 2014

UNAIDS (2014) HIV data by country. Available at: www.unaids.org/en/regionscountries/countries/. Accessed 12 Feb 2014

Vineis P, Wild CP (2014) Global cancer patterns: causes and prevention. Lancet 383:549–557

Wagner K-H, Brath H (2012) A global view on the development of non-communicable diseases. Prev Med 54(Supp):S38–S41

Wenk R, De Lima L, Eisenchlas J (2008) Palliative care research in Latin America: results of a survey within the scope of the Declaration of Venice. J Palliat Med 11:717–722

Wild CP (2012) The role of cancer research in non-communicable disease control. J Natl Cancer Inst 104:1051–1058

World Bank (nd) How we classify countries. Available at: http://data.worldbank.org/about/country-classifications. Accessed 31 Jan 2014

World Health Organization (2002) WHO definition of palliative care. www.who.int/cancer/palliative/definition/en/. Accessed 17 Jan 2014

World Health Organization (2011) NCD Country profiles, 2011. World Health Organization, Geneva

World Health Organization (2013) Global health estimates: causes of death, 2000-2011. World Health Organization, Geneva

Wright M, Clark D (2006) Hospice and palliative care in Africa: a review of developments and challenges. Oxford University Press, Oxford

Part VI

Ethical Aspects

Emergencies in Oncology and Crises in Palliative Care

16

Bernd Alt-Epping and Friedemann Nauck

Contents

16.1   Introduction

It belongs to the distinguishing features of cancer that its disease trajectory and its causative treatment implicate numerous critical situations and emergencies that lead to life-threatening situations, and in a significant proportion of patients, these emergencies (instead of the tumour manifestations themselves) will be life-limiting. Therefore, the care of patients suffering from cancer as well as the respective anti-cancer treatment requires profound expertise in oncology and in emergency care.

In very advanced stages and when the end-of-life approaches, management of these emergency situations will differ from the curative setting, and the normative dimensions of clinical decision-making will have to be taken into account in a more pronounced way.

B. Alt-Epping, MD (✉) • F. Nauck, MD
Department of Palliative Medicine, University Medical Center, Göttingen, Germany
e-mail: bernd.alt-epping@med.uni-goettingen.de; friedemann.nauck@med.uni-goettingen.de

© Springer-Verlag Berlin Heidelberg 2015
B. Alt-Epping, F. Nauck (eds.), *Palliative Care in Oncology*,
DOI 10.1007/978-3-662-46202-7_16

This chapter describes emergencies in the oncology setting and in palliative care. It takes into consideration why emergencies in oncology also apply to palliative care team members and explains the characteristics of the palliative care approach in emergencies in end-of-life care.

16.2   Emergencies in the Oncology Setting

16.2.1 Cancer-Related Emergencies

Several mechanisms that are caused by the underlying disease itself can lead to sudden, unexpected, and potentially life-threatening clinical situations. Cancer patients access the emergency department for a vast number of clinical problems (e.g. febrile neutropenia, pain, respiratory distress, and GI issues), and more than half of these visits result in hospital admissions (Mayer et al. 2011; Vandyk et al. 2012). In a large population study on cancer patients who had to visit the emergency department, lung cancer was the leading diagnosis, followed by breast, prostate, and colorectal cancer (26.9, 6.3, 6, and 7.7 % of visits, respectively; Mayer et al. 2011).

Most, but by far not all of these emergencies are caused by structural pathologic conditions, such as the mechanical compression or infiltration of organs or vessels by the primary tumour or its metastases, with resulting destructive organ failure, obstruction, or perforation. Other emergencies are even caused by disorders of haemostasis; immunological, inflammatory, or metabolic disturbances; or other 'paraneoplastic' (cancer-associated) syndromes (Cervantes and Chirivella 2004; Krych and Hiddemann 2005; Higdon and Higdon 2006; Lawrie 2007).

The term paraneoplastic syndrome refers to a broad spectrum of endocrine, neurological, haematological, dermatological, organ-related, or systemic phenomena that are caused or at least associated with concurrent malignant disease (Berger et al. 2010; Pelosof and Gerber 2010). In some cases, these clinical phenomena can precede the first diagnosis of cancer by months (Trousseau 1865); it is estimated that up to 20 % of cancer patients will suffer from paraneoplastic syndromes (depending also on whether more prevalent findings such as cachexia or fever are defined as 'paraneoplastic' or not).

Table 16.1 gives examples of emergency situations in the oncology setting. All of these scenarios have in common that immediate action is required, including the activation of the emergency medical system (EMS) or intensive care, to overcome these life-threatening situations and to achieve full clinical restoration.

16.2.2 Cancer Therapy-Related Emergencies

Table 16.1 also provides some examples of cancer *therapy*-related emergencies. Febrile neutropenia belongs to the most prevalent treatment-related morbidities and must be judged as an emergency because of its possible septic propagation, depending on the duration of neutropenia, the underlying disease entity, and on other

Table 16.1 Emergencies in the oncology setting (examples)

(Structural) cancer-related emergencies	Cancer-associated (paraneoplastic) emergencies	Cancer therapy-related emergencies
Superior vena cava syndrome	Malignant hypercalcaemia	Febrile neutropenia
Acute airway obstruction	Inappropriate secretion of	Bleeding complications
Spinal cord compression	antidiuretic hormone/hyponatraemia	Tumour lysis syndrome
Pericardial tamponade	Disorders of haemostasis	Anaphylactic reactions
Increased intracranial pressure	Cerebellar degeneration, limbic encephalitis, Lambert-Eaton syndrome, and other neuromuscular syndromes	Haemorrhagic cystitis
Urinary obstruction	Vasculitis and other dermatological syndromes	Neurological or cardiotoxic side effects
Malignant bowel obstruction	…	Extravasation of chemotherapy
Massive haemoptysis		…
Hyperleucocytosis		
Hyperviscosity syndrome		
…		

aspects of immunocompetence. Extravasation of chemotherapy is clearly an emergency, depending of the applied substances and their local toxic properties, that requires full attention of the oncologist and all possible preventive efforts. Especially in haematology, where a high number of malignant cells will be lysed by first application of chemotherapy, the effects of abundant cell destruction will lead to a complex tumour lysis syndrome, including multi-organ failure.

Thanks to recent developments in modern oncology, the spectrum of anticancer therapies has increased substantially towards 'targeted' substances, including antibodies (with their possible anaphylactic properties) and multikinase inhibitors (with their complex spectrum of side effects, including epidermal and mucosal damage, disorders of haemostasis, extravasation of fluids, and others). Here, it might be particularly difficult to differentiate between the effects of the underlying malignancy versus possible treatment-related morbidity.

16.2.3 What a Palliative Care Physician Should Know About Them

Thanks to the increasing recognition of complex demands and symptoms of cancer patients even early in the course of an incurable disease, a palliative care concept that integrates best possible symptom control and psychosocial support early in the course of the disease is pursued (see Chap. 13). Furthermore, the expanded spectrum and availability of highly active anticancer substances, their (mostly) more favourable toxicity profile, and the recent improvements in supportive therapy extend the time span when patients may receive anticancer therapy even to the very late stages of their disease. These aspects have increased the likelihood that members of specialised palliative care teams will take care of patients that are still receiving anticancer treatment. Even more, palliative home care teams or community-based palliative care teams with their low-threshold 24-h accessibility might be the first professionals encountering an emergency situation that is related to progressive disease, to cancer-associated (paraneoplastic) effects, or to treatment-related toxicity. Therefore it seems to be imperative that palliative care team members also have a basic knowledge of how to detect and manage these emergency situations and when/how/how urgently the oncologist in charge and even the emergency medical system (EMS) have to be called.

16.2.4 Emergencies in Cancer Patients That Are Unrelated to Cancer

As the overall prevalence of cancer is rising because of the increasing age of patients, especially in western societies, cancer patients often suffer not only from their malignant disease or its respective treatment but also from several comorbidities. Preexisting cardiac comorbidities such as ischaemic heart disease or heart failure might decompensate in the oncology setting because of anaemia, cardiotoxic substances (especially anthracyclines), or congestive syndromes. Preexisting pulmonary disease such as COPD might be acutely exaggerated by immunosuppression and infection or obstructive growth of pulmonary metastases. Preexisting renal disease might deteriorate into a uraemic state because of fluid imbalances, nephrotoxic chemotherapy, or other substances (e.g. nonsteroidal anti-inflammatory drugs).

> **Case Example**
> A 48-year-old male patient, suffering from advanced nasopharyngeal carcinoma that was progressive after repeated multimodal treatment, presents at the emergency department for dull thoracic pain and dyspnea. ECG shows anterior wall ST segment elevations; lab results reveal markedly increased troponin T levels (98.0 ng/l). After discussing all treatment options with the patient, his relatives and among the multi-professional team, no invasive or medical reperfusion therapy was initiated, and the patient was transferred to the palliative care unit for symptom control. There, he died from acute heart failure 2 days later.

Cardiac complications in cancer patients, in particular, imply that numerous medical as well as ethical aspects need to be considered. Because acute rhythm disorders, cardiac ischaemia, or pulmonary oedema are associated with thoracic pain, dyspnea, and acute anxiety, these conditions need to be treated vigorously and under consideration of intensive care support even in quite advanced stages. This corresponds to the finding that foregoing emergency efforts and even cardiopulmonary resuscitation in patients suffering from advanced cancer might not necessarily be in the interest of the patients themselves. Seventy-five patients suffering from cancer (only 11 of them in localised stages, 9 being treated under curative intent) were asked about their wishes towards cardiopulmonary resuscitation; 58 % of them asked that a CPR be performed in case of cardiocirculatory arrest, and 'only 32 % of patients and 28 % relatives wanted doctors to make the final decision, indicating that shared decision-making may be important' (Ackroyd et al. 2007).

Some oncologists (and palliative care physicians) experience and describe a subtle but generalised reluctance by intensive care physicians to treat cancer patients suffering from acute (cardiac) conditions. A tendency to avoid ICU admissions of cancer patients in acute (and potentially reversible) conditions such as cardiac rhythm disorders or pulmonary oedema would be even more problematic because the lifetime prognosis for patients with metastasised cancer is in general not worse than for patients suffering from non-cancer diseases such as heart failure (who are certainly offered to be admitted to ICU) (Stewart et al. 2001). In case series, oncological patients had resuscitation success rates comparable to patients without cancer (Hendrick et al. 1990).

For some patients in palliative conditions, however, foregoing cardiac therapy might correspond to the explicit wish of the patient, as in the above-stated case example, depending on age, stage of the disease, biology, disease-related experience, individual normative values, and others.

16.3 A Palliative Care Approach to Emergencies in Cancer Patients

16.3.1 A Concept of 'Crisis' Instead of 'Emergency'

In addition to the above-described, (mostly) unforeseeable, complicating emergencies in the oncology setting, with a clear mandate to act immediately ('What has to be done?') to restore a potentially reversible clinical situation, there is another understanding of 'emergency' that comes into consideration later in the course of an incurable disease. Then, maintaining or restoring best possible quality of life (or just making the disease endurable for the patient and his/her relatives) may become the main objectives of therapy. This palliative care approach to emergencies tries to embed clinical decision-making into the altered clinical circumstances, respecting the limited therapeutic options ('What is appropriate?') and endeavours to anticipate critical situations, to communicate them, and to prepare the patient and his/her relatives for the situations that might come ('How can we prepare to make this not feel like an emergency?') (Nauck and Alt-Epping 2008).

This anticipatory approach is possible because many of the emergencies in end-of-life care are foreseeable, given the rather linear course of cancer at that stage. From clinical experience, it may well be anticipated that:

- A patient with lung cancer and bilateral pulmonary metastases will suffer from dyspnea at some point of his/her disease.
- A patient with relapsed glioblastoma multiforme might develop some degree of mental disturbances and restlessness.
- A severely affected, elderly patient with acute leukaemia might develop a life-limiting septic infection while being cared for at home.
- The social and nursing support system will fail at some point when an elderly man suffering from prostate cancer and bone metastases becomes bedridden or develops a sleeping disorder.
- Many patients will develop moist respiration during the last hours of life ('death rattle') even when the preceding course of disease has been uneventful.
- A patient with exulcerating tumour of the neck might acutely die from catastrophic bleeding.

This (of course incomplete) list of scenarios implies that in the palliative care setting, 'emergencies' can be understood as acuminated clinical manifestations of a progressive, undamped disease. Therefore, major efforts are being made in the palliative care setting to reduce the 'emergency character' of these situations and instead create an understanding of experiencing a 'crisis', a foreseen and expected climax of the advancing disease. Several tools and strategies have proven helpful for this anticipatory approach:

- Obtaining sufficient *information* and understanding of the underlying cancer manifestations and their entity-specific biological properties
- Therapeutic *experience* in identifying possible crises
- Open *communication* (e.g. about diagnosis, prognosis, and expected or possible crises; involvement of relatives in the decision-making process)
- Exploring the *patient's wishes*, for instance, towards treatment intensity, hospital admission behaviour, preferred place of death, and care after death
- Reflecting *appropriateness* of possible therapeutic procedures in case they occur, and avoiding futile (and therefore not indicated) measures
- *On-demand (p.r.n.) medication* for the majority of possible crises
- *Low-threshold 24-h accessibility* to palliative care services
- Clear and accessible *documentation* of the decision-making process

16.3.2 Advance Care Planning

This anticipatory approach (or at least the communicative and documentary aspects of systematically determining the will of a patient in case of clinical frailty or deterioration) has been conceptualised as regional implementation programmes in several places (Hickman et al. 2010; Molloy et al. 2000; In der Schmitten et al. 2014). Accompanying research was able to prove that systematic implementation efforts successfully increased the percentage of persons (for instance, those living in nursing homes) who accomplished an advance directive, a power of attorney, or other predetermining documents. But to date, clear evidence for a resulting clinical

Table 16.2 'Emergencies' in palliative care (examples)

Breakthrough pain crises
Acute dyspnoea
Inability to swallow (medication/fluids)
Malignant bowel obstruction
Decompensation of social support systems
Massive wound bleeding
Cerebral fits
Agitation and cognitive impairment
Moist respiration/'death rattle'
…

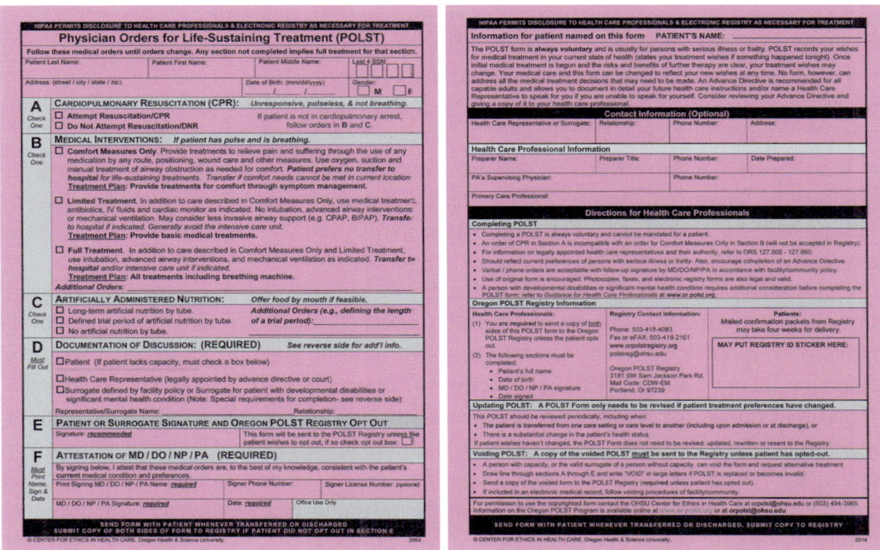

Fig. 16.1 Physician order for life-sustaining treatment www.orpolst.org (with permission)

benefit is still lacking, for instance, with respect to a reduction in unwanted hospital admissions. Furthermore, anticipating the end of life and preparing for clinical crises imply much more than just documenting one's own will; it also entails medical, nursing-related, or psychosocial aspects in the future.

On the other hand, these structured and vigorous implementation efforts that are being performed, for instance, in several US states, Canada, and Europe, might well prove to be a valuable part within a comprehensive approach in end-of-life care. Figure 16.1 shows the Oregon physician order for life-sustaining treatment (POLST) as an example for a written order, documenting the medical perspective, of the patient's presumed will in critical clinical scenarios. Although these forms were originally conceptualised for the nursing home setting, they are being increasingly used in the palliative care setting as well.

At our own institution, for example, we use a very brief informative sheet in bright yellow colours that specifically addresses the preclinical EMS team (physicians and paramedics), who are familiar with this document. This lists a brief diagnosis, a DNR status report, and all relevant telephone numbers (including the 24-h palliative care number, Wiese et al. 2007).

16.3.3 Avoiding 'Aggressive Care'?

Despite all these anticipatory efforts, a longitudinal study of Earle (Earle et al. 2008; Ho et al. 2011) demonstrated that 'aggressive care' at the end of life has increased over the years instead of decreasing. The authors defined 'aggressive care' as:

- Last dose of chemotherapy received within 14 days of death
- More than one emergency department visit within 30 days of death
- More than one hospitalisation within 30 days of death
- At least one intensive care unit (ICU) admission within 30 days of death

Current and future efforts in advance care planning will have to demonstrate whether the suggested concept of assisted, anticipatory, and documented decision-making will be able to prevent 'aggressive care' such as emergency readmissions and intensive care shortly before the patient's death.

Furthermore, end-of-life decision in patients suffering from cancer will become increasingly more complex, especially with respect to emergency situations: the developments in modern oncology described above (and in previous chapters) with their abundance of new and (in part) highly active substances will change our previous understanding of linear disease trajectories in cancer. Medical journals describe case reports of severely affected cancer patients who would have had an extremely limited prognosis until a few years ago but who have come into partial or complete remission due to extreme response to new targeted substances, resulting from the successful achievements, for instance, in genomic medicine (McDermott et al. 2011). Therefore, another feature of prolonged and versatile modern oncological treatment is that prognosticating death becomes increasingly more complex and difficult. It will be more difficult in the future to decide the point in time at which a patient has reached a stage where definitely no further anticancer option is indicated or where no more effort can be made to reverse a critical situation even by a controlled use of intensive care measures. This dilemma will be one of our foremost future challenges and duties for an integrated oncology and palliative care approach to patients suffering from incurable and advanced cancer.

References

Ackroyd R, Russon L, Newell R (2007) Views of oncology patients, their relatives and oncologists on cardiopulmonary resuscitation (CPR): questionnaire-based study. Palliat Med 21:139–144

Berger DP, Engelhardt R, Mertelsmann R (eds) (2010) Das Rote Buch – Hämatologie und Internistische Onkologie, 4th edn. ecomed MEDIZIN, Heidelberg/München/Landsberg/Frechen/Hamburg

Cervantes A, Chirivella I (2004) Oncological emergencies. Ann Oncol 15(suppl 4):299–306

Earle CC, Landrum MB, Souza JM, Neville BA, Weeks JC, Ayanian JZ (2008) Aggressiveness of cancer care near the end of life: is it a quality-of-care issue? J Clin Oncol 26:3860–3866

Hendrick JM, Pijls NH, van der Werf T, Crul JF (1990) Cardiopulmonary resuscitation on the general ward: no category of patients should be excluded in advance. Resuscitation 20:163

Hickman SE, Nelson CA, Perrin NA, Moss AH, Hammes BJ, Tolle SW (2010) A comparison of methods to communicate treatment preferences in nursing facilities: traditional practices versus the physician orders for life-sustaining treatment program. J Am Geriatr Soc 58:1241–1248

Higdon ML, Higdon JA (2006) Treatment of oncologic emergencies. Am Fam Physician 74: 1873–1880

Ho TH, Barbera L, Saskin R, Lu H, Neville BA, Earle CC (2011) Trends in the aggressiveness of end-of-life cancer care in the Universal Health Care System of Ontario, Canada. J Clin Oncol 29:1587–1591

In der Schmitten J, Lex K, Mellert C, Rothärmel S, Wegscheider K, Marckmann G (2014) Implementing an advance care planning program in German nursing homes results of an inter-regionally controlled intervention trial. Dtsch Arztebl Int 111(4):50–57

Krych M, Hiddemann W (2005) Oncological emergencies. Internist 46:7–8

Lawrie I (2007) Handbook of oncological emergencies. Eur J Cancer Care 16:392

Mayer DK, Travers D, Wyss A, Leak A, Waller A (2011) Why do patients with cancer visit emergency departments? Results of a 2008 population study in North Carolina. J Clin Oncol 29: 2683–2688

McDermott U, Downing JR, Stratton MR (2011) Genomics and the continuum of cancer care. N Engl J Med 364:340–350

Molloy DW, Guyatt GH, Russo R, Goeree R, O'Brien BJ, Bédard M, Willan A, Watson J, Patterson C, Harrison C, Standish T, Strang D, Darzins PJ, Smith S, Dubois S (2000) Systematic implementation of an advance directive program in nursing homes: a randomized controlled trial. JAMA 283(11):1437–1444

Nauck F, Alt-Epping B (2008) Crises in palliative care – a comprehensive approach. Lancet Oncol 9(11):1086–1091

Pelosof LC, Gerber DE (2010) Paraneoplastic syndromes: an approach to diagnosis and treatment. Mayo Clin Proc 85(9):838–854

POLST: https://static.squarespace.com/static/52dc687be4b0322209172e33e/t/53378c92e4b0d7d8 daacaaa6/1396149394118/Printing-POLST.pdf. Accessed 5 May 2014

Stewart S, MacIntyre K, Hole DJ, Capewell S, McMurray JJ (2001) More 'malignant' than cancer? Five-year survival following a first admission for heart failure. Eur J Heart Fail 3(3):315–322

Trousseau AT (1865) Phlegmasia alba dolens. Clinique Medicale d'Hotel-Dieu de Paris. JB Balliere et Fils 2:654–712

Vandyk AD, Harrison MB, Macartney G, Ross-White A, Stacey D (2012) Emergency department visits for symptoms experienced by oncology patients: a systematic review. Support Care Cancer 20(8):1589–1599

Wiese C, Bartels U, Geyer A, Graf B, Hanekop G (2007) Palliative and emergency medicine: teamwork through communication. Z Palliativmed 8:35–39

Palliative Care for Patients Participating in Experimental or Clinical Oncology Studies

17

Eva C. Winkler and Jan Schildmann

Contents

E.C. Winkler, MD, PhD (✉)
Medical Oncology, Program for Ethics and Patient-Oriented Care in Oncology,
National Center for Tumor Diseases (NCT), University of Heidelberg, Heidelberg, Germany

J. Schildmann, MD
Institute for Medical Ethics and History of Medicine, Ruhr University Bochum,
Bochum, Germany

© Springer-Verlag Berlin Heidelberg 2015
B. Alt-Epping, F. Nauck (eds.), *Palliative Care in Oncology*,
DOI 10.1007/978-3-662-46202-7_17

17.1   Introduction

The topic of palliative care in patients with advanced cancer who participate in clinical trials, or may do so in the future, raises a number of issues that are of interest from a medical ethics perspective. For the purpose of this chapter, we define "medical ethics perspective" as an interdisciplinary methodological approach that aims to detect and analyze the values that underlie medical practice by means of normative and empirical methods. Furthermore, we focus our empirical-ethical analysis on a distinct situation in the context of clinical trial and palliative care: the situation in which a patient with cancer, for whom there are no further established cancer-directed treatment options, may either receive treatment in line with the principles of best supportive and palliative care or enter a clinical trial in which cancer-directed treatment is tested.[1]

The values that guide our practice are often implicit. Usually, we do not consciously reflect on every decision or action in terms of whether it is right or wrong, good or bad. However, situations in which standard cancer treatment has failed and patients are confronted with the decision whether to enter a phase 1 study or to receive the best supportive care cause us to think about the right or wrong way, about the better or worse way of spending the last phase of life. The aim of this chapter is to outline and structure ethically relevant issues in the context of making decisions about palliative care versus enrollment in early phase clinical trials for advanced cancer patients and to explore some of the identified issues in more depth. In the first step we introduce different moral points of view from which one can analyze the issues related to our question, which may be coined in an abbreviated form as that of "phase 1 trial or palliative care." Then we explore in more detail the topics of disclosure about end-of-standard treatment and informed consent process for phase I/II trials (1) and conflict of obligations (2) as well as conflicts of interest (3) in the context of end-of-life care. The chapter concludes with an outlook on possible strategies and limitations to reconcile a clinical research-oriented and palliative care perspective with regard to patients with advanced cancer.

17.2   Phase 1 Trial or Palliative Care in Advanced Cancer? A View from Medical Ethics Perspectives

When faced with the question whether enrollment in a clinical trial or palliative care is the best choice for a patient with advanced cancer, several approaches can be taken to analyze the issue from a medical ethics perspective. The first relevant distinction here is whether to explore the issue either from an *individual ethics perspective* or a *societal ethics perspective*. From the individual ethics point of view,

---

[1] While we do not view the question of "palliative care versus phase 1 trial" as one to which there are only mutually exclusive answers, we pursue this dichotomy for most parts of the article because in our experience this reflects the perception of many patients and clinicians who are faced with the situation in current clinical practice.

we might ask, for example, which ethical principles and values are particularly relevant when analyzing the situation of an individual patient with cancer near the end of life? We might also consider the values and views of other individuals involved, such as physicians, nurses, relatives, and other caregivers. From this perspective, we can discuss the meaning of the principle of autonomy in such situations, for instance. Take the situation of a patient who desires cancer-directed treatment in a situation in which from the physician's perspective any other conventional treatment is not likely to provide any benefit and may even cause considerable harm. Would it be acceptable if the physician were to offer further treatment only as part of a clinical trial? Another conflict between ethical principles on an individual level, which we explore in more detail in Sect. 3.2 of this chapter, is that of providing the best possible care to the individual patient in a clinical trial versus acceptance of limitations regarding this aim that are due to the research design.

From a societal ethics point of view, we might ask which ethical principles come into play when we consider the relevance of palliative care and/or clinical research at the end of life. An example would be to explore the ethical acceptability of incentives a society might provide for participating in research trials for patients with cancer compared with offering palliative care services. Related to incentives is the question of allocation of resources. We might envision a society that prioritizes research on cancer-directed substances or one in which the optimal supportive and palliative care of patients near the end of life has the highest priority. Given that in theory there are no limits for investments with regard to both aims (and with regard to many more within and outside medicine), it is necessary for a society with a limited budget to set priorities in this respect and to justify them on moral grounds.

Next to the distinction between the individual and societal ethics perspectives, we can rely on *different normative theories* that can support us when we analyze the ethical issues related to the question of clinical research versus palliative care near the end of life. A widely used theoretical account in medical ethics is the theory of principlism by Beauchamp and Childress (Beauchamp and Childress 2013). According to this approach, most ethical problems in medicine can be described and analyzed by conflicts between four mid-level principles: *non-maleficence, beneficence, respect for patient autonomy*, and *justice*. Depending on the concrete ethical conflict, the four principles need to be specified to come to an ethically informed decision. When a patient with advanced cancer is confronted with the end of established cancer treatment, for instance, we need to define the meaning of the principle of autonomy in this situation to answer our question. Furthermore, the different principles need to be weighed or balanced: we need to determine, for example, at which point the principle of avoiding harm outweighs the principle of (future) benefit generated by clinical research in a phase 1 trial.

Next to principlism as presented by Beauchamp and Childress, there are other ethical theories that can inform our analysis. A relevant example in the context of end-of-life care is the theory of *virtue ethics*, which focuses on the character or character traits of a moral agent (Pellegrino 2006). We may, for example, ask about the important virtues physicians and other healthcare professionals should have when confronted with situations in which they discuss with their patients about the options of palliative care or participation in a clinical trial during the last phase of life. According to this account of ethics, physicians should possess and develop dispositions and attitudes to be able to act in a way that does not give precedence to their own (secondary) interests, such as financial or academic interests, but which takes into account legitimate (primary) interests, such as the increase of scientific knowledge or the protection of patients near the end of life.

We illustrate the ethical issue related to the question of clinical trials versus palliative care using paradigmatic situations in the context of clinical research and palliative care. To do this, we begin with situations that cause some moral discomfort – we have the lingering impression that they could have been solved in a better way and that questions of ethical value were involved. Such situations might be the following:

1. "The crossroads." Entering a phase 1 trial or starting best supportive or palliative care
2. Conflicts of obligation. When to stop trial participation and start with the best supportive care
3. Conflicting interests. How to deal with secondary interests of individuals and institutions in a medical research environment

The above list of situations is neither systematic nor a complete account of situations with ethical challenges in the context of palliative care and clinical cancer research. However, for the purpose of this article, it shall guide us with regard to a more detailed ethical analysis.

17.3 Selected Ethical Issues

17.3.1 "The Crossroads." Entering a Phase 1 Trial or Starting Palliative Care

Consider the following situation: a patient is suffering from metastatic colorectal cancer and has been treated with chemo-immunotherapy for more than 2 years. In the last staging exam, it was discovered that, unfortunately, he has developed progressive disease predominantly in liver and lymph nodes under the last-line treatment with a multikinase inhibitor. He is suffering from loss of appetite and some pain due to hepatic enlargement. From a clinical point of view, there are no more promising options of tumor-specific therapy, and the care should focus on symptom control. In addition, the patient should contact the home palliative care team, since symptom control can be provided close to where he lives, and more visits at the cancer center that is at a distance of 1 h are not necessarily warranted. The oncologist who discloses the imaging results of the disease progression also knows about a phase 1 trial with a new pathway inhibitor that the patient would be eligible for. This trial just opened at the cancer center. However, for patients who participate in the trial, a tissue biopsy is mandatory for the accompanying biomarker study. Furthermore, to administer the drug for the first dosage, an inpatient stay and weekly patient visits for the consecutive application at the cancer center would be scheduled. How should the oncologist present the different options: palliative home care or enrollment in an experimental trial?

Decision-making against cancer-specific chemotherapy and planning for the last phase of the disease trajectory are challenging for patients and their oncologists (Hancock et al. 2007). It implies talking about valuable goals for the last weeks or months of life. It also means dealing with the patients' feelings of hopelessness and disappointment. However, when performed well and in a timely fashion, communication about withdrawal of chemotherapy toward the end of life is an important prerequisite of high-quality patient-oriented care. We know from the literature that about one-third of patients with advanced cancer disease and a prognosis for a median survival of 6–12 months prefer a treatment that focuses on comfort care, one-third prefer to gain lifetime at any costs, and the last third is ambivalent (Winkler et al. 2009). Especially for patients who prefer intensive treatment, it is crucial that their wishes are based on a realistic assessment of their situation. Otherwise, a coping strategy of denial may result in overtreatment. Hence, for patient-centered care especially at the end of life, it is crucial to start talking about the best- and worst-case scenarios early on so that patients have time to adapt their expectations to the dynamic and prognosis of the disease and decide about the intensity and preferences for treatment (Fallowfield et al. 2002). Patients who had conversations with oncologists about their preferred care goals in case of disease progression were referred earlier to hospices and received less aggressive treatment near death; they also showed less anxiety and depression. In one study less aggressive therapy was even associated with a gain in survival time (Temel et al. 2010). Interestingly, in this study foregoing tumor-specific therapy was possible for a much higher percentage in the group of patients who were or became realistic about their own prognosis. Hence, preparing the patient early on seems to be key for patients to develop a realistic understanding of their situation and thereby prepare end-of-life decision-making. Nevertheless, clinical evidence shows that oncologists are overwhelmingly reluctant to provide patients with prognostic information and to address the change from tumor-specific therapy to the best supportive care (Clayton et al. 2005).

In this context phase I/II trials come into play, because these are the very patients who also qualify for phase I/II clinical trials since one inclusion criterion often is that all standard therapeutic lines of chemotherapy have been exhausted. For this reason, the patients who qualify for the best supportive care and for inclusion into a phase 1 trial overlap to a significant degree. The aim of phase I/II trials is to evaluate the safety and toxicity of new therapeutic agents, to learn about the pharmacokinetic properties of these agents, and to determine a safe dose for subsequent testing. The medical benefit for the patient is not the primary goal of these trials, although in the latest meta-analysis about the benefits of phase 1 oncology trials (1995–2002) at least the overall response rate in these trials was improving by 10 % compared with previous data and might be even higher today. Still, the response rate is a surrogate parameter that does not necessarily translate into clinical benefit, and entering a phase I trial compared to the best supportive care is also associated with a toxicity-related death rate of 0.5 % and grade 4 toxic events in 14 % (Horstmann et al. 2005).

It often also requires extra tests and travel, and patients may be treated in a larger cancer center instead of arranging the best supportive care at home.

All these considerations make it an imperative ethical requirement to inform patients about the experimental nature, the slim prospects of medical benefit, the additional burdens, and the symptomatic care option to justify phase I oncology trials. However, studies on the quality of informed consent in general show that patients have a poor understanding of numerous aspects of trials (Jefford and Moore 2008). With respect to phase 1 oncology trials, studies show that many patients do not recognize the unproven nature of the treatment, the potential for incremental risk from participation, the uncertainty of benefits to self, or that trials are conducted mainly to benefit future patients (Joffe et al. 2001). These so-called therapeutic misconceptions or mistaken beliefs of patients that the experimental treatment aims primarily at their clinical benefit have first been addressed by Appelbaum and collaborators, who reported about patients participating in psychiatric trials 1982 (Appelbaum et al. 1987). Since then, this was recognized as a serious problem for informed consent in clinical research and challenged the validity of patient's consent. In fact, several studies examining the informed consent process between oncologists and patients showed important omissions, including discussion of prognosis and ensuring patient understanding about supportive care options (Jenkins et al. 2011).

From an ethical point of view, an accurate understanding of patients about the risks, prospects for benefits, and alternatives to trial participation is therefore necessary. As Fallowfield suggests: "Ideally, prior to any discussion about trial entry, putative early-phase-trial patients should have had a clear "end of treatment" interview with their physician during which understanding of their prognosis was established and the positive aims and benefits of good palliative care and symptom control were discussed." She also showed that communication of oncologists and subsequent understanding of patients can be improved by an intensive workshop on communication skills (Fallowfield et al. 2012). Key elements of the informed consent discussion should include the following:

- Establish patient's knowledge of prognosis (check if patient understands)
- Discuss available other options (check if patient understands)
- Discuss aims of trial, for example, dose escalation
- Suggest that there is a chance (slim) of medical benefit
- Explain extra tests/travel involved with the trial
- Discuss that screening tests would be conducted first to check eligibility
- Discuss explicitly unknown side effects
- Explain that participation is voluntary
- Encourage patient to take time to decide
- Discuss the right to withdraw (modified from Table 1 of Fallowfield et al. 2012)

We know from patients with cancer that at least one-third often prefer tumor-specific treatment even in advanced stages of the disease (Winkler et al. 2009). As a result, if the patient is accurately informed, patients may reasonably decide to enroll in phase 1 oncology trials in hopes of obtaining benefit, after considering the anticipated risks and available clinical alternatives.

17.3.2 "The Right Moment." When to stop Trial Participation Conflicts of Obligation

Consider the following situation: a physician is taking care of a patient with advanced cancer who has consented to participate in a phase 1 trial, knowing that this is most likely to generate knowledge and that there is only a slim chance that she herself will benefit from it. The patient was assured when she enrolled in the study that she would receive appropriate symptom control also as a participant in the trial. During the course of the study, the patient is stable with regard to the cancer, and the tumor even appears to have shrunken slightly. However, the patient is increasingly burdened by a particular symptom. The substances tried for symptom relief did not work so far. The treating physician considers one further option of symptom control. However, because of interactions with the study medication, this would mean that the patient could no longer be part of the trial. What to do?

According to Morreim, a conflict of obligation exists in situations "…in which one's obligation to one person or group conflict with one's obligation to some other person or group" (Morreim 1995). Such a conflict needs to be distinguished from the currently much debated "conflicts of interest," which distinguish between primary and secondary interests; these conflicts are discussed in the following section. Hence, the above-described situation is a conflict of obligations. Conflicts of obligation in medical research often refer to burdens of a clinical trial versus the contribution to society through the benefits based on research. In general, the concept of accepting some risk of harm for the individual in exchange for scientific benefit has been viewed as ethically permissible in major codes of ethics, including the Belmont Report and the Declaration of Helsinki (Emanuel et al. 2000). One prerequisite for such balancing of possible harm for the individual against societal benefit is of course that the patient is informed. As we have just seen in the preceding section, it is far from simple to facilitate informed decision-making given the situation of patients with advanced cancer. Moreover, after having entered a trial, patients are likely to follow the suggestions of their treating physician, who at the same time is a researcher. In this situation the physician/researcher needs to cautiously investigate the risk of harm in a specific situation and decide whether continuation of trial is justified or not. The situation becomes more complex when, in addition to legitimate primary interests, we take into account that individual as well as institutional actions are also guided by secondary interests, which leads us to the already mentioned problem of conflict of interest.

17.3.3 Medical Research and Conflict of Interests

Consider a second situation of conflict: a physician is working in a large comprehensive cancer center. She is caring for a patient with advanced cancer who is eligible for a clinical trial that up to this time suffers from a rather low recruitment rate. On the ward round the day before, the patient has explicitly requested to discuss the options for the best possible care given the current situation. The physician and patient have agreed to speak about this topic in detail today. Just this morning, the clinical director pointed out to the whole team that recruitment of patients in clinical trials is of utmost importance because of the relevance of trial recruitment for the academic standing of the department, but also because of the funding associated with the number of recruited patients by the sponsors. Bearing this in mind, the physician enters the room and hopes that she can persuade the patient to enter the trial.

We assume that a majority of readers will find it easier to solve this conflict than the one described in Sect. 3.2. It seems rather obvious that we need to inform the patient about all available options and accept his or her wishes. The reason is that most of us would view the interest to enroll patients for research as less acceptable than informing the patient about all available options. The distinction between different interests within medicine has been captured in the widely used definition of conflict of interest by Thompson et al. (1993): "A conflict of interest is a set of conditions in which professional judgment concerning a primary interest (such as a patient's welfare or validity of research) tends to be unduly influenced by a secondary interest (such as financial gain)." According to this definition, patient welfare as well as producing knowledge that benefits future patients are examples for primary interests of medicine. These interests can be affected by secondary interests. While financial interests, as mentioned in the above definition, are the focus of the current debate on conflicts of interest, there are also a number of other secondary interests, such as to promote one's career and enhancing the reputation of the institution and others.

However, the question remains in the above situation how far we can go to persuade the patient to participate in a trial. How much weight should we put on the side of securing an institution's academic standing and finances in comparison with empowering an autonomous decision of the patient? Secondary interests, such as to aim for a high number of patients recruited into phase 1 trials, are not per se bad interests. In fact, such a goal can contribute considerably to advances in medicine. However, these interests should be subordinated to primary interests, not least because of the vulnerability of patients and related duties on the side of healthcare professionals. This means that any institutional interest in patient recruitment for trials should be weighed against patients' interest to receive appropriate non-biased information about available options in a situation of advanced cancer. One may request, for example, that those with the least direct interest in clinical research should discuss the options with the patient. However, a drawback of this strategy might be that these persons are not the best informed parties to explain to the patient which trials are currently available. Any physician conducting such discussions should not only be aware of available guidelines (compare Sect. 3.1), but also have taken part in experimental training sessions, which have been shown to be most effective with regard to teaching the relevant professional skills for information and decision-making in difficult situations (Fallowfield et al. 2002).

17.4 The Best of Two Worlds? How to reconcile the Oncology Research and Palliative Care Paradigm

So far, we have presented the discussion as a dichotomy of early-phase clinical trial versus palliative care and gave an account of how this discussion is framed in the literature and often also in oncology practice. It seems true that for the patient at the crossroads, balanced information about the additional burdens and the scale of potential benefits that come with the enrollment in an early-phase clinical trial need to be openly discussed (as laid out in Sect. 3.1). However, research and the palliative care paradigm should not be viewed as mutually exclusive – neither conceptually nor practically. To the contrary, palliative care has evolved as a discipline that focuses on the improvement of the quality of life of cancer patients and families through early identification and treatment of symptoms. Thus, timely referral to palliative care is important and an indicator of quality of care, since patients gain access to multidimensional care early in the trajectory of illness (Ferris et al. 2009). Since patients enrolled in phase 1 trials have a median survival and burden of symptoms similar to patients not enrolled, they clearly should have access to palliative care evaluation and treatment (Penel et al. 2010). They might not embrace the offer, since studies show that patients participating in phase 1 trials are less likely to consider palliative care and home care services (Finlay et al. 2009). But we do not know the reasons for their reluctance – it might well be that these patients perceive palliative care and research participation as incommensurable paradigms also because this is the way these two worlds are presented to them. On the other hand, many studies investigating the barriers to trial accrual at cancer centers find patient refusal to be the one main barrier. Many patients who are eligible and decide against participation in a clinical trial do so because they are worried about the quality of life and additional burdens that come with trial participation (Ho et al. 2006). Such worries might be alleviated if patients were reassured that they will receive the same support from palliative care specialists and the same focus on symptom control and quality of life as patients in standard care.

It is therefore crucial to reconcile these two paradigms and to try to offer the best of two worlds to cancer patients in an advanced stage of their disease. One important step in this direction – integrating palliative care into oncology practice – has successfully been taken by some cancer centers: MD Anderson with the group of Eduardo Bruera are a flagship and example for an advanced program. He conceptualized an integrated care model in which the oncologist routinely refers patients to palliative care for their supportive care needs (Bruera and Hui 2012). In this model all patients are screened for distress. If a high demand due to distress is detected, patients are referred to palliative care for a comprehensive assessment of their symptoms, communication, and decision-making needs with consecutive appropriate management. While it seems to be a successful model for integrating palliative care into oncology practice, it is interesting that the group of patients enrolled in clinical trials is not explicitly mentioned as a separate group to be targeted. This is all the more surprising since MD Anderson is a research institution with a strong record of early-phase clinical trials. However, the palliative care group showed that patients' referrals to palliative care by phase 1 oncologists were not delayed compared with referral by non-phase 1 oncologists. Hence, the spirit of structured supportive care seems to be transported to all parts of the organization.

Conceptually, however, a structured evaluation of supportive or palliative care needs of patients under investigational therapy would be the logical next step in reconciling the two worlds. This has been proposed as "simultaneous care" and was realized by a palliative care nurse and a social worker, who focused on supportive care needs of the patient with the aim to improve the quality of life for accompanied patients (Meyers et al. 2004).

17.5 Key Elements for Reconciling Supportive Care and Investigational Trials

From our analysis of the portrayed paradigmatic situations and the discussion about early integration of palliative care in the literature, we summarize the following points as ethically and clinically important aspects when patients with advanced cancer enroll in early-phase clinical trials:

17.5.1 Prevent Therapeutic Misconception by Aiming at a Truly Informed Consent

The literature suggests that patients on phase I trials are not psychologically prepared for transition to end of life (Agrawal et al. 2006). From an ethical point of view, it seems reasonable to choose an investigational therapy instead of the best supportive care if this decision is based on a realistic understanding of prognosis, alternative options (best supportive care), and potential burdens and benefits due to the investigational therapy. In contrast, it seems ethically questionable to enroll patients in clinical trials without a clear statement about the end of conventional therapy and the different nature of investigational studies. Preventing a therapeutic misconception is a key goal of the informed consent discussion.

17.5.2 Investigational Trials and Palliative Care need to be offered Simultaneously in a Structured Program

Although the best supportive care is often the "standard arm" compared with the investigational arm, we should not present these as alternatives. Instead, a focus on supportive or palliative care needs of patients who participate in clinical trials should be standard with respect to the quality of care. To realize this integration, it is important to bring together the two worlds of research and palliation not only conceptually, but also structurally. For example, since many patients in oncology are outpatients, it is necessary to establish outpatient palliative care services more broadly.

17.5.3 Define Palliative and Supportive Care

Notably, one essential part of the conceptual framework of the above-described integrated care program is a clear distinction of the terms "hospice care," which is part of "palliative care," which in turn is part of the broader term "supportive care." While "palliative care" addresses the needs of patients with advanced cancer, "supportive care" encompasses a broader range of services "for patients throughout various stages of the disease, including diagnosis, active treatment, end-of-life, and survivorship" (Bruera and Hui 2012).[2] Accordingly, data show that oncologists are more likely to refer patients earlier in their disease trajectory to "supportive care service," while the term "palliative care" is reserved for end-stage cancer patients (Fadul et al. 2009). A consecutive name change from palliative to supportive care resulted in a dramatic increase of mainly inpatient referrals and earlier referrals in the outpatient setting (Dalal et al. 2011).

17.5.4 Address the Conflict of Obligations/Conflict of Interest Adequately

Offering clinical trials to patients near the end of life might be associated with conflicts of obligations and conflicts of interests. The problem is not their existence, but the lack of awareness that would enable one to deal with these conflicts. While there has been a strong development to conduct ethical case conferences, ethics consultation, and comparable interventions in difficult treatment situations, the topic of research ethics – according to our experience – is mostly dealt with in a bureaucratic way at the time of research ethics approval. However, why not initiate a case conference in situations in which we are confronted with conflict of obligation or interest related to clinical research and end-of-life care? This could be done in a rather informal way, such as gathering a group of professionals who know the patient for a structured discussion or in terms of a more formal request of an ethicist (provided that one is available) (Schildmann and Vollmann 2011).

---

[2] Page 1265.

References

Agrawal M, Grady C, Fairclough DL, Meropol NJ, Maynard K, Emanuel EJ (2006) Patients' decision-making process regarding participation in phase I oncology research. J Clin Oncol 24(27):4479–4484. doi:10.1200/jco.2006.06.0269

Appelbaum PS, Roth LH, Lidz CW, Benson P, Winslade W (1987) False hopes and best data: consent to research and the therapeutic misconception. Hastings Cent Rep 17(2):20–24

Beauchamp TL, Childress JF (2013) Principles of biomedical ethics, 7th edn. Oxford University Press, New York [u.a.]

Bruera E, Hui D (2012) Conceptual models for integrating palliative care at cancer centers. J Palliat Med 15(11):1261–1269. doi:10.1089/jpm.2012.0147

Clayton JM, Butow PN, Tattersall MH (2005) When and how to initiate discussion about prognosis and end-of-life issues with terminally ill patients. J Pain Symptom Manage 30(2):132–144. doi:10.1016/j.jpainsymman.2005.02.014

Dalal S, Palla S, Hui D, Nguyen L, Chacko R, Li Z, Fadul N, Scott C, Thornton V, Coldman B, Amin Y, Bruera E (2011) Association between a name change from palliative to supportive care and the timing of patient referrals at a comprehensive cancer center. Oncologist 16(1):105–111. doi:10.1634/theoncologist. 2010-0161

Emanuel EJ, Wendler D, Grady C (2000) What makes clinical research ethical? JAMA 283(20):2701–2711

Fadul N, Elsayem A, Palmer JL, Del Fabbro E, Swint K, Li Z, Poulter V, Bruera E (2009) Supportive versus palliative care: what's in a name?: a survey of medical oncologists and midlevel providers at a comprehensive cancer center. Cancer 115(9):2013–2021. doi:10.1002/cncr.24206

Fallowfield LJ, Jenkins VA, Beveridge HA (2002) Truth may hurt but deceit hurts more: communication in palliative care. Palliat Med 16(4):297–303

Fallowfield LJ, Solis-Trapala I, Jenkins VA (2012) Evaluation of an educational program to improve communication with patients about early-phase trial participation. Oncologist 17(3):377–383. doi:10.1634/theoncologist. 2011-0271

Ferris FD, Bruera E, Cherny N, Cummings C, Currow D, Dudgeon D, Janjan N, Strasser F, von Gunten CF, Von Roenn JH (2009) Palliative cancer care a decade later: accomplishments, the need, next steps – from the American Society of Clinical Oncology. J Clin Oncol 27(18):3052–3058. doi:10.1200/jco.2008.20.1558

Finlay E, Lu HL, Henderson HR, O'Dwyer PJ, Casarett DJ (2009) Do phase 1 patients have greater needs for palliative care compared with other cancer patients? Cancer 115(2):446–453. doi:10.1002/cncr.24025

Hancock K, Clayton JM, Parker SM, der Wal S, Butow PN, Carrick S, Currow D, Ghersi D, Glare P, Hagerty R, Tattersall MH (2007) Truth-telling in discussing prognosis in advanced life-limiting illnesses: a systematic review. Palliat Med 21(6):507–517. doi:10.1177/0269216307080823

Ho J, Pond GR, Newman C, Maclean M, Chen EX, Oza AM, Siu LL (2006) Barriers in phase I cancer clinical trials referrals and enrollment: five-year experience at the Princess Margaret Hospital. BMC Cancer 6:263. doi:10.1186/1471-2407-6-263

Horstmann E, McCabe MS, Grochow L, Yamamoto S, Rubinstein L, Budd T, Shoemaker D, Emanuel EJ, Grady C (2005) Risks and benefits of phase 1 oncology trials, 1991 through 2002. N Engl J Med 352(9):895–904. doi:10.1056/NEJMsa042220

Jefford M, Moore R (2008) Improvement of informed consent and the quality of consent documents. Lancet Oncol 9(5):485–493. doi:10.1016/s1470-2045(08)70128-1

Jenkins V, Solis-Trapala I, Langridge C, Catt S, Talbot DC, Fallowfield LJ (2011) What oncologists believe they said and what patients believe they heard: an analysis of phase I trial discussions. J Clin Oncol 29(1):61–68. doi:10.1200/jco.2010.30.0814

Joffe S, Cook EF, Cleary PD, Clark JW, Weeks JC (2001) Quality of informed consent in cancer clinical trials: a cross-sectional survey. Lancet 358(9295):1772–1777. doi:10.1016/s0140-6736(01)06805-2

Meyers FJ, Linder J, Beckett L, Christensen S, Blais J, Gandara DR (2004) Simultaneous care: a model approach to the perceived conflict between investigational therapy and palliative care. J Pain Symptom Manage 28(6):548–556. doi:10.1016/j.jpainsymman.2004.03.002

Morreim EM (1995) Conflict of interest. In: Reich WT (ed) Encyclopedia of bioethics. Free Press, New York, pp 459–465 [u.a.]

Pellegrino ED (2006) Toward a reconstruction of medical morality. Am J Bioeth 6(2):65–71. doi:10.1080/15265160500508601

Penel N, Delord JP, Bonneterre ME, Bachelot T, Ray-Coquard I, Blay JY, Pascal LB, Borel C, Filleron T, Adenis A, Bonneterre J (2010) Development and validation of a model that predicts early death among cancer patients participating in phase I clinical trials investigating cytotoxics. Invest New Drugs 28(1):76–82. doi:10.1007/s10637-009-9224-x

National Commission for the Protection of Human Subjects of Biomedical and Behavioral Research, The Belmont Report (DHEW pub. no. (OS) 78-0012). Washington, DC: United States Government Printing Office.

Schildmann J, Sandow V, Vollmann J (2011) Interessenkonflikte – ethische Aspekte. In: Lieb K (ed) Interessenkonflikte in der Medizin: Hintergründe und Lösungsmöglichkeiten. Springer, Berlin/Heidelberg, pp 47–59

Temel JS, Greer JA, Muzikansky A, Gallagher ER, Admane S, Jackson VA, Dahlin CM, Blinderman CD, Jacobsen J, Pirl WF, Billings JA, Lynch TJ (2010) Early palliative care for patients with metastatic non-small-cell lung cancer. N Engl J Med 363(8):733–742. doi:10.1056/NEJMoa1000678

Thompson DF (1993) Understanding financial conflicts of interest. N Engl J Med 329:573–576

Winkler EC, Reiter-Theil S, Lange-Riess D, Schmahl-Menges N, Hiddemann W (2009) Patient involvement in decisions to limit treatment: the crucial role of agreement between physician and patient. J Clin Oncol 27(13):2225–2230. doi:10.1200/jco.2008.17.9515

Part VII

Perspectives

The Future of Oncology Palliative Care

18

Stein Kaasa and Jon Håvard Loge

Contents

S. Kaasa, MD, PhD (✉)
Department of Cancer Research and Molecular Medicine, Faculty of Medicine,
European Palliative Care Research Centre (PRC),
Norwegian University of Science and Technology (NTNU), Trondheim, Norway

St. Olavs Hospital, Trondheim University Hospital, Trondheim, Norway

Cancer Clinic, St. Olavs Hospital, Trondheim University Hospital, Trondheim, Norway
e-mail: stein.kaasa@ntnu.no

J.H. Loge, MD, PhD
Department of Cancer Research and Molecular Medicine, Faculty of Medicine,
European Palliative Care Research Centre (PRC),
Norwegian University of Science and Technology (NTNU), Trondheim, Norway

Regional Centre for Excellency in Palliative Care, South-East Norway,
Oslo, Norway

University Hospital, Oslo, Norway
e-mail: j.h.loge@medisin.uio.no

© Springer-Verlag Berlin Heidelberg 2015
B. Alt-Epping, F. Nauck (eds.), *Palliative Care in Oncology*,
DOI 10.1007/978-3-662-46202-7_18

18.1 Introduction

The previous chapters of this book have described the diversity of palliative care aspects when caring for patients suffering from incurable cancer. These aspects underline the need for better integrating palliative care and oncology.

During the last decade, it has become a "hot topic" in contemporary oncology and palliative care what is to be understood by "integration," how this can be achieved at different levels of the health care system, and what further implications of this integration process might result.

18.2 Background: The Oncology Perspective

Cancer incidence and prevalence figures are increasing. In 2012, 3.45 million new cancer cases were diagnosed in 40 European countries, and 1.75 million patients died from cancer (Ferlay et al. 2013). Death caused by cancer is frequently protracted by active and complex anticancer treatment that may provide benefit to patients early in the disease trajectory even when the disease is incurable. However, fragile patients with advanced cancer will often not tolerate chemotherapy, and its side effects may outweigh its potentially beneficial effects. This practice also results in increased use of acute care hospital services, outpatient consultations, and expensive examinations. Therefore, a recent report suggested that systemic anticancer therapy should not be used in cancer patients with a WHO performance score of 3–4 (Kelly and Smith 2014; Wright et al. 2008), who had no benefit from prior evidence-based interventions, and who are not eligible for a clinical trial and when no strong evidence supports the clinical value of further anticancer treatment (Schnipper et al. 2012).

Furthermore, a surprisingly high percentage of patients (up to 75 %) are unaware of their prognosis and their limited remaining life span, particularly outside of North America (Applebaum et al. 2014).

The growing complexity of treatment and costs related, for instance, to the increasing use of chemo- and radiotherapy and advanced imaging (e.g., CT, MRI, PET), is another concern in modern oncology and threatens the sustainability of the present services (Schnipper et al. 2012; Kelly et al. 2014; Kelly and Smith 2014). Estimates show that 40 % of cancer treatment costs in the last year of life are spent during the last month (Emanuel and Emanuel 1994). At present, cancer care accounts for about 5 % of the total health care costs in Europe (Sullivan et al. 2011). The rise in demand for treatment is expected to increase further, with estimates of a 600 % increase in costs in the next three decades (Mariotto et al. 2011).

18.3 The Palliative Care Perspective

On this background, alternative approaches for good care have been asked for (Kelly and Smith 2014). Palliative care (PC) is a comprehensive approach aiming to maintain or improve the individual patient's quality of life (QoL) and to support the caregivers by providing optimal symptom assessment and management throughout the disease trajectory (Kaasa et al. 2008). This might be even more valuable, as inadequate symptom assessment is recognized a major obstacle for adequate symptom treatment (Meuser et al. 2001). Further, patient-reported outcomes (PROs), providing subjective information on symptoms, functioning, and well-being, are not routinely used in clinical practice or in randomized controlled trials (Zikos et al. 2014), although they may help in guiding anticancer treatment decisions as well.

Despite the rapid development of PC services during the last 15–20 years, there is still a distinct separation between oncology and PC in most, if not all, European countries. This infers that the potential for optimal care during end of life (EoL) has not been fully explored. Therefore, new approaches and models need to be developed and implemented into the healthcare systems.

18.4   The Value of Palliative Care in the Oncology Setting

Several studies have demonstrated the effects of PC on cancer care and during EoL. These trials were performed in patient populations with different cancer diagnoses, were single- or multicenter, and had different endpoints, so that direct comparison of results remains difficult. Nevertheless, they may provide guidance on how to develop and implement new models of cancer palliative care.

The Norwegian trial (Jordhøy et al. 2000) was the first randomized trial (cluster-randomized) evaluating the effect of a PC program and was conducted by Kaasa's group in Trondheim. More patients of the intervention group died at home compared to the control group. No significant differences in patients' QoL were found, but the relatives' QoL was significantly better in the interventional arm (Ringdal et al. 2004).

The Boston trial (Temel et al. 2010) included patients with newly diagnosed metastatic non-small cell lung cancer that were randomly assigned to receive either early PC, combined with standard oncologic care, or standard oncologic care alone. Patients in the PC arm had better QoL, less depression, and longer median survival.

The Italian trial (Costantini et al. 2014) was a cluster-randomized trial testing the Liverpool Care Pathway (LCP: a palliative care pathway for patients in the final days/hours of life). Sixteen Italian general medical hospital wards were randomly assigned to implement LCP or continue standard practice. No significant difference in QoL was found.

The Japanese trial (Morita et al. 2013) used surveys and in-depth interviews to assess changes in the quality of PC after a complex intervention with education, support, and networking in four Japanese cities. The proportion of home deaths increased significantly, and patient and family-reported quality of care was significantly better after these interventions (Kelly and Smith 2014).

The Canadian trial (Zimmermann et al. 2014) was performed at medical oncology departments at a Canadian cancer center. Patients were cluster-randomized to

Table 18.1 Workflow on how to implement structural changes

Develop and agree upon an organizational model of oncology palliative care
Policy and administrative tasks
Structure and responsibilities
Resources (allocated/prioritized)
Develop the content of the program
Symptom management
Referral criteria
Assure the practical, clinical implementation of the program
Implementation plan
Communication and information
Measure key indicators of success
At patient level
At hospital level
At regional/national level

PC with monthly follow-up or standard cancer care. There were significant improvements in all outcomes at 4 months.

Hence, these studies clearly demonstrate that:

1. Randomized intervention studies that evaluate the integration of oncology and PC are feasible.
2. A PC approach at an early stage in patients with unfavorable prognosis may improve the patients' QoL and even prolong survival (Temel et al. 2010).

These and related findings have made several international stakeholders advocate a stronger integration of oncology and PC for patients with incurable cancer.

But how can this integration be planned and realized in complex organizational structures?

18.5   Implementing Structural Changes

Table 18.1 outlines a practical workflow which might be helpful to implement structural changes in health care in general and in oncology palliative care in particular.

Figure 18.1 illustrates three organizational levels that may operate independently. Ideally, national concepts should influence regional concepts, and those should be implemented locally. Also, recommendations and clinical structures may be influenced at a supernational level (e.g., the EU, the Council of Europe or other bodies across Europe, organizations such as the European Society of Medical Oncology (ESMO), the European Association for Palliative Care (EAPC), and the European CanCer Organization (ECCO), together with national representatives and individual clinicians and researchers).

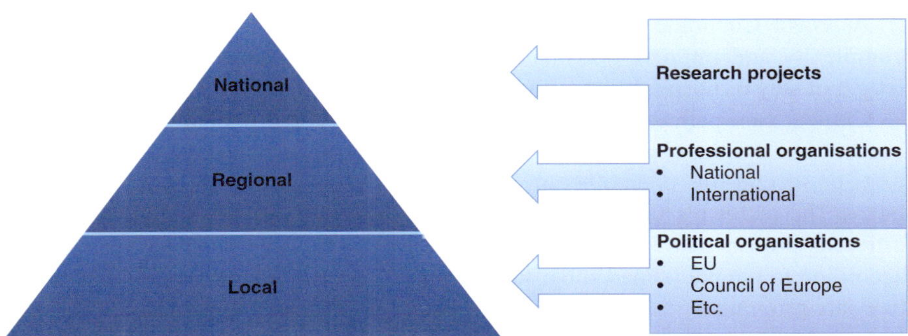

Fig. 18.1 Organizational levels and influencing factors

18.6   Integrating Oncology and Palliative Care

For implementing a concept of "integrated" oncology palliative care, the term "integration" needs to be described in further detail (Hui et al. 2014). Who should be in charge of the integration process? Who should be addressed? What is the content of integration? How to define the concept of integration? What type of organizational structure is needed in order to succeed?

In this context, three levels of integration were proposed by Leutz in 1999:

- Linkage
- Coordination
- Full integration

"Linkage" may be understood as a flow of information that is provided when needed. It may also involve a concept of response to individual needs. "Coordination" goes one step further by information sharing, often based on a system of predefined responses. Points of friction, confusion, and discontinuity between systems are solved, and processes are established to solve these issues. "Full integration" implies, for instance, shared patient records as a part of daily practice. New programs or units may be established where resources from multiple systems are pooled.

18.7   The "Integrated Program": Clinical Pathways as a Tool to Promote Integrated Care

Clinical pathways are structured multidisciplinary care plans that can facilitate a process how palliative care and oncology can be integrated in a given setting. Such pathways will provide a process plan, provide a time frame, describe the type of expertise needed at any step in the process, and describe the resources needed during the trajectory. The effects of this pathway must be evaluated by key indicators.

A recent Cochrane review concluded that clinical pathways reduce hospital complexity and improve documentation without having any negative impact on length of stay or hospital cost (Rotter et al. 2010).

Clinical care pathways for an integrated oncology and palliative care program need to be flexible, covering, for instance, patients with metastatic disease during first- or second-line chemotherapy or focusing on patients with short life expectancy. The pathways should therefore reflect different needs, different goals, and different professional competences, and several pathways need to be available according to the predefined subgroups of patients in an integrated oncology palliative care program.

> In order to classify or diagnose a patient, predefined criteria should be used, like in the ICD-11 and DSM-5 systems. Referral criteria to palliative care are not standardized in the same way as in oncology care. The European Association for Palliative Care (EAPC) and the European Palliative Care Research Centre (PRC) initiated a common platform to collect key clinical indicators that can be useful in this respect. This system, the EAPC Basic Dataset, describes medical indicators of palliative care patients (Sigurdardottir et al. 2014). This may aid to describe and report patients in clinical practice as well as in research.

18.8   A Framework of Integration

How can these care pathways contribute to the concepts of integrated care?

Figure 18.2 illustrates how a patient with known locally advanced prostate cancer, diagnosed 4 years ago, is seen by his general practitioner (GP) due to back pain (step 1). The GP concludes that the patient may have bone metastases from his prostate cancer. According to a given integrated care pathway that connects primary care, oncology, and palliative care, the patient is referred to the hospital for a diagnostic workup, which is coordinated (preplanned) by an oncologist and a secretary (step 2A). Decisions are made according to the care pathway. The next step is a standardized diagnostic workup (step 2B), according to the plan. The test results can be handled either in a coordinated patient record system, or in a fully integrated system. The consultation thereafter may be either coordinated or fully integrated. If step 3 is conducted fully integrated, the multidisciplinary team (MDT, consisting of oncologists, palliative care specialists, and nurses, for instance) will meet with or without the patient.

This example also illustrates that a fully integrated pathway at the outpatient clinic does not imply full integration at every further step. Linkage, coordination, and full integration may be adapted according to the content of each step, the patient's needs, and the available treatment options.

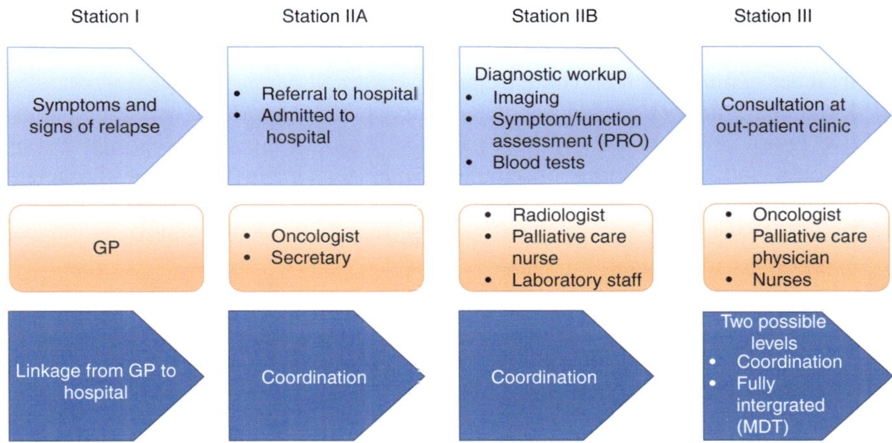

Fig. 18.2 A framework of integration. Advanced prostate cancer – bone metastases. *PRO* Patient Reported Outcomes

18.9   Resource Allocation

Another challenge within a process of implementing a new program toward integration of oncology and palliative care is to provide and to allocate resources. Without resources at the "to-do level" (nurses, doctors, and other healthcare providers), without a place to be (i.e., buildings, outpatient clinics, inpatient wards, etc.), without a given content (i.e., knowledge and skills of the individuals), or without the patients that are being addressed by the program, integration will be a challenging conduct.

Providing resources may include:

- To gather new resources
- To allocate resources from other ongoing activities
- To reorganize the existing amount of resources according to the integration concept

Often, a combination of these alternatives may be required.

A newly conceptualized model for integrated oncology palliative care will have to be prioritized within the respective organization. For this, the benefits of an integrated approach will have to be demonstrated:

- Place of care: more diseased patients will have the opportunity to stay at home with their family (or to remain in nursing homes or hospices) instead of being admitted to the hospital.
- Type of care: oncology shifts its focus from unrealistic therapeutic goals of cure and prolongation of life to symptom management and quality of life. By this, futile and intensive chemotherapy may be prevented.

- End-of-life care: by focusing on the last month(s), weeks, and days of life, patients and their families will experience a better quality of care, which also includes coping, grief, and bereavement.
- Improved symptom control: by pursuing a combined approach including palliative radio- or chemotherapy with palliative care consultations, optimal use of opioids, and other options of symptom management, including psychological and spiritual care.
- Reduced costs: by treating and caring for the patients outside highly specialized units, costs are reduced, and benefits are achieved as well.

18.10 Key Indicators of Success

A recent systematic review on the integration of oncology and palliative care highlighted 38 clinical, educational, research, and administrative aspects of integration in a total of 101 publications on the topic (Hui et al. 2014). Many of these aspects are also candidate indicators for integrated care.

Structural indicators (e.g., how many palliative care services exist within a geographical area) do not necessarily imply a truly integrated concept of oncology and palliative care. Also, availability of palliative care services is a prerequisite for integration but does not imply that integration actually takes place. The above described three level model of integration can therefore be enlarged by a fourth level: the availability of palliative care services. Structural indicators can be proposed along the whole continuum of integration (Table 18.2).

While structural indicators are static and do not measure integration per se, process (or procedural) indicators should reflect the actual integration of PC and oncology (Table 18.3).

Which indicators should be chosen depends on which level of integration is to be assessed, on the development of PC within that particular level, and how integration is defined.

Table 18.2 Examples of structural indicators of integration	National level	A PC policy and reimbursement
		PC in undergraduate curriculum
		Recognition of PC as a medical specialty
		PC research funding
	Regional level	PC services available at hospitals and communities
		Tailored educational programs in PC
		Presence of professorships and chairs in PC
		PC research funding
	Local level	PC teams are available at the oncological departments
		PC is routinely taught in educational programs
		Research is performed and published

Table 18.3 Examples of process (or procedural) indicators of integration

Explicit referral criteria – both ways
Number of referrals – both ways
Cancer treatment possible under PC ("simultaneous care")
Use of identical symptom screening methods
Use of evidence-based guidelines for symptom management
Common multidisciplinary boards/rounds
Common, continuous medical education
Agreed-upon clinical pathways
Research projects involving both services
Research endpoints reflecting major aims of PC (i.e., quality of life and symptom relief)

Conclusions

Caring for patients with advanced, incurable cancer requires a comprehensive approach, covering oncological treatment as well as palliative care aspects. This chapter proposed different models for integration of oncology and palliative care and provided general considerations on how to succeed in changing healthcare processes and outcome parameters for a successful implementation process.

But the future of palliative cancer care will not only depend on those most welcomed structural and procedural changes, but also on whether we will succeed in further disseminating the ideas and the attitude of palliative care into our society in general, and into the oncology setting in particular.

References

Applebaum AJ, Kolva EA, Kulikowski JR, Jacobs JD, DeRosa A, Lichtenthal WG et al (2014) Conceptualizing prognostic awareness in advanced cancer: a systematic review. J Health Psychol 19(9):1103–1119

Costantini M, Romoli V, Leo SD, Beccaro M, Bono L, Pilastri P et al (2014) Liverpool Care Pathway for patients with cancer in hospital: a cluster randomised trial. Lancet 383(9913):226–237

Emanuel EJ, Emanuel LL (1994) The economics of dying. The illusion of cost savings at the end of life. N Engl J Med 330(8):540–544

European Association for Palliative Care (EAPC) [cited 2014 02.12.14]. Available from: http://www.eapcnet.eu

Ferlay J, Steliarova-Foucher E, Lortet-Tieulent J, Rosso S, Coebergh JW, Comber H et al (2013) Cancer incidence and mortality patterns in Europe: estimates for 40 countries in 2012. Eur J Cancer 49(6):1374–1403

Hui D, Kim YJ, Park JC, Zhang Y, Strasser F, Cherny N et al (2015) Integration of Oncology and Palliative Care: a systematic review. Oncologist 20(1):77–83

Jordhøy MS, Fayers P, Saltnes T, Ahlner-Elmqvist M, Jannert M, Kaasa S (2000) A palliative-care intervention and death at home: a cluster randomised trial. Lancet 356(9233):888–893

Kaasa S, Loge JH, Fayers P, Caraceni A, Strasser F, Hjermstad MJ et al (2008) Symptom assessment in palliative care: a need for international collaboration. J Clin Oncol 26(23):3867–3873

Kelly RJ, Smith TJ (2014) Delivering maximum clinical benefit at an affordable price: engaging stakeholders in cancer care. Lancet Oncol 15(3):e112–e118

Kelly RJ, Hillner BE, Smith TJ (2014) Cost effectiveness of crizotinib for anaplastic lymphoma kinase-positive, non-small-cell lung cancer: who is going to blink at the cost? J Clin Oncol 32(10):983–985

Leutz WN (1999) Five laws for integrating medical and social services: lessons from the United States and the United Kingdom. Milbank Q 77(1):77–110, iv–v

Mariotto AB, Yabroff KR, Shao Y, Feuer EJ, Brown ML (2011) Projections of the cost of cancer care in the United States: 2010–2020. J Natl Cancer Inst 103(2):117–128

Meuser T, Pietruck C, Radbruch L, Stute P, Lehmann KA, Grond S (2001) Symptoms during cancer pain treatment following WHO-guidelines: a longitudinal follow-up study of symptom prevalence, severity and etiology. Pain 93(3):247–257

Morita T, Miyashita M, Yamagishi A, Akiyama M, Akizuki N, Hirai K et al (2013) Effects of a programme of interventions on regional comprehensive palliative care for patients with cancer: a mixed-methods study. Lancet Oncol 14(7):638–646

Ringdal GI, Ringdal K, Jordhøy MS, Ahlner-Elmqvist M, Jannert M, Kaasa S (2004) Health-related quality of life (HRQOL) in family members of cancer victims: results from a longitudinal intervention study in Norway and Sweden. Palliat Med 18(2):108–120

Rotter T, Kinsman L, James E, Machotta A, Gothe H, Willis J et al (2010) Clinical pathways: effects on professional practice, patient outcomes, length of stay and hospital costs. Cochrane Database Syst Rev (Online) (3):CD006632

Schnipper LE, Smith TJ, Raghavan D, Blayney DW, Ganz PA, Mulvey TM et al (2012) American Society of Clinical Oncology identifies five key opportunities to improve care and reduce costs: the top five list for oncology. J Clin Oncol 30(14):1715–1724

Sigurdardottir KR, Kaasa S, Rosland JH, Bausewein C, Radbruch L, Haugen DF (2014) The European Association for Palliative Care basic dataset to describe a palliative care cancer population: results from an international Delphi process. Palliat Med 28(6):463–473

Sullivan R, Peppercorn J, Sikora K, Zalcberg J, Meropol NJ, Amir E et al (2011) Delivering affordable cancer care in high-income countries. Lancet Oncol 12(10):933–980

Temel JS, Greer JA, Muzikansky A, Gallagher ER, Admane S, Jackson VA et al (2010) Early palliative care for patients with metastatic non-small-cell lung cancer. N Engl J Med 363(8):733–742

The European Palliative Care Research Centre (PRC) [cited 2014 02.12.14]. Available from: http://www.ntnu.edu/prc

Wright AA, Zhang B, Ray A, Mack JW, Trice E, Balboni T et al (2008) Associations between end-of-life discussions, patient mental health, medical care near death, and caregiver bereavement adjustment. JAMA 300(14):1665–1673

Zikos E, Ghislain I, Coens C, Ediebah DE, Sloan E, Quinten C et al (2014) Health-related quality of life in small-cell lung cancer: a systematic review on reporting of methods and clinical issues in randomised controlled trials. Lancet Oncol 15(2):e78–e89

Zimmermann C, Swami N, Krzyzanowska M, Hannon B, Leighl N, Oza A et al (2014) Early palliative care for patients with advanced cancer: a cluster-randomised controlled trial. Lancet 383(9930):1721–1730

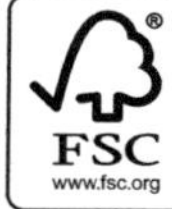

MIX
Papier aus verantwortungsvollen Quellen
Paper from responsible sources
FSC® C105338

If you have any concerns about our products,
you can contact us on
ProductSafety@springernature.com

In case Publisher is established outside the EU,
the EU authorized representative is:
Springer Nature Customer Service Center GmbH
Europaplatz 3, 69115 Heidelberg, Germany

Printed by Libri Plureos GmbH
in Hamburg, Germany